Teen Health Series

Drug Information For Teens,
Fifth Edition

Drug Information For Teens, Fifth Edition

Health Tips About The Physical And Mental
Effects Of Substance Abuse

Including Information About Alcohol, Tobacco,
Marijuana, Prescription And Over-The-Counter Drugs,
Club Drugs, Hallucinogens, Stimulants, Opiates,
Steroids, And More

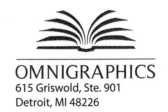

OMNIGRAPHICS
615 Griswold, Ste. 901
Detroit, MI 48226

Bibliographic Note
Because this page cannot legibly accommodate all the copyright notices, the Bibliographic Note portion of the Preface constitutes an extension of the copyright notice.

* * *

OMNIGRAPHICS
Angela L. Williams, *Managing Editor*

* * *

Library of Congress Cataloging-in-Publication Data

Names: Omnigraphics, Inc., issuing body.

Title: Drug information for teens: health tips about the physical and mental effects of substance abuse including information about alcohol, tobacco, marijuana, prescription and over-the-counter drugs, club drugs, hallucinogens, stimulants, opiates, steroids, and more.

Description: Fifth edition. | Detroit, MI: Omnigraphics, Inc., [2018] | Series: Teen health series | Audience: Grade 9 to 12. | Includes bibliographical references and index.

Identifiers: LCCN 2018021589 (print) | LCCN 2018021651 (ebook) | ISBN 9780780816398 (eBook) | ISBN 9780780816381 (hardcover: alk. paper)

Subjects: LCSH: Teenagers--Drug use--United States. | Teenagers--Alcohol use--United States. | Teenagers--Health and hygiene--United States. | Drugs--Physiological effect. | Drug abuse--United States--Prevention. | Alcoholism--United States--Prevention.

Classification: LCC HV5824.Y68 (ebook) | LCC HV5824.Y68 D774 2018 (print) | DDC 613.8--dc23

LC record available at https://lccn.loc.gov/2018021589

This book is printed on acid-free paper meeting the ANSI Z39.48 Standard. The infinity symbol that appears above indicates that the paper in this book meets that standard.

Printed in the United States

Table Of Contents

Part Four: Marijuana

Part Five: Abuse Of Legally Available Substances

Part Six: Abuse Of Illegal Substances

Part Seven: Other Drug-Related Health Concerns

Part Eight: Treatment For Addiction

Part Nine: If You Need More Information

Preface

About This Book

Recent scientific research shows that teenagers' brains are wired in a way that makes them prone to take risks. Because the part of the brain that is responsible for weighing consequences (the prefrontal cortex) is still developing, teenagers sometimes make choices based on their emotions or whims rather than the possible outcome of a situation. This is one reason why some teens experiment with drugs and alcohol. "Most kids don't really 'plan' to use drugs," says Professor Laurence Steinberg of Temple University, "at least not the first time. They are more likely to experiment on the spur of the moment, particularly when influenced by others [peer pressure]." Many factors can influence this impulsive decision: the desire to look cool or have fun, the desire to fit in with a particular group of people, or the desire to escape life's stressors.

Although recent studies show that overall teenage substance use is steadily declining, many teenagers still make the choice to use drugs and alcohol. A recent survey reports, people aged 12 to 20 years consume about one-tenth of all alcohol consumed in the United States, about half of 9th through 12th grade students reported ever having used marijuana, about 4 in 10—9th through 12th grade students reported having tried cigarettes, among 12th graders, close to 2 in 10 reported using prescription medicine without a prescription. Adolescent substance use puts teenagers at increased risk for traffic accidents, risky sexual behaviors, and violence. It can also lead to addiction—a chronic condition caused by changes in brain chemistry—which can lead to health challenges during adulthood, including infectious diseases, organ damage, and cancer.

Drug Information for Teens, Fifth Edition provides updated facts about drug use, abuse, and addiction. It describes the physical and psychological effects of alcohol, marijuana, prescription drugs, inhalants, club drugs, stimulants, and many other drugs and chemicals that are commonly abused. It includes information about drug-related health concerns, such as human immunodeficiency virus (HIV) infection, drug-facilitated rape, depression, and suicide. A section on substance abuse treatment describes care options and provides resources for helping yourself, a family member, or a friend recover from addiction. Resource directories provide contact information for national organizations, hotlines and helplines, and other sources of support.

How To Use This Book

This book is divided into parts and chapters. Parts focus on broad areas of interest; chapters are devoted to single topics within a part.

Part One: General Information About Addiction And Substance Abuse defines substance abuse and addiction, explains why people get addicted and how drugs affect brain chemistry. It provides information on preventing drug abuse, including peer pressure, statistics on teen drug use, and the Drug Enforcement Administration's Controlled Substances Act which categorizes drugs according to their legal status, medicinal qualities, and harmful effects.

Part Two: Alcohol presents facts about the use and abuse of alcohol, underage drinking statistics, and recent trends in teen drinking. It also discusses reasons, risks, and prevention for underage drinking. Binge drinking, alcohol use and health risks, family history of alcoholism, and coping with an alcoholic parent are also discussed.

Part Three: Tobacco, Nicotine, And E-Cigarettes presents facts on several forms of tobacco use, including cigarettes, smokeless tobacco, and secondhand smoke. The latest information on e-cigarettes is also provided. Various health risks associated with smoking are discussed in detail. Information on the benefits of quitting—and how to quit—is also provided.

Part Four: Marijuana includes facts about marijuana, marijuana abuse among teens, and associated health effects of marijuana including mental illness, respiratory problems, and changes in brain chemistry. Information about medical marijuana and the related federal and state laws is also included.

Part Five: Abuse Of Legally Available Substances includes facts about the abuse of prescription and over-the-counter medications, including commonly abused pain relievers, depressants, sedatives and tranquilizers, and cold and cough medicines. Information about other legally available substances—such as inhalants, steroids and sports supplements, and caffeine—are also included.

Part Six: Abuse Of Illegal Substances offers basic information about some of the most commonly abused illegal substances, including ecstasy, and other club drugs; LSD, PCP, and other hallucinogens; methamphetamine, cocaine, and other stimulants; heroin and other opiates.

Part Seven: Other Drug-Related Health Concerns covers some important topics that are associated with drug use but not necessarily related to the direct effects of the substances themselves. These include mental illness and suicide risks associated with drugs, risky sexual behavior, the spread of infectious diseases via drug paraphernalia, violence due to drug abuse, and drugged driving.

Part Eight: Treatment For Addiction discusses how to deal with addiction, the principles of treatment, the various types of treatment, and the process of recovery. It offers encouragement for those teens who need to seek help themselves and provides tips for helping friends and loved ones who may have a substance abuse problem.

Part Nine: If You Need More Information includes a directory of national organizations that provide drug-related information and a directory of places providing support services, including hotline and helpline phone numbers. A state-by-state list of referral services will help readers find local information.

Bibliographic Note

This volume contains documents and excerpts from publications issued by the following government agencies: Centers for Disease Control and Prevention (CDC); Child Welfare Information Gateway; The Cool Spot; Get Smart About Drugs; National Highway Traffic Safety Administration (NHTSA); National Institute on Alcohol Abuse and Alcoholism (NIAAA); National Institute on Drug Abuse (NIDA); National Institute on Drug Abuse (NIDA) for Teens; National Institutes of Health (NIH); Office of Dietary Supplements (ODS); Office of the Surgeon General (OGS); Substance Abuse and Mental Health Services Administration (SAMHSA); U.S. Department of Health and Human Services (HHS); U.S. Department of Justice (DOJ); U.S. Department of Veterans Affairs (VA); U.S. Drug Enforcement Administration (DEA); U.S. Food and Drug Administration (FDA); and U.S. House of Representatives.

The photograph on the front cover is © solominviktor/Shutterstock.

Medical Review

Omnigraphics contracts with a team of qualified, senior medical professionals who serve as medical consultants for the *Teen Health Series*. As necessary, medical consultants review reprinted and originally written material for currency and accuracy. Citations including the phrase "Reviewed (month, year)" indicate material reviewed by this team. Medical consultation services are provided to the *Teen Health Series* editors by:

Dr. Vijayalakshmi, MBBS, DGO, MD
Dr. Senthil Selvan, MBBS, DCH, MD
Dr. K. Sivanandham, MBBS, DCH, MS (Research), PhD

About The Teen Health Series

At the request of librarians serving today's young adults, the *Teen Health Series* was developed as a specially focused set of volumes within Omnigraphics' *Health Reference Series*. Each volume deals comprehensively with a topic selected according to the needs and interests of people in middle school and high school. Teens seeking preventive guidance, information about disease warning signs, medical statistics, and risk factors for health problems will find answers to their questions in the *Teen Health Series*. The *Series*, however, is not intended to serve as a tool for diagnosing illness, in prescribing treatments, or as a substitute for the physician/patient relationship. All people concerned about medical symptoms or the possibility of disease are encouraged to seek professional care from an appropriate healthcare provider.

If there is a topic you would like to see addressed in a future volume of the *Teen Health Series*, please write to:

Editor
Teen Health Series
Omnigraphics
615 Griswold, Ste. 901
Detroit, MI 48226

A Note About Spelling And Style

Teen Health Series editors use *Stedman's Medical Dictionary* as an authority for questions related to the spelling of medical terms and the *Chicago Manual of Style* for questions related to grammatical structures, punctuation, and other editorial concerns. Consistent adherence is not always possible, however, because the individual volumes within the *Series* include many documents from a wide variety of different producers and copyright holders, and the editor's primary goal is to present material from each source as accurately as is possible following the terms specified by each document's producer. This sometimes means that information in different chapters may follow other guidelines and alternate spelling authorities. For example, occasionally a copyright holder may require that eponymous terms be shown in possessive forms (Crohn's disease vs. Crohn disease) or that British spelling norms be retained (leukaemia vs. leukemia).

Part One
General Information About Addiction And Substance Abuse

Chapter 1

The Science Of Addiction

For much of the past century, scientists studying drug abuse labored in the shadows of powerful myths and misconceptions about the nature of addiction. When scientists began to study addictive behavior in the 1930s, people addicted to drugs were thought to be morally flawed and lacking in willpower. Those views shaped society's responses to drug abuse, treating it as a moral failing rather than a health problem, which led to an emphasis on punishment rather than prevention and treatment. Today, thanks to science, our views and our responses to addiction and other substance use disorders have changed dramatically. Groundbreaking discoveries about the brain have revolutionized our understanding of compulsive drug use, enabling us to respond effectively to the problem. As a result of scientific research, we know that addiction is a disease that affects both the brain and behavior. We have identified many of the biological and environmental factors and are beginning to search for the genetic variations that contribute to the development and progression of the disease. Scientists use this knowledge to develop effective prevention and treatment approaches that reduce the toll drug abuse takes on individuals, families, and communities.

What Is Addiction?

Addiction is defined as a chronic, relapsing brain disease that is characterized by compulsive drug seeking and use, despite harmful consequences. Addiction is a lot like other diseases, such as heart disease. Both disrupt the normal, healthy functioning of the underlying organ, have serious harmful consequences, and are preventable and treatable, but if left untreated, can

About This Chapter: This chapter includes text excerpted from "Drugs, Brains, And Behavior: The Science Of Addiction," National Institute on Drug Abuse (NIDA), July 2014. Reviewed July 2018.

last a lifetime. Addiction is considered a brain disease because drugs change the brain—they change its structure and how it works. These brain changes can be long-lasting, and can lead to the harmful behaviors seen in people who abuse drugs.

Why Do People Take Drugs?

In general, people begin taking drugs for a variety of reasons:

- **To feel good.** Most abused drugs produce intense feelings of pleasure. This initial sensation of euphoria is followed by other effects, which differ with the type of drug used. For example, with stimulants such as cocaine, the "high" is followed by feelings of power, self-confidence, and increased energy. In contrast, the euphoria caused by opiates such as heroin is followed by feelings of relaxation and satisfaction.

- **To feel better.** Some people who suffer from social anxiety, stress-related disorders, and depression begin abusing drugs in an attempt to lessen feelings of distress. Stress can play a major role in beginning drug use, continuing drug abuse, or relapse in patients recovering from addiction.

- **To do better.** Some people feel pressure to chemically enhance or improve their cognitive or athletic performance, which can play a role in initial experimentation and continued abuse of drugs such as prescription stimulants or anabolic/androgenic steroids.

- **Curiosity and "because others are doing it."** In this respect, adolescents are particularly vulnerable because of the strong influence of peer pressure. Teens are more likely than adults to engage in risky or daring behaviors to impress their friends and express their independence from parental and social rules.

If Taking Drugs Makes People Feel Good Or Better, What's The Problem?

When they first use a drug, people may perceive what seem to be positive effects; they also may believe that they can control their use. However, drugs can quickly take over a person's life. Over time, if drug use continues, other pleasurable activities become less pleasurable, and taking the drug becomes necessary for the user just to feel "normal." They may then compulsively seek and take drugs even though it causes tremendous problems for themselves and their loved ones. Some people may start to feel the need to take higher or more frequent doses, even in the early stages of their drug use. These are the telltale signs of an addiction. Even relatively moderate drug use poses dangers. Consider how a social drinker can become intoxicated, get behind the wheel of a car, and quickly turn a pleasurable activity into a tragedy that affects many lives.

Is Continued Drug Abuse A Voluntary Behavior?

The initial decision to take drugs is typically voluntary. However, with continued use, a person's ability to exert self-control can become seriously impaired; this impairment in self-control is the hallmark of addiction. Brain imaging studies of people with addiction show physical changes in areas of the brain that are critical to judgment, decision making, learning and memory, and behavior control. Scientists believe that these changes alter the way the brain works and may help explain the compulsive and destructive behaviors of addiction.

Why Study Drug Abuse And Addiction?

Abuse of and addiction to alcohol, nicotine, and illicit and prescription drugs cost Americans more than $700 billion a year in increased healthcare costs, crime, and lost productivity. Every year, illicit and prescription drugs and alcohol contribute to the death of more than 90,000 Americans, while tobacco is linked to an estimated 480,000 deaths per year. (Hereafter, unless otherwise specified, drugs refers to all of these substances.)

People of all ages suffer the harmful consequences of drug abuse and addiction.

- Babies exposed to drugs in the womb may be born premature and underweight. This exposure can slow the child's intellectual development and affect behavior later in life.

- Adolescents who abuse drugs often act out, do poorly academically, and drop out of school. They are at risk for unplanned pregnancies, violence, and infectious diseases.

- Adults who abuse drugs often have problems thinking clearly, remembering, and paying attention. They often develop poor social behaviors as a result of their drug abuse, and their work performance and personal relationships suffer.

- Parents' drug abuse often means chaotic, stress-filled homes, as well as child abuse and neglect. Such conditions harm the well-being and development of children in the home and may set the stage for drug abuse in the next generation.

How Does Science Provide Solutions For Drug Abuse And Addiction?

Scientists study the effects that drugs have on the brain and on people's behavior. They use this information to develop programs for preventing drug abuse and for helping people recover from addiction. Further research helps transfer these ideas into practice in our communities.

Chapter 2

Risk Factors For Addiction

What Are The Early Signs Of Risk That May Predict Later Drug Abuse?

Some signs of risk can be seen as early as infancy or early childhood, such as aggressive behavior, lack of self-control, or difficult temperament. As the child gets older, interactions with family, at school, and within the community can affect that child's risk for later drug abuse.

Children's earliest interactions occur in the family; sometimes family situations heighten a child's risk for later drug abuse, for example, when there is:

- A lack of attachment and nurturing by parents or caregivers

- Ineffective parenting

- A caregiver who abuses drugs

But families can provide protection from later drug abuse when there is:

- A strong bond between children and parents

- Parental involvement in the child's life

- Clear limits and consistent enforcement of discipline

About This Chapter: Text under the heading "What Are The Early Signs Of Risk That May Predict Later Drug Abuse?" is excerpted from "Preventing Drug Use Among Children And Adolescents (In Brief)," National Institute on Drug Abuse (NIDA), October 2003. Reviewed July 2018; Text beginning with the heading "Why Do Some People Become Addicted To Drugs, While Others Do Not?" is excerpted from "Drugs, Brains, And Behavior: The Science Of Addiction," National Institute on Drug Abuse (NIDA), July 2014. Reviewed July 2018.

Interactions outside the family can involve risks for both children and adolescents, such as:

- Poor classroom behavior or social skills

- Academic failure

- Association with drug-abusing peers

Other factors—such as drug availability, trafficking patterns, and beliefs that drug abuse is generally tolerated—are risks that can influence young people to start abusing drugs.

Why Do Some People Become Addicted To Drugs, While Others Do Not?

As with any other disease, vulnerability to addiction differs from person to person, and no single factor determines whether a person will become addicted to drugs. In general, the more risk factors a person has, the greater the chance that taking drugs will lead to abuse and addiction. Protective factors, on the other hand, reduce a person's risk of developing addiction. Risk and protective factors may be either environmental (such as conditions at home, at school, and in the neighborhood) or biological (for instance, a person's genes, their stage of development, and even their gender or ethnicity).

Table 2.1. Risk And Protective Factors For Drug Abuse And Addiction

Risk Factors	Protective Factors
Aggressive behavior in childhood	Good self-control
Lack of parental supervision	Parental monitoring and support
Poor social skills	Positive relationships
Drug experimentation	Academic competence
Availability of drugs at school	School antidrug policies
Community poverty	Neighborhood pride

What Environmental Factors Increase The Risk Of Addiction?

- **Home and family.** The influence of the home environment, especially during childhood, is a very important factor. Parents or older family members who abuse alcohol or drugs, or who engage in criminal behavior, can increase children's risks of developing their own drug problems.

- **Peer and school.** Friends and acquaintances can have an increasingly strong influence during adolescence. Drug-using peers can sway even those without risk factors to try drugs for the first time. Academic failure or poor social skills can put a child at further risk for using or becoming addicted to drugs.

What Biological Factors Increase Risk Of Addiction?

Scientists estimate that genetic factors account for between 40 and 60 percent of a person's vulnerability to addiction; this includes the effects of environmental factors on the function and expression of a person's genes. A person's stage of development and other medical conditions they may have are also factors. Adolescents and people with mental disorders are at greater risk of drug abuse and addiction than the general population.

What Other Factors Increase The Risk Of Addiction?

- **Early use.** Although taking drugs at any age can lead to addiction, research shows that the earlier a person begins to use drugs, the more likely he or she is to develop serious problems. This may reflect the harmful effect that drugs can have on the developing brain; it also may result from a mix of early social and biological vulnerability factors, including unstable family relationships, exposure to physical or sexual abuse, genetic susceptibility, or mental illness. Still, the fact remains that early use is a strong indicator of problems ahead, including addiction.

- **Method of administration.** Smoking a drug or injecting it into a vein increases its addictive potential. Both smoked and injected drugs enter the brain within seconds,

The brain continues to develop into adulthood and undergoes dramatic changes during adolescence. One of the brain areas still maturing during adolescence is the prefrontal cortex—the part of the brain that enables us to assess situations, make sound decisions, and keep our emotions and desires under control. The fact that this critical part of an adolescent's brain is still a work in progress puts them at increased risk for making poor decisions (such as trying drugs or continuing to take them). Also, introducing drugs during this period of development may cause brain changes that have profound and long-lasting consequences.

producing a powerful rush of pleasure. However, this intense "high" can fade within a few minutes, taking the abuser down to lower, more normal levels. Scientists believe this starkly felt contrast drives some people to repeated drug taking in an attempt to recapture the fleeting pleasurable state.

Chapter 3

How Drugs Affect The Brain

The human brain is the most complex organ in the body. This three-pound mass of gray and white matter sits at the center of all human activity—you need it to drive a car, to enjoy a meal, to breathe, to create an artistic masterpiece, and to enjoy everyday activities. In brief, the brain regulates your body's basic functions; enables you to interpret and respond to everything you experience; and shapes your thoughts, emotions, and behavior.

The brain is made up of many parts that all work together as a team. Different parts of the brain are responsible for coordinating and performing specific functions. Drugs can alter important brain areas that are necessary for life-sustaining functions and can drive the compulsive drug abuse that marks addiction. Brain areas affected by drug abuse include:

- **The brainstem**, which controls basic functions critical to life, such as heart rate, breathing, and sleeping.

- **The cerebral cortex**, which is divided into areas that control specific functions. Different areas process information from our senses, enabling us to see, feel, hear, and taste. The front part of the cortex, the frontal cortex or forebrain, is the thinking center of the brain; it powers our ability to think, plan, solve problems, and make decisions.

- **The limbic system**, which contains the brain's reward circuit. It links together a number of brain structures that control and regulate our ability to feel pleasure. Feeling pleasure motivates us to repeat behaviors that are critical to our existence. The limbic system is activated by healthy, life-sustaining activities such as eating and socializing—but it is also activated by drugs of abuse. In addition, the limbic system is responsible for our

About This Chapter: This chapter includes text excerpted from "Drugs And The Brain," National Institute on Drug Abuse (NIDA), July 2014. Reviewed June 2018.

perception of other emotions, both positive and negative, which explains the mood-altering properties of many drugs.

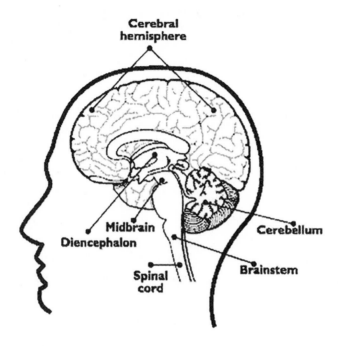

Figure 3.1. Parts Of Brain *(Source: "Brain Anatomy," National Institute on Drug Abuse (NIDA) for Teens.)*

How Do The Parts Of The Brain Communicate?

The brain is a communications center consisting of billions of neurons, or nerve cells. Networks of neurons pass messages back and forth among different structures within the brain, the spinal cord, and nerves in the rest of the body (the peripheral nervous system). These nerve networks coordinate and regulate everything we feel, think, and do.

• **Neuron to Neuron**

Each nerve cell in the brain sends and receives messages in the form of electrical and chemical signals. Once a cell receives and processes a message, it sends it on to other neurons.

• **Neurotransmitters—The Brain's Chemical Messengers**

The messages are typically carried between neurons by chemicals called neurotransmitters.

- **Receptors—The Brain's Chemical Receivers**

  The neurotransmitter attaches to a specialized site on the receiving neuron called a receptor. A neurotransmitter and its receptor operate like a "key and lock," an exquisitely specific mechanism that ensures that each receptor will forward the appropriate message only after interacting with the right kind of neurotransmitter.

- **Transporters—The Brain's Chemical Recyclers**

  Located on the neuron that releases the neurotransmitter, transporters recycle these neurotransmitters (that is, bring them back into the neuron that released them), thereby shutting off the signal between neurons.

How Do Drugs Work In The Brain?

Drugs are chemicals that affect the brain by tapping into its communication system and interfering with the way neurons normally send, receive, and process information. Some drugs, such as marijuana and heroin, can activate neurons because their chemical structure mimics that of a natural neurotransmitter. This similarity in structure "fools" receptors and allows the drugs to attach onto and activate the neurons. Although these drugs mimic the brain's own

Changes In Brain Development And Function From Drug Abuse

Most kids grow dramatically during the adolescent and teen years. Their young brains, particularly the prefrontal cortex that is used to make decisions, are growing and developing, until their mid-20's.

Long-term drug use causes brain changes that can set people up for addiction and other problems. Once a young person is addicted, his or her brain changes so that drugs are now the top priority. He or she will compulsively seek and use drugs even though doing so brings devastating consequences to his or her life, and for those who care about him.

Alcohol can interfere with developmental processes occurring in the brain. For weeks or months after a teen stops drinking heavily, parts of the brain still struggle to work correctly. Drinking at a young age is also associated with the development of alcohol dependence later in life.

(Source: "How Drugs Alter Brain Development And Affect Teens," Get Smart About Drugs, U.S. Drug Enforcement Administration (DEA).)

chemicals, they don't activate neurons in the same way as a natural neurotransmitter, and they lead to abnormal messages being transmitted through the network. Other drugs, such as amphetamine or cocaine, can cause the neurons to release abnormally large amounts of natural neurotransmitters or prevent the normal recycling of these brain chemicals. This disruption produces a greatly amplified message, ultimately disrupting communication channels.

How Do Drugs Work In The Brain To Produce Pleasure?

Most drugs of abuse directly or indirectly target the brain's reward system by flooding the circuit with dopamine. Dopamine is a neurotransmitter present in regions of the brain that regulate movement, emotion, motivation, and feelings of pleasure. When activated at normal levels, this system rewards our natural behaviors. Overstimulating the system with drugs, however, produces euphoric effects, which strongly reinforce the behavior of drug use—teaching the user to repeat it.

How Does Stimulation Of The Brain's Pleasure Circuit Teach Us To Keep Taking Drugs?

Our brains are wired to ensure that we will repeat life-sustaining activities by associating those activities with pleasure or reward. Whenever this reward circuit is activated, the brain notes that something important is happening that needs to be remembered, and teaches us to do it again and again without thinking about it. Because drugs of abuse stimulate the same circuit, we learn to abuse drugs in the same way.

Why Are Drugs More Addictive Than Natural Rewards?

When some drugs of abuse are taken, they can release 2–10 times the amount of dopamine that natural rewards such as eating and sex do. In some cases, this occurs almost immediately (as when drugs are smoked or injected), and the effects can last much longer than those produced by natural rewards. The resulting effects on the brain's pleasure circuit dwarf those produced by naturally rewarding behaviors. The effect of such a powerful reward strongly motivates people to take drugs again and again. This is why scientists sometimes say that drug abuse is something we learn to do very, very well.

What Happens To Your Brain If You Keep Taking Drugs?

For the brain, the difference between normal rewards and drug rewards can be described as the difference between someone whispering into your ear and someone shouting into a microphone. Just as we turn down the volume on a radio that is too loud, the brain adjusts to the overwhelming surges in dopamine (and other neurotransmitters) by producing less dopamine or by reducing the number of receptors that can receive signals. As a result, dopamine's impact on the reward circuit of the brain of someone who abuses drugs can become abnormally low, and that person's ability to experience any pleasure is reduced.

This is why a person who abuses drugs eventually feels flat, lifeless, and depressed, and is unable to enjoy things that were previously pleasurable. Now, the person needs to keep taking drugs again and again just to try and bring his or her dopamine function back up to normal—which only makes the problem worse, like a vicious cycle. Also, the person will often need to take larger amounts of the drug to produce the familiar dopamine high—an effect known as tolerance.

How Does Long-Term Drug Taking Affect Brain Circuits?

We know that the same sort of mechanisms involved in the development of tolerance can eventually lead to profound changes in neurons and brain circuits, with the potential to severely compromise the long-term health of the brain. For example, glutamate is another neurotransmitter that influences the reward circuit and the ability to learn. When the optimal concentration of glutamate is altered by drug abuse, the brain attempts to compensate for this change, which can cause impairment in cognitive function. Similarly, long-term drug abuse can trigger adaptations in habit or nonconscious memory systems. Conditioning is one example of this type of learning, in which cues in a person's daily routine or environment become associated with the drug experience and can trigger uncontrollable cravings whenever the person is exposed to these cues, even if the drug itself is not available. This learned "reflex" is extremely durable and can affect a person who once used drugs even after many years of abstinence.

What Other Brain Changes Occur With Drug Abuse?

Chronic exposure to drugs of abuse disrupts the way critical brain structures interact to control and inhibit behaviors related to drug use. Just as continued abuse may lead to tolerance or the need for higher drug dosages to produce an effect, it may also lead to addiction, which can drive a user to seek out and take drugs compulsively. Drug addiction erodes a person's self-control and ability to make sound decisions, while producing intense impulses to take drugs.

Chapter 4

Peer Pressure: Its Influence On Teens And Decision Making

What Is Peer Pressure?

Friends can influence an adolescent's attitudes and behaviors in ways that matter across multiple domains of health and well-being, well into adulthood. We often hear about this in the form of peer pressure, which refers more explicitly to the pressure adolescents feel from their friends or peer group to behave in certain ways, good or bad. It can take the form of encouragement, requests, challenges, threats, or insults. Sometimes, peer pressure is unspoken—an adolescent may feel pressured to do something simply because their friends are doing it.

Generally, young adolescents are the most susceptible to peer pressure, and recent research indicates that popular adolescents may be under higher pressure than other youth to conform to peer behaviors. While popular adolescents often possess a wider range of social skills and better knowledge about themselves than other youth, popularity can be associated with higher rates of alcohol and substance use, vandalism, and shoplifting.

About This Chapter: Text under the heading "What Is Peer Pressure?" is excerpted from "Peer Pressure," U.S. Department of Health and Human Services (HHS), February 7, 2018; Text beginning with the heading "Peer Pressure And The Brain" is excerpted from "Why Does Peer Pressure Influence Teens To Try Drugs?" National Institute on Drug Abuse (NIDA) for Teens, May 8, 2012. Reviewed July 2018; Text under the heading "Alcohol: The Friend Factor" is excerpted from "Alcohol: The Friend Factor," National Institute on Drug Abuse (NIDA) for Teens, June 18, 2014. Reviewed July 2018; Text under the heading "Tactful Tips For Resisting Peer Pressure To Use Drugs And Alcohol" is excerpted from "6 Tactful Tips For Resisting Peer Pressure To Use Drugs And Alcohol," National Institute on Drug Abuse (NIDA) for Teens, March 9, 2015.

Peer Pressure And The Brain

Peer pressure can influence teens' choices about a lot of things. New research shows that, when making a decision, teens think about both the risks and rewards of their actions and behaviors—but, unlike adults, teens are more likely to ignore the risk in favor of the reward. In a National Institute on Drug Abuse (NIDA)-funded study, teens driving with their friends in the car were more likely to take risks—like speeding through yellow lights—if they knew that two or more of their friends were watching. Teens were also significantly more likely to act this way than adults in the same experiment. Researchers monitored the brain activity of all the teen drivers in the study. Results showed that just knowing friends were watching activated brain regions linked with reward, especially when the teen drivers made risky decisions.

Taking Control Of Your Choices

So, be aware: The desire to impress your friends may override your fear of taking risks. This could also apply to deciding whether to try drugs or alcohol—your decision might be influenced by who's around and if you think they'd be impressed. Tell us: When you already know the risks, yet you want to impress your friends, do you run the light or slow down and stop? Do you accept a drink or turn it down? Do you go with the crowd or be your own person and impress others with your individuality? What are some ways you could put the brakes on long enough to think twice before making a decision to do something you know is risky?

Alcohol: The Friend Factor

Have you ever said "It's not me, it's my friends?" Turns out, this reasoning may not fly since what your friends do can have a big impact on you. Research studies show that teens whose best friends drink alcohol are twice as likely to try alcohol themselves. And, if teens get alcohol from friends, they're more likely to start drinking at a younger age.

It's a big deal. We know that a person who drinks alcohol early is more likely to abuse alcohol when he or she gets older. So, if your friends drink and you don't want to, what are you supposed to do? Get a whole new set of friends? It depends. You may find that some people believe drinking alcohol is the only way to have fun. But lots of people find other ways to enjoy themselves. If you're not ready to give up on your friends just yet, take some time to learn a few key strategies for dealing with peer pressure.

Remember:

- **It's brave to stand up for yourself.** Be that guy or girl who doesn't drink. It might be hard at first, but eventually, people will respect you for sticking to your beliefs. You might even start to influence some of your friends to stay away from alcohol too.

- **Not everyone is doing it.** In fact, according to NIDA's Monitoring the Future survey, nearly 75 percent of 10th graders reported NOT using alcohol in the past month.

- **It's okay to make up an excuse.** If someone is really hounding you, dodge the issue—you could say that you took medicine that will make you sick if you drink.

If you've said no and your friends still don't respect your choices, you have to ask yourself—are they really that good a friend?

Tactful Tips For Resisting Peer Pressure To Use Drugs And Alcohol

Even when you are confident in your decision not to use drugs or alcohol, it can be hard when it's your friend who is offering. A lot of times, a simple "no thanks" may be enough. But sometimes it's not. It can get intense, especially if the people who want you to join in on a bad idea feel judged. If you're all being "stupid" together, then they feel less self-conscious and don't need to take all the responsibility. But knowing they are just trying to save face doesn't end the pressure, so here are a few tips that may come in handy.

1. Offer to be the designated driver. Get your friends home safely, and everyone will be glad you didn't drink or take drugs.

2. If you're on a sports team, you can say you are staying healthy to maximize your athletic performance—besides, no one would argue that a hangover would help you play your best.

3. "I have to (study for a big test/go to a concert/visit my grandmother/babysit/march in a parade, etc.). I can't do that after a night of drinking/drugs."

4. Keep a bottled drink like a soda or iced tea with you to drink at parties. People will be less likely to pressure you to drink alcohol if you're already drinking something. If they still offer you something, just say "I'm covered."

5. Find something to do so that you look busy. Get up and dance. Offer to disc jockey (DJ).

6. When all else fails...blame your parents. They won't mind! Explain that your parents are really strict, or that they will check up on you when you get home.

If your friends aren't having it—then it's a good time to find the door. Nobody wants to leave the party or their friends, but if your friends won't let you party without drugs, then it's not going to be fun for you. Sometimes these situations totally surprise us. But sometimes we know that the party we are going to has alcohol or that people plan to do drugs at a concert. These are the times when asking yourself what you could do differently is key to not having to go through this weekend after weekend.

Teach Your Teen To Stand Up To Peer Pressure

While you might have talked to your kids at length about the dangers of drug use, it's still normal for most teen or preteens to want to fit in with their peers.

Having a genuine relationship with your teen is a key component of any drug prevention strategy. But here are a few other ways you can help your child withstand the peer pressure to use drugs.

- **Act it out:** Starting at an early age, role-playing (acting out the realistic situations your child may encounter) can be a useful way for your child to develop the skills needed to resist peer pressure.

- **Encourage your teen's talent:** Whether it's dance, music, sports, or martial arts—make sure you encourage whatever activities your teen may be interested in. Such activities can become a source of positive self-esteem for your teen and make them less susceptible to negative peer pressure.

- **Drug use and consequences:** Educate your teen about the ugly, and at times deadly consequences of becoming addicted to drugs.

(Source: "Teach Your Teen To Stand Up To Peer Pressure," Get Smart About Drugs, U.S. Drug Enforcement Administration (DEA).)

Chapter 5

Preventing Drug Abuse

Why Is Adolescence A Critical Time For Preventing Drug Addiction?

Early use of drugs increases a person's chances of developing addiction. Remember, drugs change brains—and this can lead to addiction and other serious problems. So, preventing early use of drugs or alcohol may go a long way in reducing these risks. If we can prevent young people from experimenting with drugs, we can prevent drug addiction.

Risk of drug abuse increases greatly during times of transition. For an adult, a divorce or loss of a job may lead to drug abuse; for a teenager, risky times include moving or changing schools. In early adolescence, when children advance from elementary through middle school, they face new and challenging social and academic situations. Often during this period, children are exposed to abusable substances such as cigarettes and alcohol for the first time. When they enter high school, teens may encounter greater availability of drugs, drug use by older teens, and social activities where drugs are used.

At the same time, many behaviors that are a normal aspect of their development, such as the desire to try new things or take greater risks, may increase teen tendencies to experiment with drugs. Some teens may give in to the urging of drug-using friends to share the experience with them. Others may think that taking drugs (such as steroids) will improve their appearance or their athletic performance or that abusing substances such as alcohol or 3,4-methylenedioxymethamphetamine (MDMA) (ecstasy or Molly) will ease their anxiety in social

About This Chapter: This chapter includes text excerpted from "Preventing Drug Abuse: The Best Strategy," National Institute on Drug Abuse (NIDA), July 2014. Reviewed July 2018.

situations. A growing number of teens are abusing prescription attention deficit hyperactivity disorder (ADHD) stimulants such as Adderall® to help them study or lose weight. Teens' still-developing judgment and decision-making skills may limit their ability to accurately assess the risks of all of these forms of drug use.

Using abusable substances at this age can disrupt brain function in areas critical to motivation, memory, learning, judgment, and behavior control. So, it is not surprising that teens who use alcohol and other drugs often have family and social problems, poor academic performance, health-related problems (including mental health), and involvement with the juvenile justice system.

> National drug use surveys indicate some children are already abusing drugs by age 12 or 13.

Can Research-Based Programs Prevent Drug Addiction In Youth?

Yes. The term "research-based" means that these programs have been rationally designed based on scientific evidence, rigorously tested, and shown to produce positive results. Scientists have developed a broad range of programs that positively alter the balance between risk and protective factors for drug abuse in families, schools, and communities.

How Do Research-Based Prevention Programs Work?

These prevention programs work to boost protective factors and eliminate or reduce risk factors for drug use. The programs are designed for various ages and can be designed for individual or group settings, such as the school and home. There are three types of programs:

- Universal programs address risk and protective factors common to all children in a given setting, such as a school or community.

- Selective programs target groups of children and teens who have factors that put them at increased risk of drug use.

- Indicated programs are designed for youth who have already begun using drugs.

Are All Prevention Programs Effective In Reducing Drug Abuse?

When research-based substance use prevention programs are properly implemented by schools and communities, use of alcohol, tobacco, and illegal drugs is reduced. Such programs help teachers, parents, and healthcare professionals shape youths' perceptions about the risks of substance use. While many social and cultural factors affect drug use trends, when young people perceive drug use as harmful, they reduce their level of use. Prevention is the best strategy. Cigarette smoking among teens is at its lowest point since National Institute on Drug Abuse (NIDA) began tracking it in 1975. But marijuana use has increased over the past several years as perception of its risks has declined.

Chapter 6

Drug Use Among U.S. Teens

Monitoring The Future Survey: High School And Youth Trends

Monitoring the Future (MTF) survey of drug use and attitudes among 8th, 10th, and 12th graders in hundreds of schools across the country continues to report promising trends, with past-year use of illicit drugs other than marijuana holding steady at the lowest levels in over two decades—5.8 percent among 8th graders, 9.4 percent among 10th graders, and 13.3 percent among 12th graders. This is down from peak rates of 13.1 percent for 8th graders in 1996, 18.4 percent for 10th graders in 1996, and 21.6 percent for 12th graders in 2001.

Use of many substances reached the lowest levels since the survey's inception (or since the survey began asking about them) and held steady in 2017, or in some cases, dropped even more. Substances at historic low levels of use include alcohol and cigarettes, heroin, prescription opioids, 3,4-methylenedioxymethamphetamine (MDMA) (ecstasy or Molly), methamphetamine, amphetamines, and sedatives. Other illicit drugs showed five-year declines, such as synthetic marijuana, hallucinogens other than lysergic acid diethylamide (LSD), and over-the-counter (OTC) cough and cold medications. Five-year trends, however, did reveal an increase in LSD use among high school seniors, although use still remains lower compared to its peak in 1996.

The survey also found a general decline in perceived risk of harm from using a number of substances and declining disapproval of people who use them. For example, the percentage of 8th

About This Chapter: This chapter includes text excerpted from "Monitoring The Future Survey: High School And Youth Trends," National Institute on Drug Abuse (NIDA), December 2017.

graders who think that occasional use of synthetic marijuana or OTC cough and cold medications is less than it was last year and in prior years. Among 10th graders, there was a decrease in the proportion of students who perceive a risk of harm when trying inhalants, powder cocaine, or OTC cough and cold medications once or twice. High school seniors reported reduced perception of harm in occasional cocaine, heroin, and steroid use, and reduced disapproval of trying LSD.

Opioids

Despite the continued rise in opioid and overdose deaths and high levels of opioid misuse among adults, lifetime, past-year, and past-month misuse of prescription opioids (narcotics other than heroin) dropped significantly over the last five years in 12th graders (the only grade surveyed in this category). Vicodin use notably dropped by 51 percent in 8th graders, 67 percent in 10th graders and 74 percent in 12th graders. Interestingly, teens also think these drugs are not as easy to get as they used to be. Only 35.8 percent of 12th graders said they were easily available in the 2017 survey, compared to more than 54 percent in 2010.

Marijuana

Past-year marijuana use declined among 10th graders and remains unchanged among 8th and 12th graders compared to five years ago, despite the changing state marijuana laws. Past-year use of marijuana reached its lowest levels in more than two decades among 8th and 10th graders in 2016; the one slight increase in 2017 was past-month use among 10th graders, which returned to 2014–2015 levels after a decrease in 2016. Daily use of marijuana has declined among 8th graders over the past five years to 0.7 percent. Among 12th graders, 6 percent continue to report daily use, which corresponds to about 1 in 16 high school seniors. Among all grades, perceptions of harm and disapproval around marijuana use continue to decrease, with a smaller percentage 8th and 10th graders thinking that regular marijuana use is harmful, and fewer 10th and 12th graders disapproving of regular marijuana use. While only 29.0 percent of 12th graders report that regular marijuana use poses a great risk (half of what it was 20 years ago), disapproval among 12th graders remains somewhat high, with 64.7 percent reporting they disapprove of adults smoking marijuana regularly.

This year, daily marijuana use exceeds daily cigarette use among 8th (0.8 versus 0.6%), 10th (2.9 versus 2.2%) and 12th (5.9 versus 4.2%) graders. This is the first year in which daily marijuana use appeared to outpace daily cigarette use among 8th graders-this flip occurred in 10th graders in 2014 and in 12th graders in 2015, reflecting a steep decline in daily cigarette use and fairly stable daily marijuana use.

Alcohol

Alcohol use and binge drinking continued to show a significant five-year decline among all grades. Past month use of alcohol was reported by 8.0 percent, 19.7 percent, and 33.2 percent of 8th, 10th, and 12th graders, respectively, compared to 11.0 percent, 27.6 percent, and 41.5 percent in 2012. Daily alcohol use and binge drinking (defined as consuming five or more drinks sometime in the past two weeks) also decreased significantly among all grades between 2012 and 2017. Unlike previous years, however, there were not significant declines in alcohol use between 2016 and 2017. Also, the perception of risk of binge drinking significantly decreased in 10th graders in 2017.

The percentage of high school teens who reported ever using alcohol dropped by as much as 60 percent compared to peak years. This year's survey found that 23.1 percent of 8th graders reported ever trying alcohol, which is a 60 percent drop from the peak of 55.8 percent in 1994. Among 10th graders, lifetime use fell by 40 percent from 72.0 percent in 1997 to 42.2 percent in 2017. Among 12th graders, there was a significant 25 percent drop in lifetime alcohol use from 81.7 percent in 1997 to the current 61.5 percent.

Nicotine And Tobacco

Use of traditional cigarettes has continued to decline to the lowest levels in the survey's history. Significant five-year declines-by more than half for daily use and for use of one-half pack or more per day were reported by all grades. Daily cigarette use was reported by 0.6 percent of 8th graders, 2.2 percent of 10th graders, and 4.2 percent of 12th graders in 2017. This was down from peaks of 10.4 percent and 18.3 percent among 8th and 10th graders in 1996 and a peak of 24.6 percent of 12th graders in 1997.

Use of other tobacco products including hookah and smokeless tobacco declined among high school seniors. Among 12th graders, tobacco use with a hookah fell from 13.0 percent to 10.1 percent in the last year; past-year hookah rates have declined by 45 percent in the past five years. Lifetime and past-month use of smokeless tobacco declined in 12th graders from 2016–2017 and showed a five-year decline in all grades.

For the first time in 2017, the MTF survey asked high school students about vaping specific substances ever, in the past year, and in the past month. Past-year vaping was reported by 13.3 percent of 8th graders, 23.9 percent of 10th graders, and 27.8 percent of 12th graders. Vaping was the third most common form of substance use in high school seniors and 10th graders (after alcohol and marijuana) and the second most common among 8th graders (after alcohol).

Students were also asked what substances they had consumed via vaping nicotine, marijuana, or "just flavoring." Past-year vaping of flavoring alone was most common (reported by 11.8% of 8th graders, 19.3% of 10th graders, and 20.6% of 12th graders), followed by vaping nicotine (7.5%, 15.8%, and 18.8%) and marijuana (3.0%, 8.1%, and 9.5%).

The new survey data regarding vaping also reveal a difference in perception of harm when nicotine is specifically mentioned. While 20.3 percent of 8th graders reported thinking it is harmful to regularly use e-cigarettes, 38.2 percent reported thinking it is harmful to regularly vape an e-liquid containing nicotine. Similar differences were also seen in 10th graders (19.4 reported thinking it is harmful to use e-cigarettes regularly versus 33.3 perceiving harm in regularly vaping a liquid that contains nicotine) and 12th graders (16.1 versus 27.0%).

Synthetic Drugs

Past-year use of synthetic cannabinoids (K2/herbal incense, sometimes called "fake weed" or "synthetic marijuana") has dropped significantly in the six years since the survey began tracking use of these substances. Since 2011, reported use among 12th graders has dropped from 11.4 percent to 3.7 percent. Use has also fallen from 4.4 percent to 2.0 percent among 8th graders and from 8.8 percent to 2.7 percent among 10th graders since 2012. In recent years, use of another synthetic drug called "bath salts" (technically, synthetic cathinones) among youth has become a concern. The MTF survey began tracking past-year synthetic cathinone use in 2012, and since then, there has been a decrease among 12th graders from 1.3 percent to 0.6 percent in 2017. Use among 10th graders has declined to 0.4 percent from a peak of 0.9 percent in 2013.

Drug Use In Adolescence

Illicit drug use—which includes the abuse of illegal drugs and/or the misuse of prescription medications or household substances—is something many adolescents engage in occasionally, and a few do regularly. By the 12th grade, about half of adolescents have misused an illicit drug at least once. The most commonly used drug is marijuana, but adolescents can find many harmful substances, such as prescription medications, glues, and aerosols, in the home. Many factors and strategies can help adolescents stay drug-free: Strong positive connections with parents, other family members, school, and religion; having parents present clear limits and consistent enforcement of discipline; and reduced access in the home to illegal substances.

(Source: "Drug Use In Adolescence," Get Smart About Drugs, U.S. Drug Enforcement Administration (DEA).)

Chapter 7

The Controlled Substances Act

Controlling Drugs And Other Substances Through Formal Scheduling

The Controlled Substances Act (CSA) places all substances which were in some manner regulated under existing federal law into one of five schedules. This placement is based upon the substance's medical use, potential for abuse, and safety or dependence liability. The Act also provides a mechanism for substances to be controlled (added to or transferred between schedules) or decontrolled (removed from control). The procedure for these actions is found in Section 201 of the Act.

Proceedings to add, delete, or change the schedule of a drug or other substance may be initiated by the U.S. Drug Enforcement Administration (DEA), the U.S. Department of Health and Human Services (HHS), or by petition from any interested party, including:

- The manufacturer of a drug

- A medical society or association

- A pharmacy association

- A public interest group concerned with drug abuse

- A state or local government agency

- An individual citizen

About This Chapter: This chapter includes text excerpted from "Drugs Of Abuse," U.S. Drug Enforcement Administration (DEA), June 27, 2017.

When a petition is received by the DEA, the agency begins its own investigation of the drug. The DEA also may begin an investigation of a drug at any time based upon information received from law enforcement laboratories, state and local law enforcement and regulatory agencies, or other sources of information.

Once the DEA has collected the necessary data, the DEA Administrator, by authority of the Attorney General, requests from HHS a scientific and medical evaluation and recommendation as to whether the drug or other substance should be controlled or removed from control. This request is sent to the Assistant Secretary for Health of HHS.

The Assistant Secretary, by authority of the Secretary, compiles the information and transmits back to the DEA: a medical and scientific evaluation regarding the drug or other substance, a recommendation as to whether the drug should be controlled, and in what schedule it should be placed.

The medical and scientific evaluations are binding on the DEA with respect to scientific and medical matters and form a part of the scheduling decision.

Once the DEA has received the scientific and medical evaluation from HHS, the administrator will evaluate all available data and make a final decision whether to propose that a drug or other substance should be removed or controlled and into which schedule it should be placed.

If a drug does not have a potential for abuse, it cannot be controlled. Although the term "potential for abuse" is not defined in the CSA, there is much discussion of the term in the legislative history of the Act. The following items are indicators that a drug or other substance has a potential for abuse:

1. There is evidence that individuals are taking the drug or other substance in amounts sufficient to create a hazard to their health or to the safety of other individuals or to the community.

2. There is significant diversion of the drug or other substance from legitimate drug channels.

3. Individuals are taking the drug or other substance on their own initiative rather than on the basis of medical advice from a practitioner.

4. The drug is a new drug so related in its action to a drug or other substance already listed as having a potential for abuse to make it likely that the drug will have the same potential for abuse as such drugs, thus making it reasonable to assume that there may be significant diversions from legitimate channels, significant use contrary to or

without medical advice, or that it has a substantial capability of creating hazards to the health of the user or to the safety of the community. Of course, evidence of actual abuse of a substance is indicative that a drug has a potential for abuse.

In determining into which schedule a drug or other substance should be placed, or whether a substance should be decontrolled or rescheduled, certain factors are required to be considered. These factors are listed in Section 201 (c), of the CSA as follows:

1. The drug's actual or relative potential for abuse.

2. Scientific evidence of the drug's pharmacological effect, if known. The state of knowledge with respect to the effects of a specific drug is, of course, a major consideration. For example, it is vital to know whether or not a drug has a hallucinogenic effect if it is to be controlled due to that effect. The best available knowledge of the pharmacological properties of a drug should be considered.

3. The state of current scientific knowledge regarding the substance. Criteria 2 and 3 are closely related. However, 2 is primarily concerned with pharmacological effects and 3 deals with all scientific knowledge with respect to the substance.

4. Its history and current pattern of abuse. To determine whether or not a drug should be controlled, it is important to know the pattern of abuse of that substance.

5. The scope, duration, and significance of abuse. In evaluating existing abuse, the DEA Administrator must know not only the pattern of abuse, but also whether the abuse is widespread.

6. What, if any, risk there is to the public health. If a drug creates dangers to the public health, in addition to or because of its abuse potential, then these dangers must also be considered by the administrator.

7. The drug's psychic or physiological dependence liability. There must be an assessment of the extent to which a drug is physically addictive or psychologically habit-forming.

8. Whether the substance is an immediate precursor of a substance already controlled. The CSA allows inclusion of immediate precursors on this basis alone into the appropriate schedule and thus safeguards against possibilities of clandestine manufacture. After considering the above-listed factors, the administrator must make specific findings concerning the drug or other substance. This will determine into which schedule the drug or other substance will be placed. These schedules are established by the CSA. They are as follows:

Schedule I

- The drug or other substance has a high potential for abuse.

- The drug or other substance has no currently accepted medical use in treatment in the United States.

- There is a lack of accepted safety for use of the drug or other substance under medical supervision.

- Examples of Schedule I substances include heroin, gamma-hydroxybutyric acid (GHB), lysergic acid diethylamide (LSD), marijuana, and methaqualone.

Schedule II

- The drug or other substance has a high potential for abuse.

- The drug or other substance has a currently accepted medical use in treatment in the United States or a currently accepted medical use with severe restrictions.

- Abuse of the drug or other substance may lead to severe psychological or physical dependence.

- Examples of Schedule II substances include morphine, phencyclidine (PCP), cocaine, methadone, hydrocodone, fentanyl, and methamphetamine.

Schedule III

- The drug or other substance has less potential for abuse than the drugs or other substances in Schedules I and II.

- The drug or other substance has a currently accepted medical use in treatment in the United States.

- Abuse of the drug or other substance may lead to moderate or low physical dependence or high psychological dependence.

- Anabolic steroids, codeine products with aspirin or Tylenol, and some barbiturates are examples of Schedule III substances.

Schedule IV

- The drug or other substance has a low potential for abuse relative to the drugs or other substances in Schedule III.

- The drug or other substance has a currently accepted medical use in treatment in the United States.

- Abuse of the drug or other substance may lead to limited physical dependence or psychological dependence relative to the drugs or other substances in Schedule III.

- Examples of drugs included in Schedule IV are alprazolam, clonazepam, and diazepam.

Schedule V

- The drug or other substance has a low potential for abuse relative to the drugs or other substances in Schedule IV.

- The drug or other substance has a currently accepted medical use in treatment in the United States.

- Abuse of the drug or other substances may lead to limited physical dependence or psychological dependence relative to the drugs or other substances in Schedule IV.

- Cough medicines with codeine are examples of Schedule V drugs.

Emergency Or Temporary Scheduling

The CSA was amended by the Comprehensive Crime Control Act of 1984. This Act included a provision which allows the DEA administrator to place a substance, on a temporary basis, into Schedule I, when necessary, to avoid an imminent hazard to public safety. This emergency scheduling authority permits the scheduling of a substance which is not currently controlled, is being abused, and is a risk to public health while the formal rulemaking procedures described in the CSA are being conducted. This emergency scheduling applies only to substances with no accepted medical use. A temporary scheduling order may be issued for two years with a possible extension of up to one year if formal scheduling procedures have been initiated. The notice of intent and order are published in the federal register, as are the proposals and orders for formal scheduling.

Controlled Substance Analogues

Controlled substance analogues are substances that are not formally controlled substances, but may be found in illicit trafficking. They are structurally or pharmacologically similar to Schedule I or II controlled substances and have no legitimate medical use. A substance that meets the definition of a controlled substance analogue and is intended for human consumption may be treated under the CSA as if it were a controlled substance in Schedule I.

International Treaty Obligations

United States treaty obligations may require that a drug or other substance be controlled under the CSA, or rescheduled if existing controls are less stringent than those required by a treaty. The procedures for these scheduling actions are found in Section 201 (d) of the Act. The United States is a party to the Single Convention on Narcotic Drugs of 1961, which was designed to establish effective control over international and domestic traffic in narcotics, coca leaf, cocaine, and cannabis. A second treaty, the Convention on Psychotropic Substances of 1971, which entered into force in 1976 and was ratified by Congress in 1980, is designed to establish comparable control over stimulants, depressants, and hallucinogens.

Registration

Any person who handles or intends to handle controlled substances must obtain a registration issued by DEA. A unique number is assigned to each legitimate handler of controlled drugs such as importer, exporter, manufacturer, distributor, hospital, pharmacy, practitioner, and researcher. This number must be made available to the supplier by the customer prior to the purchase of a controlled substance, and its validity can be verified online through the Diversion Control Division website at www.DEAdiversion.usdoj.gov. Thus, the opportunity for unauthorized transactions is greatly diminished.

Penalties

The CSA provides penalties for unlawful manufacturing, distribution, and dispensing of controlled substances. The penalties are basically determined by the schedule of the drug or other substance, and sometimes are specified by drug name, as in the case of marijuana. As the statute has been amended since its initial passage in 1970, the penalties have been altered by Congress.

Part Two
Alcohol

Chapter 8

Alcoholism And Alcohol Abuse

What Is Alcohol?

Ethyl alcohol, or ethanol, is an intoxicating ingredient found in beer, wine, and liquor. Alcohol is produced by the fermentation of yeast, sugars, and starches.

How Does Alcohol Affect A Person?

Alcohol affects every organ in the body. It is a central nervous system (CNS) depressant that is rapidly absorbed from the stomach and small intestine into the bloodstream. Alcohol is metabolized in the liver by enzymes. However, the liver can only metabolize a small amount of alcohol at a time, leaving the excess alcohol to circulate throughout the body. The intensity of the effect of alcohol on the body is directly related to the amount consumed.

What Is A Standard Drink In The United States?

A standard drink is equal to 14.0 grams (0.6 ounces) of pure alcohol. Generally, this amount of pure alcohol is found in:

- 12 ounces of beer (5% alcohol content)

- 8 ounces of malt liquor (7% alcohol content)

About This Chapter: Text beginning with the heading "What Is Alcohol?" is excerpted from "Alcohol And Public Health—Frequently Asked Questions," Centers for Disease Control and Prevention (CDC), March 29, 2018; Text under the heading "Signs Of Alcoholism" is excerpted from "Alcoholism—When Drinking Becomes A Disease," The Cool Spot, National Institute on Alcohol Abuse and Alcoholism (NIAAA), February 23, 2005. Reviewed July 2018. Text under the heading "Alcohol Myths" is excerpted from "Alcohol Myths," College Drinking, National Institute on Alcohol Abuse and Alcoholism (NIAAA), August 8, 2016.

- 5 ounces of wine (12% alcohol content)

- 1.5 ounces or a "shot" of 80-proof (40% alcohol content) distilled spirits or liquor (e.g., gin, rum, vodka, whiskey)

How Do I Know If It's Okay To Drink?

According to the *2015–2020 Dietary Guidelines for Americans* (DGA), some people should not drink alcoholic beverages at all, including:

- Anyone younger than age 21

- Women who are or may be pregnant

- People who are driving, planning to drive, or are participating in other activities requiring skill, coordination, and alertness

- People taking certain prescription or over-the-counter (OTC) medications that can interact with alcohol

- People with certain medical conditions

- People who are recovering from alcoholism or who are unable to control the amount they drink

---

Moderate Drinking

- Alcohol consumption is associated with a variety of short- and long-term health risks, including motor vehicle crashes, violence, sexual risk behaviors, high blood pressure, and various cancers (e.g., breast cancer).

- The risk of these harms increases with the amount of alcohol you drink. For some conditions, like some cancers, the risk increases even at very low levels of alcohol consumption (less than 1 drink).

- To reduce the risk of alcohol-related harms, the 2015–2020 U.S. Dietary Guidelines for Americans (DGA) recommends that if alcohol is consumed, it should be consumed in moderation—up to one drink per day for women and two drinks per day for men—and only by adults of legal drinking age. This is not intended as an average over several days, but rather the amount consumed on any single day. The Guidelines also do not recommend that individuals who do not drink alcohol start drinking for any reason.

(Source: "Fact Sheets—Moderate Drinking," Centers for Disease Control and Prevention (CDC).)

The *Dietary Guidelines* also recommend that if alcohol is consumed, it should be in moderation—up to 1 drink per day for women and up to 2 drinks per day for men—and only by adults of legal drinking age. However, the Guidelines do not recommend that people who do not drink alcohol start drinking for any reason. By following the *Dietary Guidelines*, you can reduce the risk of harm to yourself or others.

What Health Problems Are Associated With Excessive Alcohol Use?

Excessive drinking both in the form of heavy drinking or binge drinking, is associated with numerous health problems, including:

- Chronic diseases such as liver cirrhosis (damage to liver cells); pancreatitis (inflammation of the pancreas); various cancers, including liver, mouth, throat, larynx (the voice box), and esophagus; high blood pressure; and psychological disorders

- Unintentional injuries, such as motor-vehicle traffic crashes, falls, drowning, burns, and firearm injuries

- Violence, such as child maltreatment, homicide, and suicide

- Harm to a developing fetus if a woman drinks while pregnant, such as fetal alcohol spectrum disorders (FASDs)

- Sudden infant death syndrome (SIDS)

- Alcohol use disorders (AUDs)

Signs Of Alcoholism

When people drink too much, with time they risk becoming addicted to alcohol. This is called alcoholism, or alcohol dependence. It's a disease, and it can happen at any age. Common signs include:

- **Craving**—a strong need or urge to drink

- **Loss of control**—not being able to stop or cut down drinking

- **Not feeling well after heavy drinking**—upset stomach, sweating, shakiness, or nervousness

- **A need to drink more**—to get the same effect as before

- **Neglecting activities**—giving up or cutting back on other activities
- **Continuing to drink**—even though alcohol is causing problems

It may be hard to imagine why people with alcoholism can't just "use a little willpower" to stop drinking. But the addiction creates an uncontrollable need for alcohol. It can be as strong as the need for food and water. People may want to stop because they know that drinking harms their health and their loved ones. But quitting is extremely difficult. Although some people are able to recover from alcoholism without help, many need assistance. With treatment and support, many stop drinking and rebuild their lives.

Alcohol Myths

Know each of the myths and facts about alcohol.

Myth 1

I can drink and still be in control.

Fact: Drinking impairs your judgment, which increases the likelihood that you will do something you'll later regret such as having unprotected sex, being involved in date rape, damaging property, or being victimized by others.

Myth 2

Drinking isn't all that dangerous.

Fact: Among college students, alcohol contributes to deaths from alcohol-related unintentional injuries, as well as assaults, sexual assaults or date rapes, and poor academic performance.

Myth 3

I can sober up quickly if I have to.

Fact: It takes about 2 hours for the adult body to eliminate the alcohol content of a single drink, depending on your weight. Nothing can speed up this process—not even coffee or cold showers.

Myth 4

It's okay for me to drink to keep up with my boyfriend.

Fact: Women process alcohol differently. No matter how much he drinks, if you drink the same amount as your boyfriend, you will be more intoxicated and more impaired.

Myth 5

Beer doesn't have as much alcohol as hard liquor.

Fact: A 12-ounce bottle of beer has the same amount of alcohol as a standard shot of 80-proof liquor (either straight or in a mixed drink) or 5 ounces of wine.

Myth 6

I'd be better off if I learn to "hold my liquor."

Fact: If you have to drink increasingly larger amounts of alcohol to get a "buzz" or get "high," you are developing tolerance. Tolerance is actually a warning sign that you're developing more serious problems with alcohol.

Myth 7

I can manage to drive well enough after a few drinks.

Fact: The effects of alcohol start sooner than people realize, with mild impairment (up to .05 BAC) starting to affect speech, memory, attention, coordination, and balance. And if you are under 21, driving after drinking any amount of alcohol is illegal and you could lose your license. The risks of a fatal crash for drivers with positive blood alcohol content (BAC) compared with other drivers (i.e., the relative risk) increase with increasing BAC, and the risks increase more steeply for drivers younger than age 21 than for older drivers.

Chapter 9

Recent Trends In Teen Drinking

Underage drinking is a serious public health problem in the United States. Alcohol is the most widely used substance of abuse among America's youth, and drinking by young people poses enormous health and safety risks. The consequences of underage drinking can affect everyone—regardless of age or drinking status. We all feel the effects of the aggressive behavior, property damage, injuries, violence, and deaths that can result from underage drinking. This is not simply a problem for some families—it is a nationwide concern.

Underage Drinking Statistics

Many Young People Drink Alcohol

- By age 15, about 33 percent of teens have had at least 1 drink.

- By age 18, about 60 percent of teens have had at least 1 drink.

- In 2015, 7.7 million young people ages 12–20 reported that they drank alcohol beyond "just a few sips" in the past month.

Youth Ages 12–20 Often Binge Drink

People ages 12 through 20 drink 11 percent of all alcohol consumed in the United States. Although youth drink less often than adults do, when they do drink, they drink more. That is

About This Chapter: Text in this chapter begins with excerpts from "Underage Drinking," National Institute on Alcohol Abuse and Alcoholism (NIAAA), February 2017; Text beginning with the heading "Drinking Levels Among Youth" is excerpted from "Fact Sheets—Underage Drinking," Centers for Disease Control and Prevention (CDC), May 10, 2018.

because young people consume more than 90 percent of their alcohol by binge drinking. Binge drinking is consuming many drinks on an occasion. Drinking alcohol and binge drinking become more prevalent as young people get older.

How Much Is A Drink?

In the United States, a standard drink is one that contains about 14 grams of pure alcohol, which is found in:

- 12 ounces of beer with about 5 percent alcohol content
- 5 ounces of wine with about 12 percent alcohol content
- 1.5 ounces of distilled spirits with about 40 percent alcohol content

The percent of "pure" alcohol, expressed here as alcohol by volume (alc/vol), varies within and across beverage types. Although the "standard" drink amounts are helpful for following health guidelines, they may not reflect customary serving sizes. A large cup of beer, an overpoured glass of wine, or a single mixed drink could contain much more alcohol than a standard drink.

Drinking Patterns Vary By Age And Gender

As adolescents get older, they tend to drink more. Prevalence of drinking by boys and girls is similar, although among older adolescents, boys binge more than girls.

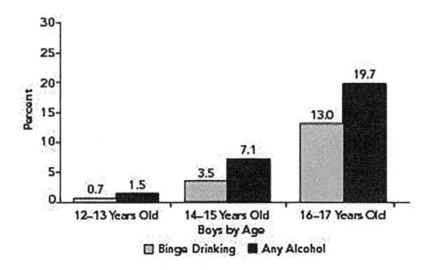

Figure 9.1. Alcohol Use Among Boys

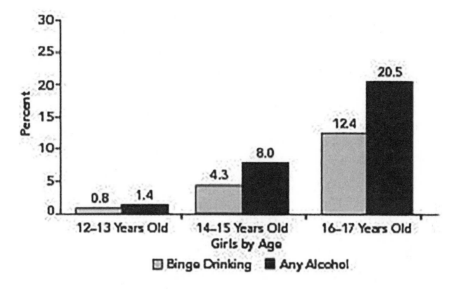

Figure 9.2. Alcohol Use Among Girls

Drinking Levels Among Youth

Alcohol is the most commonly used and abused drug among youth in the United States.

- Excessive drinking is responsible for more than 4,300 deaths among underage youth each year, and cost the United States $24 billion in economic costs in 2010.

- Although drinking by persons under the age of 21 is illegal, people aged 12–20 years drink 11 percent of all alcohol consumed in the United States. More than 90 percent of this alcohol is consumed in the form of binge drinks.

- On average, underage drinkers consume more drinks per drinking occasion than adult drinkers.

- In 2010, there were approximately 189,000 emergency rooms visits by persons under age 21 for injuries and other conditions linked to alcohol.

The 2015 Youth Risk Behavior Survey (YRBS) found that among high school students, during the past 30 days.

- 33 percent drank some amount of alcohol

- 18 percent binge drank

- 8 percent drove after drinking alcohol

- 20 percent rode with a driver who had been drinking alcohol

Other national surveys

- In 2015, the National Survey on Drug Use and Health (NSDUH) reported that 20 percent of youth aged 12–20 years drink alcohol and 13 percent reported binge drinking in the past 30 days.

- In 2015, the Monitoring the Future (MTF) Survey reported that 10 percent of 8th graders and 35 percent of 12th graders drank during the past 30 days, and 5 percent of 8th graders and 17 percent of 12th graders binge drank during the past 2 weeks.

Consequences Of Underage Drinking

Youth who drink alcohol are more likely to experience:

- School problems, such as higher absence and poor or failing grades
- Social problems, such as fighting and lack of participation in youth activities
- Legal problems, such as arrest for driving or physically hurting someone while drunk
- Physical problems, such as hangovers or illnesses
- Unwanted, unplanned, and unprotected sexual activity
- Disruption of normal growth and sexual development
- Physical and sexual assault
- Higher risk for suicide and homicide
- Alcohol-related car crashes and other unintentional injuries, such as burns, falls, and drowning
- Memory problems
- Abuse of other drugs
- Changes in brain development that may have life-long effects
- Death from alcohol poisoning

In general, the risk of youth experiencing these problems is greater for those who binge drink than for those who do not binge drink. Youth who start drinking before age 15 years are six times more likely to develop alcohol dependence or abuse later in life than those who begin drinking at or after age 21 years.

Prevention Of Underage Drinking

Reducing underage drinking will require community-based efforts to monitor the activities of youth and decrease youth access to alcohol. Recent publications by the Surgeon General and the Institute of Medicine (IOM) outlined many prevention strategies for the prevention of underage drinking, such as enforcement of minimum legal drinking age laws, national media campaigns targeting youth and adults, increasing alcohol excise taxes, reducing youth exposure to alcohol advertising, and development of comprehensive community-based programs.

Chapter 10

Underage Drinking: Reasons, Risks, And Prevention

Why Do So Many Young People Drink?

As children mature, it is natural for them to assert their independence, seek new challenges, and try taking risks. Underage drinking is a risk that attracts many developing adolescents and teens. Many want to try alcohol, but often do not fully recognize its effects on their health and behavior.

Other reasons young people drink alcohol include:

- Peer pressure

- Increased independence, or desire for it

- Stress

Prevalence Of Underage Alcohol Use

- **Prevalence of Drinking:** According to the 2015 National Survey on Drug Use and Health (NSDUH), 33.1 percent of 15-year-olds report that they have had at least 1 drink in their lives. About 7.7 million people ages 12–20 (20.3 percent of this age group) reported drinking alcohol in the past month (19.8 percent of males and 20.8 percent of females).

- **Prevalence of Binge Drinking:** According to the 2015 NSDUH, approximately 5.1 million people (about 13.4 percent) ages 12–20 (13.4 percent of males and 13.3 percent of females) reported binge drinking in the past month.

- **Prevalence of Heavy Alcohol Use:** According to the 2015 NSDUH, approximately 1.3 million people (about 3.3 percent) ages 12–20 (3.6 percent of males and 3.0 percent of females) reported heavy alcohol use in the past month.

(Source: "Alcohol Facts and Statistics," National Institute on Alcohol Abuse and Alcoholism (NIAAA).)

About This Chapter: This chapter includes text excerpted from "Underage Drinking," National Institute on Alcohol Abuse and Alcoholism (NIAAA), February 2017.

In addition, many youths may have easy access to alcohol. In 2015, among 12–14-year-olds who reported that they drank alcohol in the past month, 95.1 percent reported that they got it for free the last time they drank. In many cases, adolescents have access to alcohol through family members, or find it at home.

Underage Drinking Is Dangerous

Underage drinking poses a range of risks and negative consequences. It is dangerous because it:

Causes Many Deaths

Based on data from 2006–2010, the Centers for Disease Control and Prevention (CDC) estimates that, on average, alcohol is a factor in the deaths of 4,358 young people under age 21 each year. This includes:

- 1,580 deaths from motor vehicle crashes

- 1,269 from homicides

- 245 from alcohol poisoning, falls, burns, and drowning

- 492 from suicides

Causes Many Injuries

Drinking alcohol can cause kids to have accidents and get hurt. In 2011 alone, about 188,000 people under age 21 visited an emergency room for alcohol-related injuries.

Impairs Judgment

Drinking can lead to poor decisions about engaging in risky behavior, including drinking and driving, sexual activity (such as unprotected sex), and aggressive or violent behavior.

Increases The Risk Of Physical And Sexual Assault

Underage youth who drink are more likely to carry out or be the victim of a physical or sexual assault after drinking than others their age who do not drink.

Can Lead To Other Problems

Drinking may cause youth to have trouble in school or with the law. Drinking alcohol also is associated with the use of other drugs.

Increases The Risk Of Alcohol Problems Later In Life

Research shows that people who start drinking before the age of 15 are 4 times more likely to meet the criteria for alcohol dependence at some point in their lives.

Interferes With Brain Development

Research shows that young people's brains keep developing well into their 20s. Alcohol can alter this development, potentially affecting both brain structure and function. This may cause cognitive or learning problems and/or make the brain more prone to alcohol dependence. This is especially a risk when people start drinking young and drink heavily.

Preventing Underage Drinking

Preventing underage drinking is a complex challenge. Any successful approach must consider many factors, including:

- Genetics

- Personality

What Is "Binge Drinking?"

For adults, binge drinking means drinking so much within about 2 hours that blood alcohol concentration (BAC) levels reach 0.08 g/dL, the legal limit of intoxication. For women, this typically occurs after 4 drinks, and for men, about 5. But, according to recent research estimates, teens may reach these BAC levels after fewer drinks.

For boys:
- Ages 9–13: About 3 drinks
- Ages 14–15: About 4 drinks
- Ages 16–17: About 5 drinks

For girls:
- Ages 9–17: About 3 drinks

- Rate of maturation and development
- Level of risk
- Social factors
- Environmental factors

Several key approaches have been found to be successful. They are:

Environmental Interventions

This approach makes alcohol harder to get—for example, by raising the price of alcohol and keeping the minimum drinking age at 21. Enacting zero-tolerance laws that outlaw driving after any amount of drinking for people under 21 also can help prevent problems.

Individual-Level Interventions

This approach seeks to change the way young people think about alcohol, so they are better able to resist pressures to drink.

School-Based Interventions

These are programs that provide students with the knowledge, skills, motivation, and opportunities they need to remain alcohol free.

Family-Based Interventions

These are efforts to empower parents to set and enforce clear rules against drinking, as well as improve communication between children and parents about alcohol.

The Role Parents Play

Parents and teachers can play a big role in shaping young people's attitudes toward drinking. Parents in particular can have either a positive or negative influence.

Parents can help their children avoid alcohol problems by:

- Talking about the dangers of drinking
- Drinking responsibly, if they choose to drink
- Serving as positive role models in general

- Not making alcohol available

- Getting to know their children's friends

- Having regular conversations about life in general

- Connecting with other parents about sending clear messages about the importance of not drinking alcohol

- Supervising all parties to make sure there is no alcohol

- Encouraging kids to participate in healthy and fun activities that do not involve alcohol

Research shows that children whose parents are actively involved in their lives are less likely to drink alcohol. On the other hand, research shows that a child with a parent who binge drinks is much more likely to binge drink than a child whose parents do not binge drink.

Warning Signs Of Underage Drinking

Adolescence is a time of change and growth, including behavior changes. These changes usually are a normal part of growing up but sometimes can point to an alcohol problem. Parents and teachers should pay close attention to the following warning signs that may indicate underage drinking:

- Changes in mood, including anger and irritability

- Academic and/or behavioral problems in school

- Rebelliousness

- Changing groups of friends

- Low energy level

- Less interest in activities and/or care in appearance

- Finding alcohol among a young person's things

- Smelling alcohol on a young person's breath

- Problems concentrating and/or remembering

- Slurred speech

- Coordination problems

Chapter 11

Drinking Too Much Can Kill You

Celebrating at parties, cheering a favorite sports team, and simply enjoying a break from work are common activities throughout the year. For some people, these occasions also may include drinking—even drinking to excess. And the results can be deadly.

Although many people enjoy moderate drinking, defined as 1 drink per day for women or 2 for men, drinking too much can lead to an overdose. An overdose of alcohol occurs when a person has a blood alcohol content (or BAC) sufficient to produce impairments that increase

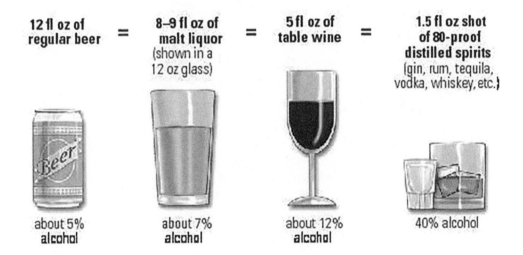

12 fl oz of
regular beer
= 8–9 fl oz of
malt liquor
(shown in a
12 oz glass)
= 5 fl oz of
table wine
= 1.5 fl oz shot
of 80-proof
distilled spirits
(gin, rum, tequila,
vodka, whiskey, etc.)

about 5%
alcohol
about 7%
alcohol
about 12%
alcohol
40% alcohol

Figure 11.1. Percent Of Pure Alcohol By Volume

About This Chapter: This chapter includes text excerpted from "Alcohol Overdose: The Dangers Of Drinking Too Much," National Institute on Alcohol Abuse and Alcoholism (NIAAA), October 2015.

the risk of harm. Overdoses can range in severity, from problems with balance and slurred speech to coma or even death. What tips the balance from drinking that has pleasant effects to drinking that can cause harm varies among individuals. Age, drinking experience, gender, the amount of food eaten, even ethnicity all can influence how much is too much. Underage drinkers may be at particular risk for alcohol overdose. Research shows that people under age 20 typically drink about 5 drinks at one time. Drinking such a large quantity of alcohol can overwhelm the body's ability to break down and clear alcohol from the bloodstream. This leads to rapid increases in BAC and significantly impairs brain function.

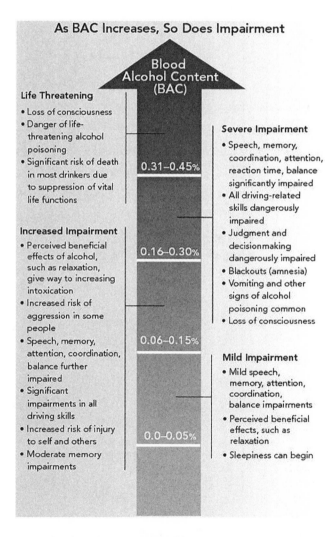

Figure 11.2. Blood Alcohol Content (BAC)

What's "At-Risk" Or "Heavy" Drinking?

For healthy adults in general, drinking more than these single-day or weekly limits is considered "at-risk" or "heavy" drinking:

- Men: More than 4 drinks on any day or 14 per week
- Women: More than 3 drinks on any day or 7 per week

About 1 in 4 people who exceed these limits already has an alcohol use disorder, and the rest are at greater risk for developing these and other problems. Again, individual risks vary. People can have problems drinking less than these amounts, particularly if they drink too quickly.

(Source: "What's "At-Risk" Or "Heavy" Drinking?" National Institute on Alcohol Abuse and Alcoholism (NIAAA).)

Alcohol Overdose Leads To Alcohol Poisoning

As BAC increases, so do alcohol's effects—as well as the risk for harm. Even small increases in BAC can decrease coordination, make a person feel sick, and cloud judgment. This can lead to injury from falls or car crashes, leave one vulnerable to sexual assault or other acts of violence, and increase the risk for unprotected or unintended sex. When BACs go even higher, amnesia (or blackouts) can occur. Continuing to drink despite clear signs of significant impairments can result in a potentially deadly type of overdose called alcohol poisoning. Alcohol poisoning occurs when there is so much alcohol in the bloodstream that areas of the brain controlling basic life support functions—such as breathing, heart rate, and temperature control—begin to shut down.

Symptoms of alcohol poisoning include:

- Confusion
- Difficulty remaining conscious
- Vomiting
- Seizures
- Trouble with breathing
- Slow heart rate
- Clammy skin
- Dulled responses, such as no gag reflex (which prevents choking)
- Extremely low body temperature

BAC can continue to rise even when a person is unconscious. Alcohol in the stomach and intestine continues to enter the bloodstream and circulate throughout the body. It is dangerous to assume that an unconscious person will be fine by sleeping it off. Alcohol acts as a depressant, hindering signals in the brain that control automatic responses such as the gag reflex.

Alcohol also can irritate the stomach, causing vomiting. With no gag reflex, a person who drinks to the point of passing out is in danger of choking on vomit, which, in turn, could lead to death by asphyxiation. Even if the drinker survives, an alcohol overdose can lead to long-lasting brain damage.

If you suspect someone has alcohol poisoning, get medical help immediately. Cold showers, hot coffee, or walking will not reverse the effects of alcohol overdose and could actually make things worse. At the hospital, medical staff will manage any breathing problems, administer fluids to combat dehydration and low blood sugar, and flush the drinker's stomach to help clear the body of toxins. The best way to avoid an alcohol overdose is to drink responsibly if you choose to drink.

According to the *Dietary Guidelines for Americans* (DGA), moderate alcohol consumption is defined as up to 1 drink per day for women and up to 2 drinks per day for men. Know that even if you drink within these limits, you could have problems with alcohol if you drink too quickly, have health conditions, or take medications. If you are pregnant or may become pregnant, you should not drink alcohol.

Heavy or at-risk drinking for women is the consumption of more than 3 drinks on any day or more than 7 per week, and for men it is more than 4 drinks on any day or more than 14 per week. This pattern of drinking too much, too often, is associated with an increased risk for alcohol use disorders. Binge drinking for women is having 4 or more drinks within 2 hours; for men, it is 5 or more drinks within 2 hours. This dangerous pattern of drinking typically results in a BAC of 0.08 percent for the average adult and increases the risk of immediate adverse consequences.

Identifying Alcohol Poisoning

Critical signs and symptoms of alcohol poisoning:

- Mental confusion, stupor, coma, or inability to wake up

- Vomiting

- Seizures

- Slow breathing (fewer than 8 breaths per minute)

- Irregular breathing (10 seconds or more between breaths)
- Hypothermia (low body temperature), bluish skin color, paleness

What Should I Do If I Suspect Someone Has Alcohol Poisoning?

- Know the danger signals
- Do not wait for someone to have all the symptoms
- Be aware that a person who has passed out may die
- If you suspect an alcohol overdose, call 911 for help

What Can Happen To Someone With Alcohol Poisoning That Goes Untreated?

- Choking on his or her own vomit
- Breathing that slows, becomes irregular, or stops
- Heart that beats irregularly or stops
- Hypothermia (low body temperature)
- Hypoglycemia (too little blood sugar), which leads to seizures
- Untreated severe dehydration from vomiting, which can cause seizures, permanent brain damage, and death

Chapter 12

Binge Drinking

Binge drinking is a serious but preventable public health problem. It is the most common, costly, and deadly pattern of excessive alcohol use in the United States. The National Institute on Alcohol Abuse and Alcoholism (NIAAA) defines binge drinking as a pattern of drinking that brings a person's blood alcohol concentration (BAC) to 0.08 grams percent or above. This typically happens when men consume 5 or more drinks or women consume 4 or more drinks in about 2 hours. Most people who binge drink are not alcohol dependent.

Who Binge Drinks?

- One in six U.S. adults binge drinks about four times a month, consuming about seven drinks per binge. This results in 17 billion total binge drinks consumed by adults annually, or 467 binge drinks per binge drinker.

- Binge drinking is most common among younger adults aged 18–34 years, but more than half of the total binge drinks are consumed by those aged 35 and older.

- Binge drinking is twice as common among men than among women. Four in five total binge drinks are consumed by men.

- Binge drinking is more common among people with household incomes of $75,000 or more and higher educational levels. Binge drinkers with lower incomes and educational levels, however, consume more binge drinks per year.

About This Chapter: This chapter includes text excerpted from "Fact Sheets—Binge Drinking," Centers for Disease Control and Prevention (CDC), March 27, 2018.

- Over 90 percent of U.S. adults who drink excessively report binge drinking in the past 30 days.

- Most people younger than age 21 who drink alcohol report binge drinking, often consuming large amounts.

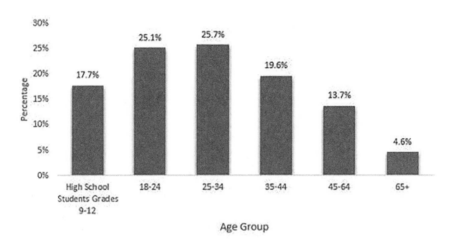

Figure 12.1. Binge Drinking Facts

Alcohol And College Students

- **Prevalence of drinking:** According to the 2015 National Survey on Drug Use and Health (NSDUH), 58.0 percent of full-time college students ages 18–22 drank alcohol in the past month compared with 48.2 percent of other persons of the same age.

- **Prevalence of binge drinking:** According to the 2015 NSDUH, 37.9 percent of college students ages 18–22 reported binge drinking in the past month compared with 32.6 percent of other persons of the same age.

- **Prevalence of heavy alcohol use:** According to the 2015 NSDUH, 12.5 percent of college students ages 18–22 reported heavy alcohol use in the past month compared with 8.5 percent of other persons of the same age.

(Source: "Alcohol Facts And Statistics," National Institute on Alcohol Abuse and Alcoholism (NIAAA).)

Binge Drinking Has Serious Risks

Binge drinking is associated with many health problems, including the following:

- Unintentional injuries such as car crashes, falls, burns, and alcohol poisoning

- Violence including homicide, suicide, intimate partner violence, and sexual assault

- Sexually transmitted diseases (STDs)

- Unintended pregnancy and poor pregnancy outcomes, including miscarriage and stillbirth

- Fetal alcohol spectrum disorders (FASDs)

- Sudden infant death syndrome (SIDS)

- Chronic diseases such as high blood pressure, stroke, heart disease, and liver disease

- Cancer of the breast, mouth, throat, esophagus, liver, and colon

- Memory and learning problems

- Alcohol dependence

Binge Drinking Costs Everyone

- Drinking too much, including binge drinking, cost the United States $249 billion in 2010, or $2.05 a drink. These costs resulted from losses in workplace productivity, healthcare expenditures, criminal justice costs, and other expenses. Binge drinking was responsible for 77 percent of these costs, or $191 billion.

Preventing Binge Drinking

The Community Preventive Services Task Force (CPSTF) recommends evidence-based interventions to prevent binge drinking and related harms. Recommended strategies include:

- Using pricing strategies, including increasing alcohol taxes

- Limiting the number of retail alcohol outlets that sell alcoholic beverages in a given area

- Holding alcohol retailers responsible for the harms caused by illegal alcohol sales to minors or intoxicated patrons (dram shop liability)

- Restricting access to alcohol by maintaining limits on the days and hours of alcohol retail sales

- Consistently enforcing laws against underage drinking and alcohol-impaired driving

- Maintaining government controls on alcohol sales (avoiding privatization)

- Screening and counseling for alcohol misuse

Chapter 13

Alcohol Use And Health Risks

Drinking too much can harm your health. Excessive alcohol use led to approximately 88,000 deaths and 2.5 million years of potential life lost (YPLL) each year in the United States from 2006–2010, shortening the lives of those who died by an average of 30 years. Further, excessive drinking was responsible for 1 in 10 deaths among working-age adults aged 20–64 years. The economic costs of excessive alcohol consumption in 2010 were estimated at $249 billion, or $2.05 a drink.

What Is A "Drink"?

In the United States, a standard drink contains 0.6 ounces (14.0 grams or 1.2 tablespoons) of pure alcohol. Generally, this amount of pure alcohol is found in:

- 12-ounces of beer (5% alcohol content)

- 8-ounces of malt liquor (7% alcohol content)

- 5-ounces of wine (12% alcohol content)

- 1.5-ounces of 80-proof (40% alcohol content) distilled spirits or liquor (e.g., gin, rum, vodka, whiskey)

About This Chapter: Text in this chapter begins with excerpts from "Fact Sheets—Alcohol Use And Your Health," Centers for Disease Control and Prevention (CDC), January 3, 2018; Text beginning with the heading "Effects On The Brain" is excerpted from "Beyond Hangovers," National Institute on Alcohol Abuse and Alcoholism (NIAAA), September 2010. Reviewed July 2018.

What Is Excessive Drinking?

Excessive drinking includes binge drinking, heavy drinking, and any drinking by pregnant women or people younger than age 21.

- Binge drinking, the most common form of excessive drinking, is defined as consuming

  - For women, 4 or more drinks during a single occasion

  - For men, 5 or more drinks during a single occasion

- Heavy drinking is defined as consuming

  - For women, 8 or more drinks per week

  - For men, 15 or more drinks per week

- Most people who drink excessively are not alcoholics or alcohol dependent.

What Is Moderate Drinking?

The *Dietary Guidelines for Americans* (DGA) defines moderate drinking as up to 1 drink per day for women and up to 2 drinks per day for men. In addition, the *Dietary Guidelines* do not recommend that individuals who do not drink alcohol start drinking for any reason.

However, there are some people who should not drink any alcohol, including those who are:

- Younger than age 21

- Pregnant or may be pregnant

- Driving, planning to drive, or participating in other activities requiring skill, coordination, and alertness

- Taking certain prescription or over-the-counter (OTC) medications that can interact with alcohol

- Suffering from certain medical conditions

- Recovering from alcoholism or are unable to control the amount they drink

By adhering to the *Dietary Guidelines*, you can reduce the risk of harm to yourself or others.

Short-Term Health Risks

Excessive alcohol use has immediate effects that increase the risk of many harmful health conditions. These are most often the result of binge drinking and include the following:

- Injuries, such as motor vehicle crashes, falls, drownings, and burns.

- Violence, including homicide, suicide, sexual assault, and intimate partner violence.

- Alcohol poisoning, a medical emergency that results from high blood alcohol levels.

- Risky sexual behaviors, including unprotected sex or sex with multiple partners. These behaviors can result in unintended pregnancy or sexually transmitted diseases (STDs), including human immunodeficiency virus (HIV).

- Miscarriage and stillbirth or fetal alcohol spectrum disorders (FASDs) among pregnant women.

Long-Term Health Risks

Over time, excessive alcohol use can lead to the development of chronic diseases and other serious problems including:

- High blood pressure, heart disease, stroke, liver disease, and digestive problems

- Cancer of the breast, mouth, throat, esophagus, liver, and colon

- Learning and memory problems, including dementia and poor school performance

- Mental health problems, including depression and anxiety

- Social problems, including lost productivity, family problems, and unemployment

- Alcohol dependence, or alcoholism

By not drinking too much, you can reduce the risk of these short- and long-term health risks.

Effects On The Brain

You're chatting with friends at a party and a waitress comes around with glasses of champagne. You drink one, then another, maybe even a few more. Before you realize it, you are laughing more loudly than usual and swaying as you walk. By the end of the evening, you are too slow to move out of the way of a waiter with a dessert tray and have trouble speaking clearly. The next morning, you wake up feeling dizzy and your head hurts. You may have a hard time remembering everything you did the night before.

These reactions illustrate how quickly and dramatically alcohol affects the brain. The brain is an intricate maze of connections that keeps our physical and psychological processes running smoothly. Disruption of any of these connections can affect how the brain works. Alcohol also can have longer-lasting consequences for the brain—changing the way it looks and works and resulting in a range of problems.

Most people do not realize how extensively alcohol can affect the brain. But recognizing these potential consequences will help you make better decisions about what amount of alcohol is appropriate for you.

Defining The Brain Changes

Using brain imaging and psychological tests, researchers have identified the regions of the brain most vulnerable to alcohol's effects. These include:

- **Cerebellum**—This area controls motor coordination. Damage to the cerebellum results in a loss of balance and stumbling, and also may affect cognitive functions such as memory and emotional response.
- **Limbic system**—This complex brain system monitors a variety of tasks including memory and emotion. Damage to this area impairs each of these functions.
- **Cerebral cortex**—Our abilities to think, plan, behave intelligently, and interact socially stem from this brain region. In addition, this area connects the brain to the rest of the nervous system. Changes and damage to this area impair the ability to solve problems, remember, and learn.

Alcohol Shrinks And Disturbs Brain Tissue

Heavy alcohol consumption—even on a single occasion—can throw the delicate balance of neurotransmitters off course. Alcohol can cause your neurotransmitters to relay information too slowly, so you feel extremely drowsy. Alcohol-related disruptions to the neurotransmitter balance also can trigger mood and behavioral changes, including depression, agitation, memory loss, and even seizures.

Long-term, heavy drinking causes alterations in the neurons, such as reductions in the size of brain cells. As a result of these and other changes, brain mass shrinks and the brain's inner cavity grows bigger. These changes may affect a wide range of abilities, including motor coordination; temperature regulation; sleep; mood; and various cognitive functions, including learning and memory.

One neurotransmitter particularly susceptible to even small amounts of alcohol is called glutamate. Among other things, glutamate affects memory. Researchers believe that alcohol interferes with glutamate action, and this may be what causes some people to temporarily "blackout," or forget much of what happened during a night of heavy drinking.

Alcohol also causes an increased release of serotonin, another neurotransmitter, which helps regulate emotional expression, and endorphins, which are natural substances that may spark feelings of relaxation and euphoria as intoxication sets in. Researchers now understand that the brain tries to compensate for these disruptions. Neurotransmitters adapt to create balance in the brain despite the presence of alcohol. But making these adaptations can have negative results, including building alcohol tolerance, developing alcohol dependence, and experiencing alcohol withdrawal symptoms.

What Factors Make A Difference?

Different people react differently to alcohol. That is because a variety of factors can influence your brain's response to alcohol. These factors include:

- **How much and how often you drink.** The more you drink, the more vulnerable your brain is.

- **Your genetic background and family history of alcoholism.** Certain ethnic populations can have stronger reactions to alcohol, and children of alcoholics are more likely to become alcoholics themselves.

- **Your physical health.** If you have liver or nutrition problems, the effects of alcohol will take longer to wear off.

Other Alcohol-Related Brain Conditions

Liver Damage That Affects The Brain

Not only does alcoholic liver disease affect liver function itself, it also damages the brain. The liver breaks down alcohol—and the toxins it releases. During this process, alcohol's byproducts damage liver cells. These damaged liver cells no longer function as well as they should and allow too much of these toxic substances, ammonia and manganese in particular, to travel to the brain. These substances proceed to damage brain cells, causing a serious and potentially fatal brain disorder known as hepatic encephalopathy.

Hepatic encephalopathy causes a range of problems, from less severe to fatal. These problems can include:

- Sleep disturbances

- Mood and personality changes

- Anxiety

- Depression

- Shortened attention span

- Coordination problems, including asterixis, which results in handshaking or flapping

- Coma

- Death

Doctors can help treat hepatic encephalopathy with compounds that lower blood ammonia concentrations and with devices that help remove harmful toxins from the blood. In some cases, people suffering from hepatic encephalopathy require a liver transplant, which generally helps improve brain function.

Fetal Alcohol Spectrum Disorders (FASDs)

Alcohol can affect the brain at any stage of development—even before birth. Fetal alcohol spectrum disorders are the full range of physical, learning, and behavioral problems, and other birth defects that result from prenatal alcohol exposure. The most serious of these disorders, fetal alcohol syndrome (FAS), is characterized by abnormal facial features and is usually associated with severe reductions in brain function and overall growth. FAS is the leading preventable birth defect associated with mental and behavioral impairment in the United States today. The brains of children with FAS are smaller than normal and contain fewer cells, including neurons. These deficiencies result in lifelong learning and behavioral problems. Current research is investigating whether the brain function of children and adults with FAS can be improved with complex rehabilitative training, dietary supplements, or medications.

Effects On The Heart

Americans know how prevalent heart disease is—about 1 in 12 of us suffer from it. What we don't always recognize are the connections heart disease shares with alcohol. On the one hand, researchers have known for centuries that excessive alcohol consumption can damage the heart. Drinking a lot over a long period of time or drinking too much on a single occasion can put your heart—and your life—at risk. On the other hand, researchers now understand that drinking moderate amounts of alcohol can protect the hearts of some people from the risks of coronary artery disease (CHD). Deciding how much, if any, alcohol is right for you can be complicated. To make the best decision for yourself, you need to know the facts and then consult your physician.

Alcoholic Cardiomyopathy

Long-term heavy drinking weakens the heart muscle, causing a condition called alcoholic cardiomyopathy. A weakened heart droops and stretches and cannot contract effectively. As a result, it cannot pump enough blood to sufficiently nourish the organs. In some cases, this blood flow shortage causes severe damage to organs and tissues. Symptoms of cardiomyopathy include shortness of breath and other breathing difficulties, fatigue, swollen legs and feet, and irregular heartbeat. It can even lead to heart failure.

Arrhythmias

Both binge drinking and long-term drinking can affect how quickly a heart beats. The heart depends on an internal pacemaker system to keep it pumping consistently and at the right speed. Alcohol disturbs this pacemaker system and causes the heart to beat too rapidly, or irregularly. These heart rate abnormalities are called arrhythmias. Two types of alcohol-induced arrhythmias are:

- **Atrial fibrillation.** In this form of arrhythmia, the heart's upper, or atrial, chambers shudder weakly but do not contract. Blood can collect and even clot in these upper chambers. If a blood clot travels from the heart to the brain, a stroke can occur; if it travels to other organs such as the lungs, an embolism, or blood vessel blockage, occurs.

- **Ventricular tachycardia.** This form of arrhythmia occurs in the heart's lower, or ventricular, chambers. Electrical signals travel throughout the heart's muscles, triggering contractions that keep blood flowing at the right pace. Alcohol-induced damage to heart muscle cells can cause these electrical impulses to circle through the ventricle too many times, causing too many contractions. The heart beats too quickly, and so does not fill up with enough blood between each beat. As a result, the rest of the body does not get enough blood. Ventricular tachycardia causes dizziness, lightheadedness, unconsciousness, cardiac arrest, and even sudden death. Drinking to excess on a particular occasion, especially when you generally don't drink, can trigger either of these irregularities. In these cases, the problem is nicknamed "holiday heart syndrome," because people who don't usually drink may consume too much alcohol at parties during the holiday season. Over the long term, chronic drinking changes the course of electrical impulses that drive the heart's beating, which creates arrhythmia.

Strokes

A stroke occurs when blood cannot reach the brain. In about 80 percent of strokes, a blood clot prevents blood flow to the brain. These are called ischemic strokes. Sometimes, blood accumulates in the brain, or in the spaces surrounding it. This causes hemorrhagic strokes.

Both binge drinking and long-term heavy drinking can lead to strokes even in people without coronary heart disease. Studies show that people who binge drink are about 56 percent more likely than people who never binge drink to suffer an ischemic stroke over 10 years. Binge drinkers also are about 39 percent more likely to suffer any type of stroke than people who never binge drink. In addition, alcohol exacerbates the problems that often lead to strokes, including hypertension, arrhythmias, and cardiomyopathy.

Hypertension

Chronic alcohol use, as well as binge drinking, can cause high blood pressure, or hypertension. Your blood pressure is a measurement of the pressure your heart creates as it beats, and the pressure inside your veins and arteries. Healthy blood vessels stretch like elastic as the heart pumps blood through them. Hypertension develops when the blood vessels stiffen, making them less flexible. Heavy alcohol consumption triggers the release of certain stress hormones that in turn constrict blood vessels. This elevates blood pressure. In addition, alcohol may affect the function of the muscles within the blood vessels, causing them to constrict and elevate blood pressure.

Effects On The Liver

Heavy drinking—even for just a few days at a time—can cause fat to build up in the liver. This condition, called steatosis, or fatty liver, is the earliest stage of alcoholic liver disease and the most common alcohol-induced liver disorder. The excessive fat makes it more difficult for the liver to operate and leaves it open to developing dangerous inflammations, like alcoholic hepatitis.

For some, alcoholic hepatitis does not present obvious symptoms. For others, though, alcoholic hepatitis can cause fever, nausea, appetite loss, abdominal pain, and even mental confusion. As it increases in severity, alcoholic hepatitis dangerously enlarges the liver, and causes jaundice, excessive bleeding, and clotting difficulties.

Another liver condition associated with heavy drinking is fibrosis, which causes scar tissue to build up in the liver. Alcohol alters the chemicals in the liver needed to break down and remove this scar tissue. As a result, liver function suffers.

If you continue to drink, this excessive scar tissue builds up and creates a condition called cirrhosis, which is a slow deterioration of the liver. Cirrhosis prevents the liver from performing critical functions, including managing infections, removing harmful substances from the blood, and absorbing nutrients.

A variety of complications, including jaundice, insulin resistance and type 2 diabetes, and even liver cancer, can result as cirrhosis weakens liver function. Risk factors ranging from genetics and gender, to alcohol accessibility, social customs around drinking, and even diet can affect a person's individual susceptibility to alcoholic liver disease. Statistics show that about one in five heavy drinkers will develop alcoholic hepatitis, while one in four will develop cirrhosis.

Effects On The Pancreas

A pancreas unaffected by alcohol sends enzymes out to the small intestine to metabolize food. Alcohol jumbles this process. It causes the pancreas to secrete its digestive juices internally, rather than sending the enzymes to the small intestine. These enzymes, as well as acetaldehyde—a substance produced from metabolizing, or breaking down the alcohol—are harmful to the pancreas. If you consume alcohol excessively over a long time, this continued process can cause inflammation, as well as swelling of tissues and blood vessels.

This inflammation is called pancreatitis, and it prevents the pancreas from working properly. Pancreatitis occurs as a sudden attack, called acute pancreatitis. As excessive drinking continues, the inflammation can become constant. This condition is known as chronic pancreatitis.

Pancreatitis is also a risk factor for the development of pancreatic cancer. A heavy drinker may not be able to detect the build-up of pancreatic damage until the problems set off an attack.

An acute pancreatic attack causes symptoms including:

- Abdominal pain, which may radiate up the back

- Nausea and vomiting

- Fever

- Rapid heart rate

- Diarrhea

- Sweating

Chronic pancreatitis causes these symptoms as well as severe abdominal pain, significant reduction in pancreatic function and digestion, and blood sugar problems. Chronic pancreatitis can slowly destroy the pancreas and lead to diabetes or even death.

While a single drinking binge will not automatically lead to pancreatitis, the risk of developing the disease increases as excessive drinking continues over time.

These risks apply to all heavy drinkers, but only about 5 percent of people with alcohol dependence develop pancreatitis. Some people are more susceptible to the disease than others, but researchers have not yet identified exactly what environmental and genetic factors play the biggest role.

Cancer Risks

Genetics, environment, and lifestyle habits can all heighten your risk of getting cancer. We can't do anything to change our genes, and we often can't do much to change our environment. But lifestyle habits are a different story.

Drinking too much alcohol is one lifestyle habit that can increase your risk of developing certain cancers. This does not mean that anyone who drinks too much will develop cancer. But numerous studies do show the more you drink, the more you increase your chances of developing certain types of cancer.

For example, a group of Italy-based scientists reviewed more than 200 studies examining alcohol's impact on cancer risk. The collective results of these studies clearly demonstrate that the more you drink, the higher your risk for developing a variety of cancers. The National Cancer Institute (NCI) identifies alcohol as a risk factor for the following types of cancer:

- Mouth

- Esophagus

- Pharynx

- Larynx

- Liver

- Breast

At least 7 out of 10 people with mouth cancer drink heavily. Drinking five or more drinks per day can also increase your risk of developing other types of cancers, including colon or rectal cancer. In fact, summary estimates from the World Cancer Research Fund (WCRF) report indicate that women who drink five standard alcohol drinks each day have about 1.2 times the risk of developing colon or rectal cancer than women who do not drink at all.

People who drink are also more likely to smoke, and the combination increases the risk significantly. Smoking alone is a known risk factor for some cancers. But smoking and drinking together intensifies the cancer-causing properties of each substance. The overall effect poses an even greater risk.

The risk of throat and mouth cancers is especially high because alcohol and tobacco both come in direct contact with those areas. Overall, people who drink and smoke are 15 times more likely to develop cancers of the mouth and throat than nondrinkers and nonsmokers.

Women And Cancer

One recent, groundbreaking study followed the drinking habits of 1.2 million middle-aged women over 7 years. The study found that alcohol increases women's chances of developing cancers of the breast, mouth, throat, rectum, liver, and esophagus. The researchers link alcohol to about 13 percent of these cancer cases.

In addition, the study concluded that cancer risk increases no matter how little or what kind of alcohol a woman drinks. Even one drink a day can raise risk, and it continues to rise with each additional drink. While men did not participate in this study, the researchers believe this risk is likely similar for men.

This study also attributes about 11 percent of all breast cancer cases to alcohol. That means that of the 250,000 breast cancer cases diagnosed in the United States in 2008, about 27,000 may stem from alcohol.

Effects On The Immune System

Germs and bacteria surround us everywhere. Luckily, our immune system is designed to protect our bodies from the scores of foreign substances that can make us sick. Drinking too much alcohol weakens the immune system, making your body a much easier target for disease.

Understanding the effect alcohol can have on your immune system can inform the decisions you make about drinking alcohol.

Alcohol suppresses both the innate and the adaptive immune systems. Chronic alcohol use reduces the ability of white blood cells to effectively engulf and swallow harmful bacteria. Excessive drinking also disrupts the production of cytokines, causing your body to either produce too much or not enough of these chemical messengers. An abundance of cytokines can damage your tissues, whereas a lack of cytokines leaves you open to infection.

Chronic alcohol use also suppresses the development of T-cells and may impair the ability of natural killer (NK) cells to attack tumor cells. This reduced function makes you more vulnerable to bacteria and viruses, and less capable of destroying cancerous cells.

With a compromised immune system, chronic drinkers are more liable to contract diseases like pneumonia and tuberculosis than people who do not drink too much. There is also data linking alcohol's damage to the immune system with an increased susceptibility to contracting HIV infection. HIV develops faster in chronic drinkers who already have the virus.

Drinking a lot on a single occasion also can compromise your immune system. Drinking to intoxication can slow your body's ability to produce cytokines that ward off infections by causing inflammations. Without these inflammatory responses, your body's ability to defend itself against bacteria is significantly reduced. A study shows that slower inflammatory cytokine production can reduce your ability to fight off infections for up to 24 hours after getting drunk.

Alcohol-Related Deaths

- An estimated 88,000 people die from alcohol-related causes annually, making alcohol the third leading preventable cause of death in the United States. The first is tobacco, and the second is poor diet and physical inactivity.

- In 2014, alcohol-impaired driving fatalities accounted for 9,967 deaths (31 percent of overall driving fatalities).

(Source: "Alcohol Facts And Statistics," National Institute on Alcohol Abuse and Alcoholism (NIAAA).)

Chapter 14

A Family History Of Alcoholism

If you are among the millions of people in this country who have a parent, grandparent, or other close relative with alcoholism, you may have wondered what your family's history of alcoholism means for you. Are problems with alcohol a part of your future? Is your risk for becoming an alcoholic greater than for people who do not have a family history of alcoholism? If so, what can you do to lower your risk?

What Is Alcoholism?

Alcoholism, or alcohol dependence, is a disease that includes four symptoms:

1. **Craving.** A strong need, or urge, to drink.

2. **Loss of control.** Not being able to stop drinking once drinking has begun.

3. **Physical dependence.** Withdrawal symptoms, such as upset stomach, sweating, shakiness, and anxiety after stopping drinking.

4. **Tolerance.** The need to drink greater amounts of alcohol to get "high."

Many scientific studies, including research conducted among twins and children of alcoholics, have shown that genetic factors influence alcoholism. These findings show that children of alcoholics are about four times more likely than the general population to develop alcohol problems. Children of alcoholics also have a higher risk for many other behavioral and emotional problems. But alcoholism is not determined only by the genes you inherit from your

---

About This Chapter: This chapter includes text excerpted from "A Family History Of Alcoholism: Are You At Risk?" National Institute on Alcohol Abuse and Alcoholism (NIAAA), June 2012. Reviewed July 2018.

parents. In fact, more than one–half of all children of alcoholics do not become alcoholic. Research shows that many factors influence your risk of developing alcoholism. Some factors raise the risk while others lower it.

Genes are not the only things children inherit from their parents. How parents act and how they treat each other and their children has an influence on children growing up in the family. These aspects of family life also affect the risk for alcoholism. Researchers believe a person's risk increases if he or she is in a family with the following difficulties:

- An alcoholic parent is depressed or has other psychological problems
- Both parents abuse alcohol and other drugs
- The parents' alcohol abuse is severe; and
- Conflicts lead to aggression and violence in the family

The good news is that many children of alcoholics from even the most troubled families do not develop drinking problems. Just as a family history of alcoholism does not guarantee that you will become an alcoholic, neither does growing up in a very troubled household with alcoholic parents. Just because alcoholism tends to run in families does not mean that a child of an alcoholic parent will automatically become an alcoholic too. The risk is higher but it does not have to happen.

Things To Do

If you are worried that your family's history of alcohol problems or your troubled family life puts you at risk for becoming alcoholic, here is some common-sense advice to help you:

Avoid underage drinking—First, underage drinking is illegal. Second, research shows that the risk for alcoholism is higher among people who begin to drink at an early age, perhaps as a result of both environmental and genetic factors.

Drink moderately as an adult—Even if they do not have a family history of alcoholism, adults who choose to drink alcohol should do so in moderation—no more than one drink a day for most women, and no more than two drinks a day for most men, according to guidelines from the U.S. Department of Agriculture (USDA) and the U.S. Department of Health and Human Services (HHS). Some people should not drink at all, including women who are pregnant or who are trying to become pregnant, recovering alcoholics, people who plan to drive or engage in other activities that require attention or skill, people taking certain medications, and people with certain medical conditions.

People with a family history of alcoholism, who have a higher risk for becoming dependent on alcohol, should approach moderate drinking carefully. Maintaining moderate drinking habits may be harder for them than for people without a family history of drinking problems. Once a person moves from moderate to heavier drinking, the risks of social problems (for example, drinking and driving, violence, and trauma) and medical problems (for example, liver disease, brain damage, and cancer) increase greatly.

Talk to a healthcare professional—Discuss your concerns with a doctor, nurse, nurse practitioner, or other healthcare provider. They can recommend groups or organizations that could help you avoid alcohol problems. If you are an adult who already has begun to drink, a healthcare professional can assess your drinking habits to see if you need to cut back on your drinking and advise you about how to do that.

> More than 10 percent of U.S. children live with a parent with alcohol problems, according to a study.
>
> *(Source: "Alcohol Facts And Statistics," National Institute on Alcohol Abuse and Alcoholism (NIAAA).)*

Chapter 15

Coping With An Alcoholic Parent

Impact Of Parental Substance Use On Children

The way parents with substance use disorders behave and interact with their children can have a multifaceted impact on the children. The effects can be both indirect (e.g., through a chaotic living environment) and direct (e.g., physical or sexual abuse). Parental substance use can affect parenting, prenatal development, and early childhood and adolescent development. It is important to recognize, however, that not all children of parents with substance use issues will suffer abuse, neglect, or other negative outcomes.

Parenting

A parent's substance use disorder may affect his or her ability to function effectively in a parental role. Ineffective or inconsistent parenting can be due to the following:

- Physical or mental impairments caused by alcohol or other drugs

- Reduced capacity to respond to a child's cues and needs

- Difficulties regulating emotions and controlling anger and impulsivity

- Disruptions in healthy parent-child attachment

- Spending limited funds on alcohol and drugs rather than food or other household needs

About This Chapter: Text beginning with the heading "Impact Of Parental Substance Use On Children" is excerpted from "Parental Substance Use And The Child Welfare System," Child Welfare Information Gateway, U.S. Department of Health and Human Services (HHS), October 2014. Reviewed July 2018; Text under the heading "Helping Children Of Addicted Parents Find Help" is excerpted from "Helping Children Of Addicted Parents Find Help," National Institute on Drug Abuse (NIDA) for Teens, February 16, 2012. Reviewed July 2018.

- Spending time seeking out, manufacturing, or using alcohol or other drugs

- Incarceration, which can result in inadequate or inappropriate supervision for children

- Estrangement from family and other social supports

Family life for children with one or both parents that abuse drugs or alcohol often can be chaotic and unpredictable. Children's basic needs—including nutrition, supervision, and nurturing—may go unmet, which can result in neglect. These families often experience a number of other problems—such as mental illness, domestic violence, unemployment, and housing instability—that also affect parenting and contribute to high levels of stress. A parent with a substance abuse disorder may be unable to regulate stress and other emotions, which can lead to impulsive and reactive behavior that may escalate to physical abuse. Different substances may have different effects on parenting and safety. For example, the threats to a child of a parent who becomes sedated and inattentive after drinking excessively differ from the threats posed by a parent who exhibits aggressive side effects from methamphetamine use. Dangers may be posed not only from use of illegal drugs, but also, and increasingly, from abuse of prescription drugs (pain relievers, antianxiety medicines, and sleeping pills). Polysubstance use (multiple drugs) may make it difficult to determine the specific and compounded effects on any individual. Further, risks for the child's safety may differ depending upon the level and severity of parental substance use and associated adverse effects.

Prenatal And Infant Development

The effects of parental substance use disorders on a child can begin before the child is born. Maternal drug and alcohol use during pregnancy have been associated with premature birth, low birth weight, slowed growth, and a variety of physical, emotional, behavioral, and cognitive problems. Research suggests powerful effects of legal drugs, such as tobacco, as well as illegal drugs on prenatal and early childhood development. Fetal alcohol spectrum disorders (FASDs) are a set of conditions that affect an estimated 40,000 infants born each year to mothers who drank alcohol during pregnancy. Children with FASD may experience mild to severe physical, mental, behavioral, and/or learning disabilities, some of which may have lifelong implications (e.g., brain damage, physical defects, attention deficits). In addition, increasing numbers of newborns—approximately 3 per 1,000 hospital births each year—are affected by neonatal abstinence syndrome (NAS), a group of problems that occur in a newborn who was exposed prenatally to addictive illegal or prescription drugs. The full impact of prenatal substance exposure depends on a number of factors. These include the frequency, timing, and type of substances used by pregnant women; co-occurring environmental deficiencies; and the extent of prenatal care. Research suggests that some of the negative outcomes of prenatal exposure can be improved by supportive home environments and positive parenting practices.

Child And Adolescent Development

Children and youth of parents who use or abuse substances and have parenting difficulties have an increased chance of experiencing a variety of negative outcomes:

- Poor cognitive, social, and emotional development

- Depression, anxiety, and other trauma and mental health symptoms

- Physical and health issues

- Substance use problems

Parental substance use can affect the well-being of children and youth in complex ways. For example, an infant who receives inconsistent care and nurturing from a parent engaged in addiction-related behaviors may suffer from attachment difficulties that can then interfere with the growing child's emotional development. Adolescent children of parents with substance use disorders, particularly those who have experienced child maltreatment and foster care, may turn to substances themselves as a coping mechanism. In addition, children of parents with substance use issues are more likely to experience trauma and its effects, which include difficulties with concentration and learning, controlling physical and emotional responses to stress, and forming trusting relationships.

> Researchers have found that children of parents with an alcohol use disorder are at greater risk for depression, anxiety disorders, problems with cognitive and verbal skills, and parental abuse or neglect. Furthermore, they are 4 times more likely than other children to develop symptoms of an alcohol use disorder themselves.
>
> *(Source: "Children Living With Parents Who Have A Substance Use Disorder," Substance Abuse and Mental Health Services Administration (SAMHSA).)*

Child Welfare Laws Related To Parental Substance Use

In response to concerns over the potential negative impact on children of parental substance abuse and illegal drug-related activities, approximately 47 States and the District of

Columbia (DC) have child protection laws that address some aspect of parental substance use. Some States have expanded their civil definitions of child abuse and neglect to include a caregiver's use of a controlled substance that impairs the ability to adequately care for a child and/or exposure of a child to illegal drug activity (e.g., sale or distribution of drugs, home-based meth labs). Exposure of children to illegal drug activity is also addressed in 33 States' criminal statutes.

Federal and state laws also address prenatal drug exposure. The Child Abuse Prevention and Treatment Act (CAPTA) requires States receiving CAPTA funds to have policies and procedures for healthcare personnel to notify child protective services (CPS) of substance-exposed newborns and to develop procedures for safe care of affected infants. As yet, there are no national data on CAPTA-related reports for substance-exposed newborns. In some State statutes, substance abuse during pregnancy is considered child abuse and/or grounds for termination of parental rights. State statutes and State and local policies vary widely in their requirements for reporting suspected prenatal drug abuse, testing for drug exposure, CPS response, forced admission to treatment of pregnant women who use drugs, and priority access for pregnant women to state-funded treatment programs.

Innovative Prevention And Treatment Approaches

While parental substance abuse continues to be a major challenge in child welfare, the past two decades have witnessed some new and more effective approaches and innovative programs to address child protection for families where substance abuse is an issue. Some examples of promising and innovative prevention and treatment approaches include the following:

- Promotion of protective factors, such as social connections, concrete supports, and parenting knowledge, to support families and buffer risks

- Early identification of at-risk families in substance abuse treatment programs and through expanded prenatal screening initiatives so that prevention services can be provided to promote child safety and well-being in the home

- Priority and timely access to substance abuse treatment slots for mothers involved in the child welfare system

- Gender-sensitive treatment and support services that respond to the specific needs, characteristics, and co-occurring issues of women who have substance use disorders

- Family-centered treatment services, including inpatient treatment for mothers in facilities where they can have their children with them and programs that provide services to each family member

- Recovery coaches or mentoring of parents to support treatment, recovery, and parenting

- Shared family care in which a family experiencing parental substance use and child maltreatment is placed with a host family for support and mentoring

Find more information on specific programs and service models:

- National Center on Substance Abuse and Child Welfare (NCSACW), Regional Partnership Grant (RPG) Program: Overview of Grantees' Services and Interventions (ncsacw.samhsa.gov/files/RPG_Program_Brief_2_Services_508_reduced.pdf)

- National Resource Center (NRC) for In-Home Services, In-Home Programs for Drug Affected Families (secure.goozmo.com/user_files/26365.pdf)

- Substance Abuse and Mental Health Services Administration's (SAMHSA) National Registry of Evidence-Based Programs and Practices (NREPP) (www.nrepp.samhsa.gov/landing.aspx)

Helping Children Of Addicted Parents Find Help

A child looks to his parents or caregivers for total support—from birth to adulthood. But what happens to a child when his parents are addicted to drugs or alcohol?

Celebrating Recovery, Offering Hope

It's estimated that 25 percent of youth under age 18 are exposed to family alcohol abuse or dependence. Research shows that children in this environment are more likely to develop depression or anxiety in adolescence and use alcohol or other drugs early on. Having a parent who is addicted to drugs or alcohol can lead to lifelong problems if the child or teen doesn't get help and support.

February 12–18, 2012, is Children of Alcoholics (COA) Week, an event to celebrate the recovery of children of all ages who have gotten the help they needed to recover from the pain they experienced as a result of a close family member's alcohol problems. The observance also offers hope to those still suffering.

Finding Support

Help is out there. Teens can talk to a school guidance counselor, coach, or trusted teacher. For those who attend religious services, a clergy member is also an option.

Teens may be reluctant to talk to an acquaintance about such a personal problem. Another good option is Alateen, a program that offers support for children of parents who are addicted. Alateen members come together in a free and confidential setting to:

- Share experiences and hope
- Discuss difficulties
- Learn effective ways to cope with problems
- Encourage one another

Another option is the National Suicide Prevention Lifeline (NSPL) at 800-273-TALK (800-273-8255). This service is also confidential, and counselors can help with substance abuse and family problems, in addition to suicide prevention.

Part Three
Tobacco, Nicotine, And E-Cigarettes

Chapter 16

Tobacco And Nicotine Addiction

What Are Tobacco And Nicotine Products?

Tobacco is a leafy plant grown around the world, including in parts of the United States. There are many chemicals found in tobacco leaves or created by burning them (as in cigarettes), but nicotine is the ingredient that can lead to addiction. Other chemicals produced by smoking, such as tar, carbon monoxide, acetaldehyde, and nitrosamines, also can cause serious harm to the body. For example, tar causes lung cancer and other serious diseases that affect breathing, and carbon monoxide can cause heart problems.

Teens who are considering smoking for social reasons should keep this in mind: Tobacco use is the leading preventable cause of disease, disability, and death in the United States. According to the Centers for Disease Control and Prevention (CDC), cigarettes cause more than 480,000 premature deaths in the United States each year—from smoking or exposure to secondhand smoke—about 1 in every 5 U.S. deaths, or 1,300 deaths every day. An additional 16 million people suffer with a serious illness caused by smoking. So, for every 1 person who dies from smoking, 30 more suffer from at least 1 serious tobacco-related illness.

Also known as:

Cigarettes: Butts, Cigs, and Smokes

Smokeless tobacco: Chew, Dip, Snuff, Snus, and Spit Tobacco

Hookah: Goza, Hubble-bubble, Narghile, Shisha, and Waterpipe

About This Chapter: This chapter includes text excerpted from "Tobacco, Nicotine, And E-Cigarettes," National Institute on Drug Abuse (NIDA) for Teens, July 2017.

How Tobacco And Nicotine Products Are Used

Tobacco and nicotine products come in many forms. People can smoke, chew, sniff, or inhale their vapors.

- Smoked tobacco products

  - **Cigarettes (regular, light, and menthol):** No evidence exists that "lite" or menthol cigarettes are safer than regular cigarettes.

  - **Cigars and pipes:** Some small cigars are hollowed out to make room for marijuana, known as "blunts." Some young people do this to attempt to hid the fact that they are smoking marijuana. either way, they are inhaling toxic chemicals.

  - **Bidis and kreteks (clove cigarettes):** Bidis are small, thin, hand-rolled cigarettes primarily imported to the United States from India and other Southeast Asian countries. Kreteks—sometimes referred to as clove cigarettes—contain about 60–80 percent tobacco and 20–40 percent ground cloves. Flavored bidis and kreteks are banned in the United States because of the ban on flavored cigarettes.

  - **Hookahs or water pipes:** Hookah tobacco comes in many flavors, and the pipe is typically passed around in groups. A recent study found that a typical hookah session delivers approximately 125 times the smoke, 25 times the tar, 2.5 times the nicotine, and 10 times the carbon monoxide as smoking a cigarette.

- Smokeless tobacco products. The tobacco is not burned with these products:

  - **Chewing tobacco.** It is typically placed between the cheek and gums.

  - **Snuff:** Ground tobacco that can be sniffed if dried or placed between the cheek and gums.

  - **Dip:** Moist snuff that is used like chewing tobacco.

  - **Snus:** A small pouch of moist snuff.

  - **Dissolvable products (including lozenges, orbs, sticks, and strips)**

What Happens In The Brain When You Use Tobacco And Nicotine?

Like other drugs, nicotine increases levels of a neurotransmitter called dopamine. Dopamine is released normally when you experience something pleasurable like good food, your favorite activity, or spending time with people you care about. When a person uses tobacco products, the release of dopamine causes similar effects. This effect wears off quickly, causing people who smoke to get the urge to light up again for more of that good feeling, which can lead to addiction.

A typical smoker will take 10 puffs on a cigarette over the period of about 5 minutes that the cigarette is lit. So, a person who smokes about 1 pack (25 cigarettes) daily gets 250 "hits" of nicotine each day.

Studies suggest that other chemicals in tobacco smoke, such as acetaldehyde, may increase the effects of nicotine on the brain. When smokeless tobacco is used, nicotine is absorbed through the mouth tissues directly into the blood, where it goes to the brain. Even after the tobacco is removed from the mouth, nicotine continues to be absorbed into the bloodstream. Also, the nicotine stays in the blood longer for users of smokeless tobacco than for smokers.

Mental health, beliefs about smoking, perception of schoolmates' smoking, and other substance use are additional factors that can influence an adolescent's risk for smoking and nicotine dependence. Emotional problems—including depression and recent negative life events—are associated with tobacco use among adolescents. Smoking among peers and within social groups is a major environmental factor that influences adolescent smoking; social smoking is a more important motivator for adolescents compared to adult smokers.

(Source: "Tobacco, Nicotine, And E-Cigarettes," National Institute On Drug Abuse (NIDA).)

What Happens To Your Body When You Use Tobacco And Nicotine?

When nicotine enters the body, it initially causes the adrenal glands to release a hormone called adrenaline. The rush of adrenaline stimulates the body and causes an increase in blood pressure, heart rate, and breathing. Most of the harm to the body is not from the nicotine, but from other chemicals in tobacco or those produced when burning it—including carbon monoxide, tar, formaldehyde, cyanide, and ammonia. Tobacco use harms every organ in the body and can cause many problems. The health effects of smokeless tobacco are somewhat different from those of smoked tobacco, but both can cause cancer.

Secondhand Smoke

People who do not smoke but live or hang out with smokers are exposed to secondhand smoke—exhaled smoke as well as smoke given off by the burning end of tobacco products.

Just like smoking, this also increases the risk for many diseases. Each year, an estimated 58 million Americans are regularly exposed to secondhand smoke and more than 42,000 non-smokers die from diseases caused by secondhand smoke exposure. One in four U.S. middle and high school students say they've been exposed to unhealthy secondhand aerosol from e-cigarettes.

The table below lists the health problems people are at risk for when smoking or chewing tobacco or as a result of exposure to secondhand smoke.

Table 16.1. Increased Risk Of Health Problems

Health Effect	Smoking Tobacco	Secondhand Smoke	Smokeless Tobacco
Cancer	**Cancers:** Cigarette smoking can be blamed for about one-third of all cancer deaths, including 90 percent of lung cancer cases. Tobacco use is also linked with cancers of the mouth, pharynx, larynx, esophagus, stomach, pancreas, cervix, kidney, ureter, bladder, and bone marrow (leukemia).	**Lung cancer:** People exposed to secondhand smoke increase their risk for lung cancer by 20–30 percent. About 7,300 lung cancer deaths occur per year among people who do not smoke.	**Cancers:** Close to 30 chemicals in smokeless tobacco have been found to cause cancer. People who use smokeless tobacco are at increased risk for oral cancer (cancers of the mouth, lip, tongue, and pharynx) as well as esophageal and pancreatic cancers.
Lung Problems	**Breathing problems:** Bronchitis (swelling of the air passages to the lungs), emphysema (damage to the lungs), and pneumonia have been linked with smoking. **Lowered lung capacity:** People who smoke can't exercise or play sports for as long as they once did.	**Breathing problems:** Secondhand smoke causes breathing problems in people who do not smoke, like coughing, phlegm, and lungs not working as well as they should.	

Table 16.1. Continued

Health Effect	Smoking Tobacco	Secondhand Smoke	Smokeless Tobacco
Heart Disease/Stroke	**Heart disease and stroke:** Smoking increases the risk for stroke, heart attack, vascular disease (diseases that affect the circulation of blood through the body), and aneurysm (a balloon-like bulge in an artery that can rupture and cause death).	**Heart disease:** Secondhand smoke increases the risk for heart disease by 25–30 percent. It is estimated to contribute to as many as 34,000 deaths related to heart disease.	**Heart disease and stroke:** Recent research shows smokeless tobacco may play a role in causing heart disease and stroke.
Other Health Problems	**Cataracts:** People who smoke can get cataracts, which is clouding of the eye that causes blurred vision. **Loss of sense** of smell and taste **Aging skin and teeth:** After smoking for a long time, people find their skin ages faster and their teeth discolor.		**Mouth problems:** Smokeless tobacco increases the chance of getting cavities, gum disease, and sores in the mouth that can make eating and drinking painful.
Pregnant Women and Children	**Pregnant women:** Pregnant women who smoke are at increased risk for delivering their baby early or suffering a miscarriage, stillbirth, or experiencing other problems with their pregnancy. Smoking by pregnant women also may be associated with learning and behavior problems in children.	**Health problems for children:** Children exposed to secondhand smoke are at an increased risk for sudden infant death syndrome, lung infections, ear problems, and more severe asthma.	

Table 16.1. Continued

Health Effect	Smoking Tobacco	Secondhand Smoke	Smokeless Tobacco
Accidental Death	**Fire-related deaths:** Smoking is the leading cause of fire-related deaths—more than 600 deaths each year.		

Can You Die If You Use Tobacco And Nicotine Products?

Yes. Tobacco use (both smoked and smokeless) is the leading preventable cause of death in the United States. It is a known cause of cancer. Smoking tobacco also can lead to early death from heart disease, health problems in children, and accidental home and building fires caused by dropped cigarettes. In addition, the nicotine in smokeless tobacco may increase the risk for sudden death from a condition where the heart does not beat properly (ventricular arrhythmias); as a result, the heart pumps little or no blood to the body's organs.

According to the CDC, cigarette smoking results in more than 480,000 premature deaths in the United States each year—about 1 in every 5 U.S. deaths, or 1,300 deaths every day. On average, smokers die 10 years earlier than nonsmokers. People who smoke are at increased risk of death from cancer, particularly lung cancer, heart disease, lung diseases, and accidental injury from fires started by dropped cigarettes. The good news is that people who quit may live longer. A 24-year-old man who quits smoking will, on average, increase his life expectancy (how long he is likely to live) by 5 years.

Are Tobacco Or Nicotine Products Addictive?

Yes. It is the nicotine in tobacco that is addictive. Each cigarette contains about 10 milligrams of nicotine. A person inhales only some of the smoke from a cigarette, and not all of each puff is absorbed in the lungs. The average person gets about 1–2 milligrams of the drug from each cigarette.

Studies of widely used brands of smokeless tobacco showed that the amount of nicotine per gram of tobacco ranges from 4.4–25.0 milligrams. Holding an average-size dip in your mouth for 30 minutes gives you as much nicotine as smoking 3 cigarettes. A 2-can-a-week snuff dipper gets as much nicotine as a person who smokes 1½ packs a day.

Whether a person smokes tobacco products or uses smokeless tobacco, the amount of nicotine absorbed in the body is enough to make someone addicted. When this happens, the person continues to seek out the tobacco even though he or she understands the harm it causes. Nicotine addiction can cause:

- **Tolerance:** Over the course of a day, someone who uses tobacco products develops tolerance—more nicotine is required to produce the same initial effects. In fact, people who smoke often report that the first cigarette of the day is the strongest or the "best."

- **Withdrawal:** When people quit using tobacco products, they usually experience uncomfortable withdrawal symptoms, which often drive them back to tobacco use. Nicotine withdrawal symptoms include:

  - Irritability

  - Problems with thinking and paying attention

  - Sleep problems

  - Increased appetite

  - Craving, which may last 6 months or longer, and can be a major stumbling block to quitting

How Many Teens Use Tobacco And Nicotine Products?

Smoking and smokeless tobacco use generally start during the teen years. Among people who use tobacco:

- Each day, nearly 3,200 people younger than 18 years of age smoke their first cigarette.

- Every day, an estimated 2,100 youth and young adults who have been occasional smokers become daily cigarette smokers.

- If smoking continues at the current rate among youth in this country, 5.6 million of Americans under the age of 18—or about 1 in every 13 young people—could die prematurely (too early) from a smoking-related illness.

- E-cigarettes are the most commonly used form of tobacco among youth in the United States.

- Young people who use e-cigarettes or smokeless tobacco may be more likely to also become smokers.

- Using smokeless tobacco remains a mostly male behavior. About 490,000 teens ages 12–17 are current smokeless tobacco users. For every 100 teens who use smokeless tobacco, 85 of them are boys.

A survey of teens in the United States shows cigarette smoking is on the decline. That could be in part due to the introduction of e-cigarettes. Teens today are more likely to smoke an e-cigarette than a regular cigarette.

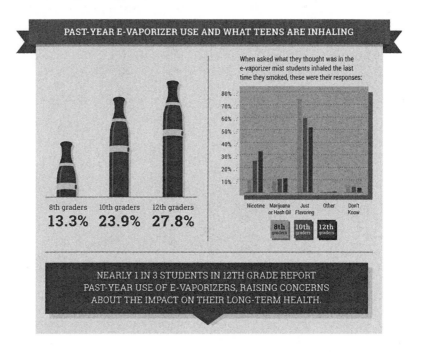

Figure 16.1. E-Vaporizer Use Among Teens

Below is a table showing the percentage of teens who use tobacco and nicotine products:

Table 16.2. Trends In Prevalence Of Various Drugs For 8th Graders, 10th Graders, And 12th Graders; 2017 (In Percent)*

Drug	Time Period	8th Graders	10th Graders	12th Graders
Cigarettes (any use)	Lifetime	9.4	15.9	26.6
	Past Month	(1.90)	5	9.7
	Daily	(0.60)	2.2	4.2
	1/2-pack+/day	0.2	0.7	1.7

Table 16.2. Continued

Drug	Time Period	8th Graders	10th Graders	12th Graders
Smokeless Tobacco	Lifetime	6.2	9.1	(11.00)
	Past Month	(1.70)	3.8	(4.90)
	Daily	0.4	0.6	2
Any Vaping	Lifetime	18.5	30.9	35.8
	Past Year	13.3	23.9	27.8
	Past Month	6.6	13.1	16.6

*Data in brackets indicate statistically significant change from the previous year.

What Do I Do If I Want To Quit Using Tobacco And Nicotine Products?

Treatments can help people who use tobacco products manage these symptoms and improve the likelihood of successfully quitting. For now, teen and young adult smokers who want to quit have good options for help. Nearly 70 percent of people who smoke want to quit. Most who try to quit on their own relapse (go back to smoking)—often within a week. Most former smokers have had several failed quit attempts before they finally succeed.

Some people believe e-cigarette products may help smokers lower nicotine cravings while they are trying to quit smoking cigarettes. But, researchers do not yet know if e-cigarettes are truly helpful for people trying to quit. There is also the possibility that they could strengthen the nicotine addiction, which would make quitting more difficult, and they can introduce nicotine to young people who have not yet tried smoking.

If you or someone you know needs more information or is ready to quit, check out these resources:

Teens
- Visit SmokeFree.gov.

Adults
- Call 800-QUIT-NOW (800-784-8669), a national toll-free number that can help people get the information they need to quit smoking.
- Visit SmokeFree.gov.

Chapter 17

Teen Tobacco Use

Youth use of tobacco in any form is unsafe. If smoking continues at the current rate among youth in this country, 5.6 million of Americans younger than 18 will die early from a smoking-related illness. That's about 1 of every 13 Americans aged 17 years or younger alive today.

Tobacco Use Among Youth

Preventing tobacco use among youth is critical to ending the tobacco epidemic in the United States.

- Tobacco use is started and established primarily during adolescence.

  - Nearly 9 out of 10 cigarette smokers first tried smoking by age 18, and 98 percent first tried smoking by age 26.

  - Each day in the United States, more than 3,200 youth aged 18 years or younger smoke their first cigarette, and an additional 2,100 youth and young adults become daily cigarette smokers.

- Flavorings in tobacco products can make them more appealing to youth.

  - In 2014, 73 percent of high school students and 56 percent of middle school students who used tobacco products in the past 30 days reported using a flavored tobacco product during that time.

About This Chapter: This chapter includes text excerpted from "Smoking And Tobacco Use—Youth and Tobacco Use," Centers for Disease Control and Prevention (CDC), March 5, 2018.

Estimates Of Current Tobacco Use Among Youth

Cigarettes

- From 2011–2016, current cigarette smoking declined among middle and high school students.

    - About 2 of every 100 middle school students (2.2%) reported in 2016 that they smoked cigarettes in the past 30 days—a decrease from 4.3 percent in 2011.

    - 8 of every 100 high school students (8.0%) reported in 2016 that they smoked cigarettes in the past 30 days—a decrease from 15.8 percent in 2011.

Electronic Cigarettes

- Current use of electronic cigarettes increased among middle and high school students from 2011–2016.

    - About 4 of every 100 middle school students (4.3%) reported in 2016 that they used electronic cigarettes in the past 30 days—an increase from 0.6 percent in 2011.

    - About 11 of every 100 high school students (11.3%) reported in 2016 that they used electronic cigarettes in the past 30 days—an increase from 1.5 percent in 2011.

Hookahs

- From 2011–2016, current use of hookahs increased among middle and high school students.

    - 2 of every 100 middle school students (2.0%) reported in 2016 that they had used hookah in the past 30 days—an increase from 1.0 percent in 2011.

    - Nearly 5 of every 100 high school students (4.8%) reported in 2016 that they had used hookah in the past 30 days—an increase from 4.1 percent in 2011.

Smokeless Tobacco

- In 2016:

    - About 2 of every 100 middle school students (2.2%) reported current use of smokeless tobacco.

    - Nearly 6 of every 100 high school students (5.8%) reported current use of smokeless tobacco.

All Tobacco Product Use

- In 2016, about 7 of every 100 middle school students (7.2%) and about 20 of every 100 high school students (20.2%) reported current use of some type of tobacco product.

- In 2013, nearly 18 of every 100 middle school students (17.7%) and nearly half (46.0%) of high school students said they had ever tried a tobacco product.

Use Of Multiple Tobacco Products Is Prevalent Among Youth

- In 2016, about 3 of every 100 middle school students (3.1%) and nearly 10 of every 100 high school students (9.6%) reported current use of two or more tobacco products in the past 30 days.

- In 2013, more than 9 of every 100 middle school students (9.4%) and more than 31 of every 100 high school students (31.4%) said they had ever tried two or more tobacco products.

Youth who use multiple tobacco products are at higher risk for developing nicotine dependence and might be more likely to continue using tobacco into adulthood.

Notes: "Current use" is determined by respondents indicating that they have used a tobacco product on at least 1 day during the past 30 days.

Table 17.1. Tobacco Use* Among High School Students In 2016

Tobacco Product	Overall	Females	Males
Any tobacco product†	20.20%	17.00%	23.50%
Electronic cigarettes	11.30%	9.50%	13.10%
Cigarettes	8.00%	6.90%	9.10%
Cigars	7.70%	5.60%	9.00%
Smokeless tobacco	5.80%	3.30%	8.30%
Hookahs	4.80%	5.10%	4.50%
Pipe tobacco	1.40%	0.90%	1.80%
Bidis	0.50%	0.30%	0.70%

*Use is determined by respondents indicating that they have used a tobacco product on at least 1 day during the past 30 days.

†Any tobacco product includes cigarettes, cigars, smokeless tobacco (including chewing tobacco, snuff, dip, snus, and dissolvable tobacco), tobacco pipes, bidis, hookah, and electronic cigarettes.

Table 17.2. Tobacco Use* Among Middle School Students In 2016

Tobacco Product	Overall	Females	Males
Any tobacco product†	7.20%	5.90%	8.30%
Electronic cigarettes	4.30%	3.40%	5.10%
Cigarettes	2.20%	1.80%	2.50%
Cigars	2.20%	1.70%	2.70%
Smokeless tobacco	2.20%	1.50%	3.00%
Hookahs	2.00%	1.90%	2.10%
Pipe tobacco	0.70%	0.60%	0.80%
Bidis	0.30%	–§	0.40%

*Use is determined by respondents indicating that they have used a tobacco product on at least 1 day during the past 30 days.

†Any tobacco product includes cigarettes, cigars, smokeless tobacco (including chewing tobacco, snuff, dip, snus, and dissolvable tobacco), tobacco pipes, bidis, hookah, and electronic cigarettes.

§Where percentages are missing, sample sizes were less than 50 or relative standard error was greater than 30 percent and thus considered unreliable.

Factors Associated With Youth Tobacco Use

Factors associated with youth tobacco use include the following:

- Social and physical environments
  - The way mass media show tobacco use as a normal activity can promote smoking among young people.
  - Youth are more likely to use tobacco if they see that tobacco use is acceptable or normal among their peers.
  - High school athletes are more likely to use smokeless tobacco than their peers who are nonathletes.
  - Parental smoking may promote smoking among young people.
- Biological and genetic factors
  - There is evidence that youth may be sensitive to nicotine and that teens can feel dependent on nicotine sooner than adults.
  - Genetic factors may make quitting smoking more difficult for young people.
  - A mother's smoking during pregnancy may increase the likelihood that her offspring will become regular smokers.

- Mental health: There is a strong relationship between youth smoking and depression, anxiety, and stress.

- Personal perceptions: Expectations of positive outcomes from smoking, such as coping with stress and controlling weight, are related to youth tobacco use.

- Other influences that affect youth tobacco use include:

  - Lower socioeconomic status, including lower income or education

  - Lack of skills to resist influences to tobacco use

  - Lack of support or involvement from parents

  - Accessibility, availability, and price of tobacco products

  - Low levels of academic achievement

  - Low self-image or self-esteem

  - Exposure to tobacco advertising

Reducing Youth Tobacco Use

National, state, and local program activities have been shown to reduce and prevent youth tobacco use when implemented together. They include the following:

- Higher costs for tobacco products (for example, through increased taxes)

- Prohibiting smoking in indoor areas of worksites and public places

- Raising the minimum age of sale for tobacco products to 21 years, which has recently emerged as a potential strategy for reducing youth tobacco use

- TV and radio commercials, posters, and other media messages targeted toward youth to counter tobacco product advertisements

- Community programs and school and college policies and interventions that encourage tobacco-free environments and lifestyles

- Community programs that reduce tobacco advertising, promotions, and availability of tobacco products

Some social and environmental factors have been found to be related to lower smoking levels among youth. Among these are:

- Religious participation

- Racial/ethnic pride and strong racial identity

- Higher academic achievement and aspirations

Continued efforts are needed to prevent and reduce the use of all forms of tobacco use among youth.

Regulations Restricting The Sale And Distribution Of Tobacco Products To Protect Children And Adolescents

Since 2009, the U.S. Food and Drug Administration (FDA) has regulated cigarettes, smokeless, and roll-your-own tobacco. In 2016, the FDA finalized a rule to regulate all tobacco products, including:

- E-cigarettes/electronic cigarettes/vaporizers
- Cigars
- Hookah (waterpipe tobacco)
- Pipe tobacco
- Nicotine gels
- Dissolvables

These rules protect children and adolescents by restricting youth access to all tobacco products by:

- Not allowing products to be sold to anyone younger than 18 and requiring age verification via photo ID
- Not allowing tobacco products to be sold in vending machines (unless in an adult-only facility)
- Not allowing the distribution of free samples of tobacco products

(Source: "Youth And Tobacco," U.S. Food and Drug Administration (FDA).)

Chapter 18

E-Cigarettes

E-cigarettes come in many shapes and sizes. Most have a battery, a heating element, and a place to hold a liquid. It produces an aerosol by heating a liquid that usually contains nicotine—the addictive drug in regular cigarettes, cigars, and other tobacco products—flavorings, and other chemicals that help to make the aerosol. Users inhale this aerosol into their lungs. Bystanders can also breathe in this aerosol when the user exhales into the air. They are known by many different names. They are sometimes called "e-cigs," "e-hookahs," "mods," "vape pens," "vapes," "tank systems," and "electronic nicotine delivery systems (ENDS)." Some e-cigarettes are made to look like regular cigarettes, cigars, or pipes. Some resemble pens, universal serial bus (USB) sticks, and other everyday items. Larger devices such as tank systems, or "mods," do not resemble other tobacco products. Using an e-cigarette is sometimes called "vaping." It can be used to deliver marijuana and other drugs.

What Is In E-Cigarette Aerosol?

The e-cigarette aerosol that users breathe from the device and exhale can contain harmful and potentially harmful substances, including:

- Nicotine

- Ultrafine particles that can be inhaled deep into the lungs

- Flavoring such as diacetyl, a chemical linked to a serious lung disease

About This Chapter: Text in this chapter begins with excerpts from "Smoking And Tobacco Use—Electronic Cigarettes," Centers for Disease Control and Prevention (CDC), April 10, 2018; Text beginning with the heading "E-Cigarettes And Young People: A Public Health Concern" is excerpted from "E-Cigarettes And Young People: A Public Health Concern," Centers for Disease Control and Prevention (CDC), January 31, 2017.

- Volatile organic compounds (VOCs)

- Cancer-causing chemicals

- Heavy metals such as nickel, tin, and lead

It is difficult for consumers to know what e-cigarette products contain. For example, some e-cigarettes marketed as containing zero percent nicotine have been found to contain nicotine.

What Are The Health Effects Of Using E-Cigarettes?

E-cigarettes are still fairly new, and scientists are still learning about their long-term health effects. Here is what we know now.

- Most e-cigarettes contain nicotine, which has known health effects.

  - Nicotine is highly addictive.

  - Nicotine is toxic to developing fetuses.

  - Nicotine can harm adolescent brain development, which continues into the early to mid-20s.

  - Nicotine is a health danger for pregnant women and their developing babies.

- Besides nicotine, e-cigarette aerosol can contain substances that harm the body.

  - This includes cancer-causing chemicals and tiny particles that reach deep into lungs. However, e-cigarette aerosol generally contains fewer harmful chemicals than smoke from burned tobacco products.

- E-cigarettes can cause unintended injuries.

  - Defective e-cigarette batteries have caused fires and explosions, some of which have resulted in serious injuries. Most explosions happened when the e-cigarette batteries were being charged.

    - The U.S. Food and Drug Administration (FDA) collects data to help address this issue. You can report an e-cigarette explosion, or any other unexpected health or safety issue with an e-cigarette, here (www.safetyreporting.hhs.gov/SRP2/en/Home.aspx?sid=73eb1e98-65b8-4ba5-ab69-2aaa4f76971f).

  - In addition, acute nicotine exposure can be toxic. Children and adults have been poisoned by swallowing, breathing, or absorbing e-cigarette liquid through their skin or eyes.

What Are The Risks Of E-Cigarettes For Youth, Young Adults, And Pregnant Women?

Most e-cigarettes contain nicotine, which is addictive and toxic to developing fetuses. Nicotine exposure can also harm adolescent brain development, which continues into the early to mid-20s. E-cigarette aerosol can contain chemicals that are harmful to the lungs. And youth e-cigarette use is associated with the use of other tobacco products, including cigarettes.

Are E-Cigarettes Less Harmful Than Regular Cigarettes?

Yes—but that doesn't mean e-cigarettes are safe. E-cigarette aerosol generally contains fewer toxic chemicals than the deadly mix of 7,000 chemicals in smoke from regular cigarettes. However, e-cigarette aerosol is not harmless. It can contain harmful and potentially harmful substances, including nicotine, heavy metals like lead, VOCs, and cancer-causing agents.

Can E-Cigarettes Help Adults Quit Smoking Cigarettes?

E-cigarettes are not currently approved by the FDA as a quit smoking aid. The U.S. Preventive Services Task Force (USPSTF), a group of health experts that makes recommendations about preventive healthcare, has concluded that evidence is insufficient to recommend e-cigarettes for smoking cessation in adults, including pregnant women.

However, e-cigarettes may help nonpregnant adult smokers if used as a complete substitute for all cigarettes and other smoked tobacco products.

- To date, the few studies on the issue are mixed. A Cochrane Review found evidence from two randomized controlled trials that e-cigarettes with nicotine can help smokers stop smoking in the long term compared with placebo (nonnicotine) e-cigarettes. However, there are some limitations to the existing research, including the small number of trials, small sample sizes, and wide margins of error around the estimates.

- A Centers for Disease Control and Prevention (CDC) study found that many adults are using e-cigarettes in an attempt to quit smoking. However, most adult e-cigarette users do not stop smoking cigarettes and are instead continuing to use both products (known as "dual use"). Dual use is not an effective way to safeguard your health, whether you're using e-cigarettes, smokeless tobacco, or other tobacco products in addition to regular cigarettes. Because smoking even a few cigarettes a day can be dangerous, quitting smoking completely is very important to protect your health.

Who Is Using E-Cigarettes?

E-cigarettes are now the most commonly used tobacco product among youth.

- In the United States, youth are more likely than adults to use e-cigarettes.

- In 2016, more than 2 million U.S. middle and high school students used e-cigarettes in the past 30 days, including 4.3 percent of middle school students and 11.3 percent of high school students.

In 2016, 3.2 percent of U.S. adults were current e-cigarette users.

- In 2015, among adult e-cigarette users overall, 58.8 percent also were current regular cigarette smokers, 29.8 percent were former regular cigarette smokers, and 11.4 percent had never been regular cigarette smokers.

- Among current e-cigarette users aged 45 years and older in 2015, most were either current or former regular cigarette smokers, and 1.3 percent had never been cigarette smokers. In contrast, among current e-cigarette users aged 18–24 years, 40.0 percent had never been regular cigarette smokers.

E-Cigarettes And Young People: A Public Health Concern

E-cigarettes, devices that typically deliver nicotine, flavorings, and other additives to users through an inhaled aerosol, are a rapidly emerging trend, and are especially popular among youth and young adults. These devices are referred to by a variety of names, including "e-cigs," "e-hookahs," "mods," "vape pens," "vapes," and "tank systems." E-cigarettes can also be used to deliver other drugs besides nicotine, such as marijuana.

Scientists are still learning more about how e-cigarettes affect health. However, there is already enough evidence to justify efforts to prevent e-cigarette use by young people. We know that the vapor from e-cigarettes is harmful because it contains harmful ingredients, including nicotine. Nicotine exposure during adolescence can cause addiction and can harm the developing brain.

Sources of e-cigarette advertisement exposure.

- 14.4 million youth are exposed to advertising in retail stores
- 10.5 million youth are exposed to advertising through the Internet
- 9.6 million youth are exposed through TV or movies
- 8 million youth are exposed through newspapers or magazines

U.S. students exposed to e-cigarette advertisements, by school type and number of sources of exposure.

A high proportion of U.S. Middle and High School students saw e-cigarette advertisements in 2014 from one or more of the following four sources:

1. Retail
2. Internet
3. TV/movies
4. Magazines/newspapers.

Overall,

- 66 percent of U.S. Middle School Students
- 71 percent of U.S. High School Students
- 69 percent U.S. Middle and High School Students

(Source: "Youth Tobacco Use Infographics," Centers for Disease Control and Prevention (CDC).)

In 2016, a U.S. Surgeon General's Report on e-cigarette use among youth and young adults became the first report issued by a federal agency that carefully reviewed the public health issue of e-cigarettes and their impact on our nation's young people. Because most tobacco use starts during adolescence, actions to protect our nation's young people from a lifetime of nicotine addiction are critical.

E-cigarettes are now the most commonly used form of tobacco by youth in the United States. And dual use, or using both e-cigarettes and conventional cigarettes, is common among youth and young adults 18–25 years of age. Reasons reported by young people for using e-cigarettes include curiosity, taste, and the belief that e-cigarettes are less harmful than other tobacco products.

Flavored e-cigarettes are very popular, especially with young adults. More than 9 of every 10 young adult e-cigarette users said they use e-cigarettes flavored to taste like menthol, alcohol, candy, fruit, chocolate, or other sweets. More than 8 of every 10 youth ages 12–17 who use e-cigarettes said they use flavored e-cigarettes.

E-cigarettes are a 2.5 billion dollar business in the United States. As of 2014, the e-cigarette industry spent $125 million a year to advertise their products, and used many of the techniques that made traditional cigarettes popular such as sexual content and customer satisfaction. We know that marketing and advertising of conventional tobacco products like cigarettes can lead youth to use tobacco, and scientists are also finding that youth who are exposed to e-cigarette advertisements are more likely to use the product than youth who are not exposed.

The following are specific actions that parents and other adults can take to reduce young people's exposure to e-cigarettes:

- **Restrict e-cigarette use around young people.** Don't let anyone use e-cigarettes or other tobacco products around young people. Not only are youth watching the behaviors of others as an example, but they're also at risk of exposure to nicotine and other chemicals that can be harmful to their health.

- **Visit tobacco-free locations.** Avoid restaurants and other locations that allow the use of tobacco products, including e-cigarettes.

- **Ensure school is tobacco-free.** Check with your school administration to ensure your child's school, college, or university is completely tobacco-free, including being free of e-cigarettes.

- **Make your home tobacco-free.** Make your home and vehicles tobacco-free by not allowing the use of any tobacco products, including e-cigarettes, by family members, friends, and guests. This is an important step to fully protect your children from exposure to secondhand cigarette smoke and secondhand aerosol from e-cigarettes.

- **Be an example.** Be an example to youth by living tobacco-free. Even if you're quitting tobacco, share the reasons why you want to be tobacco-free and ask for support in your journey.

Chapter 19

Smoking's Immediate Effects On The Body

Smoking harms nearly every organ of the body. Some of these harmful effects are immediate. Find out the health effects of smoking on different parts of your body.

> Smoking remains the leading cause of preventable death and disease in the United States, killing more than 480,000 Americans each year. Smoking causes immediate damage to your body, which can lead to long-term health problems. For every smoking-related death, at least 30 Americans live with a smoking-related illness. The only proven strategy to protect yourself from harm is to never smoke, and if you do smoke or use tobacco products, to quit.
>
> *(Source: "How To Quit," Centers for Disease Control and Prevention (CDC).)*

Brain

Nicotine from cigarettes is as addictive as heroin. Nicotine addiction is hard to beat because it changes your brain. The brain develops extra nicotine receptors to accommodate the large doses of nicotine from tobacco. When the brain stops getting the nicotine it's used to, the result is nicotine withdrawal. You may feel anxious, irritable, and have strong cravings for nicotine.

Head And Face

Ears

Smoking reduces the oxygen supply to the cochlea, a snail-shaped organ in the inner ear. This may result in permanent damage to the cochlea and mild to moderate hearing loss.

About This Chapter: This chapter includes text excerpted from "Health Effects," Smokefree.gov, U.S. Department of Health and Human Services (HHS), May 31, 2018.

Eyes

Smoking causes physical changes in the eyes that can threaten your eyesight. Nicotine from cigarettes restricts the production of a chemical necessary for you to be able to see at night. Also, smoking increases your risk of developing cataracts and macular degeneration (both can lead to blindness).

Mouth

Smoking takes a toll on your mouth. Smokers have more oral health problems than non-smokers, like mouth sores, ulcers, and gum disease. You are more likely to have cavities and lose your teeth at a younger age. You are also more likely to get cancers of the mouth and throat.

Face

Smoking can cause your skin to be dry and lose elasticity, leading to wrinkles and stretch marks. Your skin tone may become dull and grayish. By your early 30s, wrinkles can begin to appear around your mouth and eyes, adding years to your face.

Heart

Stressed Heart

Smoking raises your blood pressure and puts stress on your heart. Over time, stress on the heart can weaken it, making it less able to pump blood to other parts of your body. Carbon monoxide from inhaled cigarette smoke also contributes to a lack of oxygen, making the heart work even harder. This increases the risk of heart disease, including heart attacks.

Sticky Blood

Smoking makes your blood thick and sticky. The stickier the blood, the harder your heart must work to move it around your body. Sticky blood is also more likely to form blood clots that block blood flow to your heart, brain, and legs. Over time, thick, sticky blood damages the delicate lining of your blood vessels. This damage can increase your risk for a heart attack or stroke.

Fatty Deposits

Smoking increases the cholesterol and unhealthy fats circulating in the blood, leading to unhealthy fatty deposits. Over time, cholesterol, fats, and other debris build up on the walls of your arteries. This buildup narrows the arteries and blocks normal blood flow to the heart, brain, and legs. Blocked blood flow to the heart or brain can cause a heart attack or stroke. Blockage in the blood vessels of your legs could result in the amputation of your toes or feet.

Lungs
Scarred Lungs

Smoking causes inflammation in the small airways and tissues of your lungs. This can make your chest feel tight or cause you to wheeze or feel short of breath. Continued inflammation builds up scar tissue, which leads to physical changes in your lungs and airways that can make breathing hard. Years of lung irritation can give you a chronic cough with mucus.

Emphysema

Smoking destroys the tiny air sacs, or alveoli, in the lungs that allow oxygen exchange. When you smoke, you are damaging some of those air sacs. Alveoli don't grow back, so when you destroy them, you have permanently destroyed part of your lungs. When enough alveoli are destroyed, the disease emphysema develops. Emphysema causes severe shortness of breath and can lead to death.

Cilia And Respiratory Infections

Your airways are lined with tiny brush like hairs, called cilia. The cilia sweep out mucus and dirt so your lungs stay clear. Smoking temporarily paralyzes and even kills cilia. This makes you more at risk for infection. Smokers get more colds and respiratory infections than nonsmokers.

Deoxyribonucleic Acid (DNA)
Cancer

Your body is made up of cells that contain genetic material, or deoxyribonucleic acid (DNA), that acts as an "instruction manual" for cell growth and function. Every single puff of a cigarette causes damages to your DNA. When DNA is damaged, the "instruction manual" gets messed up, and the cell can begin growing out of control and create a cancer tumor. Your body tries to repair the damage that smoking does to your DNA, but over time, smoking can wear down this repair system and lead to cancer (like lung cancer). One-third of all cancer deaths are caused by tobacco.

Stomach And Hormones

Belly

Bigger belly. Smokers have bigger bellies and less muscle than nonsmokers. They are more likely to develop type 2 diabetes, even if they don't smoke every day. Smoking also makes it harder to control diabetes once you already have it. Diabetes is a serious disease that can lead to blindness, heart disease, kidney failure, and amputations.

Lower Estrogen Levels

Smoking lowers a female's level of estrogen. Low estrogen levels can cause dry skin, thinning hair, and memory problems. Women who smoke have a harder time getting pregnant and having a healthy baby. Smoking can also lead to early menopause, which increases your risk of developing certain diseases (like heart disease).

Erectile Dysfunction (ED)

Smoking increases the risk of erectile dysfunction (ED)—the inability to get or keep an erection. Toxins from cigarette smoke can also damage the genetic material in sperm, which can cause infertility or genetic defects in your children.

Blood And The Immune System

High White Blood Cell (WBC) Count

When you smoke, the number of white blood cells (WBCs) (the cells that defend your body from infections) stays high. This is a sign that your body is under stress—constantly fighting against the inflammation and damage caused by tobacco. A high WBC count is like a signal from your body, letting you know you've been injured. WBC counts that stay elevated for a long time are linked with an increased risk of heart attacks, strokes, and cancer.

Longer To Heal

Nutrients, minerals, and oxygen are all supplied to the tissue through the bloodstream. Nicotine causes blood vessels to tighten, which decreases levels of nutrients supplied to wounds.

As a result, wounds take longer to heal. Slow wound healing increases the risk of infection after an injury or surgery and painful skin ulcers can develop, causing the tissue to slowly die.

Weakened Immune System

Cigarette smoke contains high levels of tar and other chemicals, which can make your immune system less effective at fighting off infections. This means you're more likely to get sick. Continued weakening of the immune system can make you more vulnerable to autoimmune diseases like rheumatoid arthritis and multiple sclerosis. It also decreases your body's ability to fight off cancer!

Muscles And Bones

Tired Muscles

Muscle deterioration. When you smoke, less blood and oxygen flow to your muscles, making it harder to build muscle. The lack of oxygen also makes muscles tire more easily. Smokers have more muscle aches and pains than nonsmokers.

More Broken Bones

Ingredients in cigarette smoke disrupt the natural cycle of bone health. Your body is less able to form healthy new bone tissue, and it breaks down existing bone tissue more rapidly. Over time, smoking leads to a thinning of bone tissue and loss of bone density. This causes bones to become weak and brittle. Compared to nonsmokers, smokers have a higher risk of bone fractures, and their broken bones take longer to heal.

Chapter 20

Health Harms From Smoking And Other Tobacco Use

Why Smoking Tobacco Products Is So Deadly

The danger of smoking comes from inhaling chemical compounds, some in the tobacco and some that are created when tobacco is burned. The tobacco in cigarettes is a blend of dried tobacco leaf and tobacco sheet made from stems, ribs, and other tobacco leaf waste. The process used to make modern cigarettes includes the use of many chemicals. In all, scientists have identified more than 7,000 chemicals and chemical compounds in tobacco smoke. At least 70 of them are known specifically to cause cancer. All cigarettes are harmful, and any exposure to tobacco smoke can cause both immediate and long-term damage to the body. There is no safe level of exposure to tobacco smoke, and there is no safe cigarette. To reduce cancer risk, quitting smoking entirely is an important strategy that has been proven to work.

Smoking leads to disease and disability and harms nearly every organ of the body. More than 16 million Americans are living with a disease caused by smoking. For every person who dies because of smoking, at least 30 people live with a serious smoking-related illness. Smoking causes cancer, heart disease, stroke, lung diseases, diabetes, and chronic obstructive pulmonary disease (COPD), which includes emphysema and chronic bronchitis. Smoking also increases the risk for tuberculosis, certain eye diseases, and problems of the immune system, including rheumatoid arthritis.

(Source: "Health Effects," Centers for Disease Control and Prevention (CDC).)

About This Chapter: This chapter includes text excerpted from "Let's Make The Next Generation Tobacco-Free: Your Guide To The 50th Anniversary Surgeon General's Report On Smoking And Health," Office of the Surgeon General (OGS), July 2015.

Smoking—The Cancer Trigger

Cancer is a serious disease that happens when cells grow uncontrollably in the body. These cells grow into tumors that damage organs and can spread to other parts of the body. Smoking can cause cancer almost anywhere in the body. Nearly all lung cancer—the number-one cancer killer of both men and women—is caused by smoking. If no one in the United States smoked, we could prevent one out of three cancer deaths.

Deoxyribonucleic Acid (DNA) Damage

DNA is the "blueprint" for every cell in the human body—the cell's "instruction manual." DNA controls a cell's growth and the work each cell does. When tobacco smoke damages DNA, cells can begin growing abnormally. Typically, the body releases special cells to attack and kill cells that are growing out of control. However, toxic chemicals in cigarette smoke weaken this process and make it easier for the abnormal cells to keep growing and dividing.

Lung Cancer

Lung cancer is the number-one cause of cancer death for both men and women. Nearly 9 out of 10 lung cancers are caused by smoking. In fact, smokers today are much more likely to develop lung cancer than smokers were in 1964, when the first Surgeon General's Report on Smoking and Health linked smoking to lung cancer.

Smoking Linked To Two Additional Cancers

Evidence now proves that smoking causes liver cancer, and colorectal cancer, which is the second deadliest cancer among those that affect both men and women. Studies suggest a link between smoking and breast cancer, but the evidence is not as firm. Studies also suggest that men with prostate cancer who smoke may be more likely to die from the disease than nonsmokers.

Cancer Treatment

People who continue to smoke after being diagnosed with cancer raise their risk for future cancers and death. They're more likely to die from their original cancer, secondary cancers, and all other causes than are former smokers and people who have never smoked.

Smoking—The Breath Blocker

Respiratory Diseases

The chemicals in cigarette smoke cause immediate damage to cells and tissue in the human body, including those on the path from the mouth to the lung's air sacs—the final target of the smoke. Delicate lung tissue damaged by chemicals in cigarette smoke doesn't have a chance to heal if it is exposed to these chemicals in large amounts day after day. The result is a wide range of deadly lung conditions.

Chronic Obstructive Pulmonary Disease (COPD)

Smoking causes chronic obstructive pulmonary disease (COPD). COPD includes several underlying lung diseases, such as emphysema and chronic bronchitis, in which the airways are damaged and can never completely heal, and the lungs lose their elastic properties. People with COPD suffer from shortness of breath, coughing, difficulty exercising, air trapped in their lungs, swollen airways, and scar tissue. As a result, they may even have trouble with routine activities such as walking and dressing. Their quality of life can drop significantly. Over time, COPD causes low oxygen levels in the body. People with COPD are at high risk for many other serious diseases, including lung cancer and heart disease. The disease has no cure. Women are now dying from COPD in about the same numbers as men, and women appear more susceptible to developing severe COPD at younger ages. Women smokers in certain age groups are more than 38 times as likely to develop COPD, compared with women who have never smoked.

Tuberculosis (TB)

Tuberculosis (TB) is a common infection worldwide that usually attacks the lungs. TB is spread through the air when people with the disease cough or sneeze. It was once a leading cause of death in the United States, but advances in public health have made TB far less common here. However, it remains a serious health issue elsewhere in the world. According to the World Health Organization (WHO), TB caused 1.4 million deaths worldwide in 2011. There is now enough evidence to conclude that smoking increases a person's risk of getting TB disease and dying from it.

Other Respiratory Damage Caused By Smoking

More than 11 percent of high school students in the United States have asthma, and studies suggest that youth who smoke are more likely to develop asthma. Breathing someone else's smoke also triggers asthma attacks in nonsmokers. Children exposed to secondhand smoke have more respiratory infections than children who are not exposed.

Although the body has ways to prevent or lessen the severity of injury caused by agents inhaled into the lungs, these defenses are overwhelmed when the body is exposed to cigarette smoke over and over again. People who stop smoking begin to breathe easier, may regain higher levels of oxygen in the body, and lower their risk of respiratory disease compared to those who continue to smoke.

Smoking—The Heart Stopper

More than 16 million Americans have heart disease, almost 8 million already have had a heart attack and 7 million have had a stroke. Cardiovascular disease (CVD) is the single largest cause of all deaths in the United States, killing more than 800,000 people a year. CVD includes narrow or blocked arteries in and around the heart (coronary heart disease (CHD)), high blood pressure (hypertension), heart attack (acute myocardial infarction), stroke, and heart-related chest pain (angina pectoris). Smoking is a major cause of CVD. Even people who smoke fewer than five cigarettes a day show signs of early stages of CVD. The risk of CVD increases when more cigarettes a day are smoked, and when smoking continues for many years. Exposure to secondhand smoke can increase the risk for a heart attack or stroke. More than 33,000 nonsmokers die every year in the United States from CHD caused by exposure to secondhand smoke.

Peripheral Arterial Disease (PAD)

Blood vessels are found throughout the body and carry oxygen to every organ. The oxygen makes it possible for organs to do the work needed to keep the body healthy and working correctly. Cigarette smoke makes cells lining blood vessels swell so that the vessels become narrower, reducing the flow of blood. Even smoking every now and then, or inhaling someone else's smoke, damages blood vessels.

Atherosclerosis, or hardening of the arteries, occurs when artery walls thicken and the opening inside the artery narrows. Peripheral arterial disease (PAD) or peripheral vascular disease (PVD) occurs when arteries that supply the legs, feet, arms, or hands become narrow, reducing blood flow. Without normal blood flow, people with PAD may have pain when they walk, and cells and tissue can die from lack of oxygen. In extreme cases, gangrene can develop and the infected limb may have to be removed. Smoking is the most common preventable cause of PAD.

Coronary Heart Disease (CHD)

Components in the blood, called platelets, stick together along with proteins to form clots. Clotting prevents blood loss and infection after an injury. Chemicals in cigarette smoke cause blood to thicken and form clots inside veins and arteries, even when clotting isn't needed to prevent bleeding or infection. Smoking also promotes the formation of plaque in the walls of arteries and clots can form where there is plaque. This is especially dangerous when arteries are already narrowed from smoking, because the clots can easily block those arteries. When arteries are blocked, the oxygen to nearby organs is cut off. CHD occurs when arteries that carry blood to heart muscles are blocked by clots. This blockage can lead to a heart attack and sudden death.

Stroke

A stroke is loss of brain function caused when blood flow within the brain is interrupted. Strokes can occur when arteries that carry blood to the brain become blocked from narrowing or a clot, or when a blood vessel leaks or bursts inside the brain. Strokes can cause permanent brain damage and death. Smoking increases the risk for stroke. Deaths from strokes are more likely among smokers than among former smokers or people who have never smoked. The more cigarettes a person smokes per day, the higher his or her risk of dying from a stroke. Even exposure to secondhand smoke can cause strokes in nonsmokers.

Abdominal Aortic Aneurysm (AAA)

The aorta is the body's main artery that carries oxygen-rich blood to all parts of the body. Smoking is a known cause of early hardening of the abdominal aorta, the part of the aorta that supplies blood to the abdomen, pelvis, and legs. Autopsy studies have found that smoking during adolescence can cause this dangerous condition as early as young adulthood. Hardening of the abdominal aorta can lead to an aneurysm, or a weakened and bulging area. A ruptured abdominal aortic aneurysm (AAA) causes life-threatening bleeding and is often fatal. Almost all deaths from AAAs are caused by smoking and other tobacco use. Women smokers have a higher risk of dying from an aortic aneurysm than men who smoke.

Smoking And Reproduction

For many reasons, men and women who want to have children should not smoke. Studies suggest that smoking affects hormone production. This could make it more difficult for women smokers to become pregnant. Pregnant women who smoke or who are exposed to second-hand smoke endanger their unborn babies, as well as their own health. Babies whose mothers smoked during pregnancy or who are exposed to secondhand smoke after birth are more likely to die of sudden infant death syndrome (SIDS) than are babies who are not exposed. More than 100,000 of the smoking-caused deaths over the last 50 years were of babies who died from SIDS or other health conditions. Deadly chemicals in cigarette smoke reached these infants before they were born, or when they were exposed to cigarette smoke during infancy.

Pregnancy Complications

More than 400,000 babies born in the United States every year are exposed to chemicals in cigarette smoke before birth because their mothers smoke. Smoking is known to cause ectopic pregnancy, a condition in which the fertilized egg fails to move to the uterus and instead attaches in the fallopian tube or to other organs outside the womb. Ectopic pregnancy almost always causes the fetus to die and poses a serious risk to the health of the mother. Another possible complication from smoking during pregnancy is miscarriage.

Mothers who smoke during pregnancy are more likely to deliver their babies early. Preterm delivery is a leading cause of death, disability, and disease among newborns. Mothers who smoke during pregnancy are also more likely to deliver babies with low birth weight, even if they are full term. Carbon monoxide (CO) in tobacco smoke keeps the fetus from getting enough oxygen. Smoking during pregnancy can also cause tissue damage in the fetus, especially in the lungs and brain. This damage can last throughout childhood and into the teenage years.

Birth Defects

Smoking during pregnancy can cause birth defects. Women who smoke during early pregnancy are more likely to deliver babies with cleft lips and/or cleft palates—conditions in which the lip or palate fails to form completely. Both conditions interfere with an infant's ability to eat properly, and both must be corrected with surgery.

Male Reproduction And Sexual Function

In the United States, 18 million men over age 20 suffer from erectile dysfunction (ED). A man with ED can't have and maintain an erection that is adequate for satisfactory sexual performance, which can affect reproduction. Evidences conclude that smoking is a cause of ED. Cigarette smoke alters blood flow necessary for an erection, and smoking interferes with the healthy function of blood vessels in erectile tissue. Men need healthy sperm for fertility. Smoking damages DNA in sperm, which can lead to infertility or early fetal death.

Diabetes can cause serious health problems, including heart disease, blindness, kidney failure, and nerve and blood vessel damage of the feet and legs, which can lead to amputation. A person with diabetes who smokes is more likely to have trouble regulating insulin and controlling the disease than nonsmokers with diabetes. Both smoking and diabetes cause problems with blood flow, which raises the risk of blindness and amputations. Smokers with diabetes are also more likely to have kidney failure than nonsmokers with diabetes. Diabetes is the seventh leading cause of death in the United States.

Smoking And Diabetes

Diabetes—a disease that causes blood sugar levels in the body to be too high—is a growing health crisis around the world. In the United States, more than 25 million adults suffer from diabetes. We now know that smoking causes type 2 diabetes, also known as adult-onset diabetes. Smokers are 30–40 percent more likely to develop type 2 diabetes than nonsmokers. The more cigarettes an individual smokes, the higher the risk for diabetes. Diabetes can cause serious health problems, including heart disease, blindness, kidney failure, and nerve and blood vessel damage of the feet and legs, which can lead to amputation. A person with diabetes who smokes is more likely to have trouble regulating insulin and controlling the disease than nonsmokers with diabetes. Both smoking and diabetes cause problems with blood flow, which raises the risk of blindness and amputations. Smokers with diabetes are also more likely to have kidney failure than nonsmokers with diabetes. Diabetes is the seventh leading cause of death in the United States.

Smoking And The Immune System

The immune system is the body's way of protecting itself from infection and disease. The immune system fights everything from cold and flu viruses to serious conditions such as cancer. Smoking compromises the immune system and can make the body less successful at fighting disease. Smokers have more respiratory infections than nonsmokers, in part because the chemicals in cigarettes make it harder for their immune systems to successfully attack the viruses and bacteria that can cause respiratory infections. In fact, smokers generally are much less healthy than nonsmokers. Their overall health is worse, they need to go to the doctor more often, and they are admitted to the hospital more often. Smoking also causes autoimmune disorders. Autoimmune disorders occur when the immune system attacks the body's healthy cells.

For example, in rheumatoid arthritis, or RA, the immune system attacks the joints and tissue around the joints, causing swelling and pain. As a result, people with RA have a harder time getting around and doing normal daily activities. We now know RA can be caused by smoking, and smoking makes some RA treatments less effective. More women have RA than men.

Smoking And Eye Disease

Chemicals in cigarette smoke restrict blood flow to important organs by causing blood vessels to narrow. The eye has many tiny blood vessels that keep it healthy and working properly. Chemicals in tobacco smoke damage these blood vessels and prevent them from carrying enough oxygen throughout the eye. Smoking causes damage to delicate cells in the eye, and exposure to cigarette smoke over long periods of time means the cells do not have a chance to heal. These effects from smoking can cause serious eye diseases. Age-related macular degeneration, or AMD, is an eye disease that causes loss of vision in the center of the field of vision. The retina is a delicate tissue that lines the inside of the eye. It is sensitive to light and sends visual images to the brain. The macula is the most sensitive part of the retina and is the part of the eye that gives you sharp vision. Age-related macular degeneration damages the macula over time and can lead to loss of vision in the center of the eye. AMD is common in older people and is the leading cause of vision loss in people over age 65. Smoking is now known to cause AMD. Studies show that quitting smoking may reduce that risk, but it might take 20 or more years after smokers quit for the risk to go down. In addition to causing AMD, smoking causes cataracts. A cataract is the clouding of the eye's lens. Cataracts cause loss of vision because the clouding prevents light from passing through the lens to the retina. Cataract disease is the leading cause of blindness but can be treated with surgery. Cataracts usually occur in older adults.

Chapter 21

Facts About Smoking Cessation

Smoking remains the leading cause of preventable death and disease in the United States, killing more than 480,000 Americans each year. Smoking causes immediate damage to your body, which can lead to long-term health problems. For every smoking-related death, at least 30 Americans live with a smoking-related illness. The only proven strategy to protect yourself from harm is to never smoke, and if you do smoke or use tobacco products, to quit.

Quitting Smoking

Tobacco use can lead to tobacco/nicotine dependence and serious health problems. Quitting smoking greatly reduces the risk of developing smoking-related diseases.

Tobacco/nicotine dependence is a condition that often requires repeated treatments, but there are helpful treatments and resources for quitting. Smokers can and do quit smoking. In fact, today there are more former smokers than current smokers.

Nicotine Dependence

- Most smokers become addicted to nicotine, a drug that is found naturally in tobacco.
- More people in the United States are addicted to nicotine than to any other drug. Research suggests that nicotine may be as addictive as heroin, cocaine, or alcohol.

About This Chapter: Text in this chapter begins with excerpts from "Smoking And Tobacco Use—How To Quit," Centers for Disease Control and Prevention (CDC), December 11, 2017; Text beginning with the heading "Quitting Smoking" is excerpted from "Smoking And Tobacco Use—Quitting Smoking," Centers for Disease Control and Prevention (CDC), December 11, 2017.

- Quitting smoking is hard and may require several attempts. People who stop smoking often start again because of withdrawal symptoms, stress, and weight gain.

- Nicotine withdrawal symptoms may include:

  - Feeling irritable, angry, or anxious

  - Having trouble thinking

  - Craving tobacco products

  - Feeling hungrier than usual

Health Benefits Of Quitting

Tobacco smoke contains a deadly mix of more than 7,000 chemicals; hundreds are harmful, and about 70 can cause cancer. Smoking increases the risk for serious health problems, many diseases, and death. People who stop smoking greatly reduce their risk for disease and early death. Although the health benefits are greater for people who stop at earlier ages, there are benefits at any age. You are never too old to quit.

Stopping smoking is associated with the following health benefits:

- Lowered risk for lung cancer and many other types of cancer.

- Reduced risk for heart disease, stroke, and peripheral vascular disease (PVD) (narrowing of the blood vessels outside your heart).

- Reduced heart disease risk within 1–2 years of quitting.

- Reduced respiratory symptoms, such as coughing, wheezing, and shortness of breath. While these symptoms may not disappear, they do not continue to progress at the same rate among people who quit compared with those who continue to smoke.

- Reduced risk of developing some lung diseases (such as chronic obstructive pulmonary disease, also known as COPD, one of the leading causes of death in the United States).

- Reduced risk for infertility in women of childbearing age. Women who stop smoking during pregnancy also reduce their risk of having a low birth weight baby.

Smokers' Attempts To Quit

Among all current U.S. adult cigarette smokers, nearly 7 out of every 10 (68.0%) reported in 2015 that they wanted to quit completely.

- Since 2002, the number of former smokers has been greater than the number of current smokers.

Percentage of adult daily cigarette smokers who stopped smoking for more than 1 day in 2015 because they were trying to quit:

- More than 5 out of 10 (55.4%) of all adult smokers
- Nearly 7 out of 10 (66.7%) smokers aged 18–24 years
- Nearly 6 out of 10 (59.8%) smokers aged 25–44 years
- More than 4 out of 10 (49.6%) smokers aged 45–64 years
- About 4 out of 10 (47.2%) smokers aged 65 years or older

  Percentage of high school cigarette smokers who tried to stop smoking in the past 12 months:

- More than 4 out of 10 (45.5%) of all high school students who smoke

Ways To Quit Smoking

Most former smokers quit without using one of the treatments that scientific research has shown can work. However, the following treatments are proven to be effective for smokers who want help to quit:

- Brief help by a doctor (such as when a doctor takes 10 minutes or less to give a patient advice and assistance about quitting)
- Individual, group, or telephone counseling
- Behavioral therapies (such as training in problem solving)
- Treatments with more person-to-person contact and more intensity (such as more or longer counseling sessions)
- Programs to deliver treatments using mobile phones

Medications for quitting that have been found to be effective include the following:

- Nicotine replacement products
  - Over-the-counter (OTC) (nicotine patch (which is also available by prescription), gum, lozenge)
  - Prescription (nicotine patch, inhaler, nasal spray)
- Prescription nonnicotine medications: bupropion SR (Zyban®), varenicline tartrate (Chantix®)

Counseling and medication are both effective for treating tobacco dependence, and using them together is more effective than using either one alone.

- More information is needed about quitting for people who smoke cigarettes and also use other types of tobacco.

Complementary Health Approaches For Quitting Smoking

Some people also try complementary health approaches to help them quit smoking. Here are 5 things you should know about what the science says about several complementary health approaches for quitting smoking:

1. Current evidence suggests that several mind and body practices may help people quit smoking. A few studies have found that mind and body practices such as meditation-based therapies, yoga, and guided imagery (a relaxation technique) can help reduce cigarette use and cravings.

2. Research results on other mind and body practices, including acupuncture and hypnosis, show little evidence of benefit. A 2010 systematic review of the scientific literature concluded that hypnotherapy did not provide any greater effect on the rates of quitting than 18 other therapies or no treatment. A 2011 systematic review of acupuncture studies found no consistent evidence that acupuncture is effective for smoking cessation, but that firm conclusion can't be drawn because of the limited quality and quantity of available evidence.

3. There is no current evidence that any dietary supplement helps people quit smoking. A few studies have been conducted on the dietary supplements S-adenosyl-L-methionine (SAMe), silver acetate, lobeline (from the herb Lobelia inflata), and St. John's wort, but none has been shown to be effective. The natural product cytisine, primarily used in Central and Eastern European countries for smoking cessation, is not currently approved by the U.S. Food and Drug Administration (FDA) but has been shown to be effective in helping smokers quit.

4. The mind and body practices discussed here are generally considered safe for healthy people when they're performed appropriately. If you have any health problems, talk with both your healthcare provider and the complementary health practitioner/instructor before starting to use a mind and body practice.

5. If you are considering a dietary supplement, remember that "natural" does not necessarily mean "safe." Some supplements have side effects, and some may interact with drugs or other supplements to produce adverse effects. In particular, St. John's wort has been shown to interact with many drugs.

(Source: "5 Things To Know About Complementary Health Approaches For Quitting Smoking," National Center for Complementary and Integrative Health (NCCIH).)

Helpful Resources

Quitline Services

Call 800-QUIT-NOW (800-784-8669) if you want help quitting. This is a free telephone support service that can help people who want to stop smoking or using tobacco. Callers are routed to their state quitlines, which offer several types of quit information and services. These may include:

- Free support, advice, and counseling from experienced quitline coaches

- A personalized quit plan

- Practical information on how to quit, including ways to cope with nicotine withdrawal

- The latest information about stop-smoking medications

- Free or discounted medications (available for at least some callers in most states)

- Referrals to other resources

- Mailed self-help materials

Online Help

Get free help online, too.

- For information on quitting, go to the Quit Smoking Resources page (www.cdc.gov/tobacco/quit_smoking/how_to_quit/resources/index.htm) on Centers for Disease Control and Prevention's (CDC) website.

- Read inspiring stories about former smokers and their reasons for quitting at CDC's Tips From Former Smokers page (www.cdc.gov/tobacco/campaign/tips/).

Chapter 22

How Can I Quit Smoking?

Take Steps To Quit

Prepare To Quit

Quitting is hard. But quitting can be a bit easier if you have a plan. When you think you're ready to quit, here are a few simple steps you can take to put your plan into action.

Know Why You're Quitting

Before you actually quit, it's important to know why you're doing it. Do you want to be healthier? Save money? Keep your family safe? If you're not sure, ask yourself these questions:

- What do I dislike about smoking?

- What do I miss out on when I smoke?

- How is smoking affecting my health?

- What will happen to me and my family if I keep smoking?

- How will my life get better when I quit?

Still not sure? Different people have different reasons for quitting smoking.

About This Chapter: This chapter includes text excerpted from "Take Steps To Quit," Centers for Disease Control and Prevention (CDC), March 21, 2018.

Learn How To Handle Your Triggers And Cravings

Triggers are specific persons, places, or activities that make you feel like smoking. Knowing your smoking triggers can help you learn to deal with them.

Cravings are short but intense urges to smoke. They usually only last a few minutes. Plan ahead and come up with a list of short activities you can do when you get a craving.

Find Ways To Handle Nicotine Withdrawal

During the first few weeks after you quit, you may feel uncomfortable and crave a cigarette. This is because of withdrawal. During withdrawal, your body is getting used to not having nicotine from cigarettes. For most people, the worst symptoms of withdrawal last a few days to a few weeks. During this time, you may:

- Feel a little depressed

- Be unable to sleep

- Become cranky, frustrated, or mad

- Feel anxious, nervous, or restless

- Have trouble thinking clearly

You may be tempted to smoke to relieve these feelings. Just remember that they are temporary, no matter how powerful they feel at the time.

Fact: The worst withdrawal symptoms only last a few days to a couple of weeks. Stay strong!

One of the best ways to deal with nicotine withdrawal is to try nicotine replacement therapy (NRT). NRT can reduce withdrawal symptoms. And NRT can double your chances of quitting smoking for good. NRT comes in several different forms, including gum, patch, nasal spray, inhaler, and lozenge. Many are available without a prescription.

A lot of research has been done on NRT. It has been shown to be safe and effective for almost all smokers who want to quit, including teens. But if you have a severe medical condition or are pregnant, talk to your doctor about using NRT. If you plan to use NRT, remember to have it available on your quit day. Read the instructions on the NRT package and follow them carefully. NRT will give you the most benefit if you use it as recommended.

Explore Your Quit Smoking Options

It is difficult to quit smoking on your own, but quitting "cold turkey" is not your only choice. In fact, choosing another option may improve your chances of success. Check out:

- SmokefreeTXT (www.smokefree.gov/smokefreetxt) text message program

- QuitGuide app (www.smokefree.gov/tools-tips/apps/quitguide)

- Quitlines like 800-QUIT-NOW (800-784-8669) and 877-44U-QUIT (877-448-7848)

- Find a quit method that might be right for you.

Tell Your Family And Friends You Plan To Quit

Quitting smoking is easier when the people in your life support you. Let them know you are planning to quit and explain how they can help. Here are a few tips:

- Tell your family and friends your reasons for quitting.

- Ask them to check in with you to see how things are going.

- Ask them to help you think of smokefree activities you can do together (like going to the movies or a nice restaurant).

- Ask a friend or family member who smokes to quit with you, or at least not smoke around you.

- Ask your friends and family not to give you a cigarette—no matter what you say or do.

- Alert your friends and family that you may be in a bad mood while quitting. Ask them to be patient and help you through it.

Support is one of the keys to successfully quitting. Find more ways to get support to help you quit.

Make A Quit Plan

Having a plan can make quitting easier. Create your personalized plan to help you stay focused, confident, and motivated to quit.

Build Your Quit Plan

Have You Built A Quit Plan?

One of the keys to a successful quit is preparation. A great way to prepare to quit smoking is to create a quit plan. Quit plans:

- Combine quit smoking strategies to keep you focused, confident, and motivated to quit

- Help you identify challenges you will face as you quit and ways to overcome them

- Can improve your chances of quitting smoking for good

The following steps will help you to create your own customized quit plan. As you move through the steps, keep a record of your plan and have it readily available during your quit.

Pick A Quit Date

When it comes to choosing a quit date, sooner is better than later. Many smokers choose a date within two weeks to quit smoking. This will give you enough time to prepare. Really think about your quit date. Avoid choosing a day where you know you will be busy, stressed, or tempted to smoke (e.g., a night out with friends or days where you may smoke at work).

Next Step: Circle your quit day on your calendar. Write it out somewhere where you will see it every day. This will remind you of your decision to become smokefree and give you time to prepare to quit.

Let Loved Ones Know You Are Quitting

Quitting smoking is easier with support from important people in your life. Let them know ahead of your quit date that you are planning to quit. Explain how they can help you quit. We all need different things, so be sure you let friends and family know exactly how they can help.

Next Step: Support is one of the keys to successfully quitting. However, it can be hard to ask for help, even from the people closest to you. Review tips on getting support to make sure you get the help you need.

Remove Reminders Of Smoking

Getting rid of smoking reminders can keep you on track during your quit. Smoking reminders can include your cigarettes, matches, ashtrays, and lighters. It may also help to make things clean and fresh at work in your car and at home. Even the smell of cigarettes can cause a cigarette craving.

Next Step: Throw away all your cigarettes and matches. Give or throw away your lighters and ashtrays. Don't save one pack of cigarettes "just in case."

Identify Your Reasons To Quit Smoking

Everyone has their own reasons for quitting smoking. Maybe they want to be healthier, save some money, or keep their family safe. As you prepare to quit, think about your own reasons for quitting. Remind yourself of them every day. They can inspire you to stop smoking for good.

Next Step: Make a list of all the reasons you want to quit smoking. Keep it in a place where you can see it every day. Any time you feel the urge to smoke, review your list. It will keep you motivated to stay smokefree.

Identify Your Smoking Triggers

When you smoke, it becomes tied to many parts of your life. Certain activities, feelings, and people are linked to your smoking. When you come across these things, they may "trigger" or turn on your urge to smoke. Try to anticipate these smoking triggers and develop ways to deal with them.

Next Step: Make a list of everything that makes you feel like smoking. Now, write down one way you can deal with or avoid each item on your list. Keep this list nearby during your quit. Having trouble with your list? Find examples of ways to deal with smoking triggers on Centers for Disease Control and Prevention's (CDC) cravings page.

Develop Coping Strategies

Nicotine is the chemical in cigarettes that makes you addicted to smoking. When you stop smoking, your body has to adjust to no longer having nicotine in its system. This is called withdrawal. Withdrawal can be unpleasant, but you can get through it. Developing strategies to cope with withdrawal ahead of your quit can help ensure you stay smokefree for good!

Next Steps: Medications and behavior changes can help you manage the symptoms of withdrawal. Many quit smoking medications are available over the counter. Make sure you have them on hand prior to your quit. While medications will help, they can't do all the work for you. Develop other quit smoking strategies to use with medications. Remember that withdrawal symptoms' including cravings' will fade with every day that you stay smokefree.

Have Places You Can Turn To For Immediate Help

Quitting smoking is hardest during the first few weeks. You will deal with uncomfortable feelings, temptations to smoke, withdrawal symptoms, and cigarette cravings. Whether it is a quitline, support group, or good friend, make sure you have quit smoking support options available at all times.

Next Steps: Plan on using multiple quit smoking support options. Keep them handy in case you need them during your quit. Here a few options you may want to consider:

- **SmokefreeTXT:** A mobile text messaging service designed for adults and young adults across the United States who are trying to quit smoking.

- **Quitlines:** If you want to talk to a quit smoking counselor right away, call 800-QUIT-NOW (800-784-8669).

- **Quit smoking apps:** Mobile phone applications can help you prepare to quit, provide support, and track your progress.

- **Support groups:** Visit your county or state government's website to see if they offer quit smoking programs in your area.

- **Friends and family:** Getting support from the important people in your life can make a big difference during your quit.

- **Medications:** If you are using a quit smoking medication, such as the patch, gum, or lozenges, make sure you have them on hand.

Set Up Rewards For Quit Milestones

Quitting smoking happens one minute, one hour, one day at a time. Reward yourself throughout your quit. Celebrate individual milestones, including being 24 hours smokefree, one week smokefree, and one month smokefree. Quitting smoking is hard, be proud of your accomplishments.

Next Steps: You should be proud every time you hit a quit smoking milestone. Treat yourself with a nice dinner, day at the movies, or any other smokefree activity. Plan out your milestones ahead of time and set up a smokefree reward for each one.

Build Support To Stay Quit

Ask For Help

Getting support from the important people in your life can make a big difference when you quit smoking. Friends, family, coworkers, and others can be there for you. You are not alone. You also can connect with others and grow your support network through Smokefree's social media resources:

- Facebook (www.facebook.com/SmokefreeUS)

- Twitter (twitter.com/smokefreegov)

- Instagram (www.instagram.com/smokefreeus)

- Pinterest (www.pinterest.com/SmokefreeUS)

Give your social circle a boost by connecting with other people who share your interests. Think about the things you like to do. Then start a conversation with someone new. Chances are, you'll find you have things in common.

Make quitting easier by teaming up with a friend who wants to quit too.

Here are some tips for getting support, either in person or online.

You might like to solve problems on your own, but everyone can use a little help from time to time. It doesn't mean you're weak. If you're not sure how to ask, text a friend or send an email. You might say, "I want to quit smoking. Can you help?" Know an ex-smoker? Ask them why and how they quit.

Be Specific About What You Want

Your friends and family won't always be able to know what help you need as you quit. Be specific about what support you want and don't want. Try to be nice about it. They are just trying to do what is best for you. For example, if you're feeling stressed after a long day at work and craving a cigarette, ask a friend to help plan a smokefree night out to distract you.

Avoid Stressful Situations

Stress can make you feel like you want to smoke. Think about what stresses you most and look for ways to deal with that stress. Ask friends and family to be aware of your stressors. They can help make your life easier as you quit.

Certain places can be a trigger to smoke. Make plans to stay smokefree when you're there.

Say Thank You

Tell your friends you appreciate them, whether you speak it, text it, or show it with your actions. Saying thanks doesn't take a lot of time, so do it in the moment before you forget. Got a friend who gave up their last piece of gum to help you beat a cigarette craving? Buy some gum and give it to them with a note that says, "Thanks for helping me stay quit!" And being grateful has benefits for you too. Studies show that being grateful can improve physical health, mental health, and self-esteem. Being grateful also can reduce stress.

Focus On People Who Can Help

If a friendship doesn't feel right anymore, it might be time to let it go. Don't be afraid to try a little distance with people who aren't giving you the support you need. Letting go can be hard, but it's sometimes for the best. Then focus on spending time with people who make you feel good about yourself and want you to succeed.

Invest In Your Relationships

The relationships you encourage and support the most may be the ones that are there for you the most while you quit. You will also feel more comfortable calling on them for support if the relationship is strong. You might go to a movie your friend really wants to see, even if it's not your top choice. Or go out of your way to call a friend just to chat and see how things are going.

Support Others

Support is a two-way street. If you want others to be there for you, you have to be there for them, too. Check in with your friends and help them out when you can. Sometimes small favors mean the most. Do something to brighten someone's day. Make a friend smile by emailing or texting them a joke, get someone a small treat for their birthday, or call a family member to see how they are doing. Got a quit method or quitting tip that worked for you? Post it on social media at SmokefreeUS or Smokefree Women. Sharing your success can be a great motivator and support for others to become smokefree.

Prepare For Cravings

How To Manage Cravings

You won't be able to avoid all of your triggers. And learning how to deal with triggers takes practice. So, when a craving is triggered, it's important to have a plan to beat that urge to smoke.

Cravings typically last 5–10 minutes. It might be uncomfortable, but try to wait it out. Make a list of things you can do to get through the craving. Here are a few to try.

Get Support

- Call or text someone. You don't have to do this alone. Learn how to lean on people you trust.

- Find a local quitline. Call 800-QUIT-NOW (800-784-8669) to connect directly to your state's quitline.

- Use the National Cancer Institute's quitline. Call 877-44U-QUIT (877-448-7848) to talk with an expert for free.

- Try SmokefreeTXT. Sign up to get 24/7 support sent right to your phone.

- Chat with a counselor. Get real-time help from the National Cancer Institute (NCI).

- Use an app. The QuitGuide app allows you to track cravings and slips by time of day and location, and has many other features to help you become smokefree.

Cravings last the length of a few songs! Make a playlist to distract yourself.

Think About Your Reasons For Quitting

- Review your reasons. Remind yourself why you want to quit. This can be a powerful motivator to keep you smokefree.

- Calculate your savings. Cigarettes are expensive! Add up the money you'll save, and decide what to do with it. This is a great way to stay motivated and kill time while you let a craving pass.

Stay Busy

- Keep your mouth busy. Chew a stick of gum instead of picking up a cigarette. Keep hard candy with you. Drink more water.

- Do something else. When a craving hits, stop what you're doing immediately and switch to doing something different. Simply changing your routine might help you shake off a craving.

- Go for a walk or jog. Or go up and down the stairs a few times. Physical activity, even in short bursts, can help boost your energy and beat a craving.

- Take slow, deep breaths. Breathe through your craving. Inhale through your nose and exhale through your mouth. Repeat this 10 times or until you're feeling more relaxed.

Go To A Smokefree Zone

- Visit a public place. Most public places don't allow smoking. Go to a movie, a store, or another smokefree place where you can't smoke.

- Practice what you already do. What have you done before when you found yourself in a smokefree place? Tap into that same approach when your next craving comes along

Try Nicotine Replacement Therapy

Even if you use nicotine replacement therapy (NRT), you might have a craving that's difficult to deal with. Think about trying a short-acting NRT, such as a lozenge or gum, plus long-acting NRT, such as the patch, to get past the craving.

Do A Good Deed

Try distracting yourself for a few minutes by being helpful to a friend, family member, or coworker. This takes the focus off yourself and how you are feeling and instead allows you to think of another person's needs. It can be a helpful way to cope with a craving until it passes. Plus, doing good deeds can have positive effects on your health, like reducing stress. Managing stress can be a key part of quitting smoking.

Don't Give Up

Do whatever it takes to beat the urge to smoke. Keep trying different things until you find what works for you. Just don't smoke. Not even one puff!

Manage Withdrawal

Nicotine withdrawal is different for every smoker. Every smoker feels different during withdrawal.

The most common symptoms include:

- Having cravings for cigarettes
- Feeling down or sad
- Having trouble sleeping
- Feeling irritable' on edge' or grouchy
- Having trouble thinking clearly and concentrating
- Feeling restless and jumpy
- Having a slower heart rate
- Feeling more hungry or gaining weight

You may have tough days and easy days with these symptoms. Over time, the symptoms and cravings will fade as long as you stay smokefree. Medications and changing the things you do can help you manage withdrawal symptoms. Try some yoga*. It increases oxygen to the brain, lowers stress, calms nerves and improves your mood!

A mind and body practice with origins in ancient Indian philosophy. The various styles of yoga typically combine physical postures, breathing techniques, and meditation or relaxation.

Mood Changes

Mood changes are common after quitting smoking. Some people feel increased sadness. You might be irritable, restless, or feel down or blue. Changes in mood from quitting smoking may be part of withdrawal. Withdrawal is your body getting used to not having nicotine. Mood changes from nicotine withdrawal usually get better in a week or two. If mood changes do not get better in a couple of weeks, you should talk to your doctor. Something else, like depression, could be the reason.

Smoking may seem to help you with depression. You might feel better in the moment. But there are many problems with using cigarettes to cope with depression. There are other things you can try to lift your mood:

- **Exercise.** Being physically active can help. Start small and build up over time. This can be hard to do when you're depressed. But your efforts will pay off.

- **Structure your day.** Make a plan to stay busy. Get out of the house if you can.

- **Be with other people.** Many people who are depressed are cut off from other people. Being in touch or talking with others every day can help your mood.

- **Reward yourself.** Do things you enjoy. Even small things add up and help you feel better.

- **Get support.** If you are feeling down after quitting smoking, it may help to talk about this with friends and family. Your doctor also can help.

Nicotine Cravings

For many smokers, cravings for a cigarette last much longer than other symptoms of withdrawal. Many people are surprised when cravings sometimes happen without warning. Cravings can be set off by reminders of smoking. These reminders are often called triggers. People, places, and things can trigger a craving. This means it's important to have a plan for how you'll handle a craving when it hits.

The good news is that most cravings last for only 15–20 minutes. Finding ways to get through that short period of time is a key way to deal with cravings. Anything that can distract you and keep you busy can be helpful. Getting active also can work. A 15-minute walk can help you distract yourself until the craving passes. Most smokers who try nicotine replacement therapy find it helpful for getting through withdrawal and managing cravings.

Nicotine Withdrawal Isn't Dangerous

Withdrawal can be uncomfortable and some people may feel high levels of symptoms. But there is no health danger from nicotine withdrawal. In fact' quitting smoking is the best thing you can do for your health. Even extreme withdrawal symptoms will fade over time.

Avoid Secondhand Smoke

Quitting will make the people you care about happier and healthier. This may be one of your reasons for quitting.

Dangers Of Secondhand Smoke

The main way smoking hurts nonsmokers is through secondhand smoke. Secondhand smoke is the combination of smoke that comes from a cigarette and smoke breathed out by a smoker. When a nonsmoker is around someone smoking, they breathe in secondhand smoke.

Secondhand smoke is dangerous to anyone who breathes it in. It can stay in the air for several hours after somebody smokes. Breathing secondhand smoke for even a short time can hurt your body. Take this quiz to see how much you know about the dangers of secondhand smoke.

Health Effects Of Secondhand Smoke

Over time, secondhand smoke has been associated with serious health problems in nonsmokers:

- Lung cancer in people who have never smoked.

- More likely that someone will get heart disease' have a heart attack' and die early.

- Breathing problems like coughing' extra phlegm' wheezing' and shortness of breath.

Secondhand smoke is especially dangerous for children, babies, and women who are pregnant:

- Mothers who breathe secondhand smoke while pregnant are more likely to have babies with low birth weight.

- Babies who breathe secondhand smoke after birth have more lung infections than other babies.

- Secondhand smoke causes kids who already have asthma to have more frequent and severe attacks.

- Children exposed to secondhand smoke are more likely to develop bronchitis, pneumonia, and ear infections and are at increased risk for sudden infant death syndrome (SIDS).

The only way to fully protect nonsmokers from the dangers of secondhand smoke is to not allow smoking indoors. Separating smokers from nonsmokers (like "no smoking" sections in restaurants)' cleaning the air' and airing out buildings does not get rid of secondhand smoke.

Other Ways Smoking Affects Others

Smoking affects the people in your life in other ways, beyond their health. When you smoke, you may miss out on:

- Spending time with family and friends.

- Having more money to spend on the people you love.

- Setting a good example for your children. Children who are raised by smokers are more likely to become smokers themselves.

Steps You Can Take To Protect Your Loved Ones

The best thing you can do to protect your family from secondhand smoke is to quit smoking. Right away, you get rid of their exposure to secondhand smoke in your home and car, and reduce it anywhere else you go together.

Make sure your house and car remain smokefree. Kids breathe in secondhand smoke at home more than any other place. The same goes for many adults. Don't allow anyone to smoke in your home or car. Setting this rule will:

- Reduce the amount of secondhand smoke your family breathes in.

- Help you quit smoking and stay smokefree.

- Lower the chance of your child becoming a smoker.

When you're on the go, you can still protect your family from secondhand smoke:

- Make sure caretakers like nannies, babysitters, and daycare staff do not smoke.

- Eat at smokefree restaurants.

- Avoid indoor public places that allow smoking.

- Teach your children to stay away from secondhand smoke.

Part Four
Marijuana

Chapter 23

What Is Marijuana?

Marijuana, which can also be called weed, pot, dope, or cannabis, is the dried flowers and leaves of the cannabis plant. It contains mind-altering (e.g., psychoactive) compounds like tetrahydrocannabinol, or THC, as well as other active compounds like cannabidiol, or CBD, that are not mind-altering.

How Is Marijuana Used?

There are many ways of using marijuana, and each one affects users differently. Marijuana can be rolled up and smoked like a cigarette (a joint) or a cigar (a blunt). Marijuana can also be smoked in a pipe. Sometimes people mix it in food and eat it or brew it as a tea (edibles). Smoking oils, concentrates, and extracts from the marijuana plant are on the rise. People who use this practice call it "dabbing."

Marijuana use is widespread among adolescents and young adults. According to the Monitoring the Future survey—an annual survey of drug use and attitudes among the Nation's middle and high school students—most measures of marijuana use by 8th, 10th, and 12th graders peaked in the mid-to-late 1990s and then began a period of gradual decline through the mid-2000s before leveling off. Most measures showed some decline again in the past 5 years. Teens' perceptions of the risks of marijuana use have steadily declined over the past decade, possibly related to increasing public debate about legalizing or loosening restrictions on marijuana for medicinal and recreational use.

(Source: "Marijuana," National Institute on Drug Abuse (NIDA).)

About This Chapter: This chapter includes text excerpted from "Marijuana And Public Health—Frequently Asked Questions," Centers for Disease Control and Prevention (CDC), March 7, 2018.

What Determines How Marijuana Affects A Person?

Like any other drug, marijuana's effects on a person depends on a number of factors, including the person's previous experience with the drug or other drugs, biology (e.g., genes), gender, how the drug is taken, and how strong it is.

Is Marijuana Medicine?

The marijuana plant has chemicals that may help symptoms for some health problems. More and more states are making it legal to use the plant as medicine for certain conditions. But there isn't enough research to show that the whole plant works to treat or cure these conditions. Also, the U.S. Food and Drug Administration (FDA) has not recognized or approved the marijuana plant as medicine.

Because marijuana is often smoked, it can damage your lungs and cardiovascular system (e.g., heart and blood vessels). These and other damaging effects on the brain and body could make marijuana more harmful than helpful as a medicine. Another problem with marijuana as a medicine is that the ingredients aren't exactly the same from plant to plant. There's no way to know what kind and how much of a chemical you're getting.

Two medicines have been made as pills from a chemical that's like tetrahydrocannabinol (THC), one of the chemicals found in the marijuana plant that makes people feel "high." These two medicines can treat nausea if you have cancer and make you hungry if you have acquired immunodeficiency syndrome (AIDS) and don't feel like eating. But the chemical used to make these medicines affects the brain also, so it can do things to your body other than just working as medicine.

Another marijuana chemical that scientists are studying, called cannabidiol (CBD), doesn't make you high because it acts on different parts of the nervous system than THC. Scientists think this chemical might help children who have a lot of seizures (when your body starts twitching and jerking uncontrollably) that can't be controlled with other medicines. Some studies have started to see whether it can help.

Is It Possible For Someone To Become Addicted To Marijuana?

Yes, about 1 in 10 marijuana users will become addicted. For people who begin using younger than 18, that number rises to 1 in 6.

How Do I Know If I Am Addicted To Marijuana?

Some of the signs that someone might be addicted to marijuana include:

- Trying but failing to quit using marijuana

- Giving up important activities with friends and family in favor of using marijuana

- Using marijuana even when it is known that it causes problems at home, school, or work.

Compared to marijuana users who are not addicted, people who are addicted to marijuana are at a higher risk of the negative consequences of using the drug, such as problems with attention, memory, and learning.

Is It Possible To "Overdose" Or Have A "Bad Reaction" To Marijuana?

A fatal overdose is unlikely, but that doesn't mean marijuana is harmless. The signs of using too much marijuana are similar to the typical effects of using marijuana but more severe. These signs may include extreme confusion, anxiety, paranoia, panic, fast heart rate, delusions or hallucinations, increased blood pressure, and severe nausea or vomiting. In some cases, these reactions can lead to unintentional injuries such as a motor vehicle crash, fall, or poisoning.

What Are The Effects Of Mixing Marijuana With Alcohol, Tobacco, Or Prescription Drugs?

Using alcohol and marijuana at the same time is likely to result in greater impairment than when using either one alone. Using marijuana and tobacco at the same time may also lead to increased exposure to harmful chemicals, causing greater risks to the lungs, and the cardiovascular system. Also, be aware that marijuana may change how prescription drugs work. Always talk with your doctor about any medications you are taking or thinking about taking and possible side effects when mixed with other things like marijuana.

How Harmful Is K2/Spice (Synthetic Marijuana Or Synthetic Cannabinoids)?

Synthetic cannabinoids (e.g., synthetic marijuana, K2, Spice, Spike)—or plants sprayed with unknown chemicals—are dangerous and unpredictable. Synthetic cannabinoids are not marijuana, but like THC, they bind to the same cannabinoid receptors in the brain and other organs. Research shows that synthetic cannabinoids affect the brain much more powerfully than marijuana creating unpredictable and, in some cases, life-threatening effects including nausea, anxiety, paranoia, brain swelling, seizures, hallucinations, aggression, heart palpitations, and chest pains.

Does Marijuana Use Lead To Other Drug Use?

The majority of people who use marijuana do not go on to use other, "harder" substances. More research is needed to understand if marijuana is a "gateway drug"—a drug that is thought to lead to the use of more dangerous drugs (such as cocaine or heroin).

Is It Safe For A Breastfeeding Mom To Use Marijuana?

Chemicals from marijuana can be passed to your baby through breast milk. THC is stored in fat and is slowly released over time, meaning that your baby could still be exposed even after you stop using marijuana. However, data on the effects of marijuana exposure to the infant or baby through breastfeeding are limited and conflicting. To limit potential risk to the infant, breastfeeding mothers should reduce or avoid marijuana use.

Can Secondhand Marijuana Smoke Affect Nonsmokers, Including Children?

Secondhand marijuana smoke contains THC, the chemical responsible for most of marijuana's psychological effects, and many of the same toxic chemicals in smoked tobacco. Smoked marijuana has many of the same cancer-causing substances as smoked tobacco, but there are still a lot of unanswered questions around secondhand marijuana smoke exposure and its impact on chronic diseases such as heart disease, cancer, and lung diseases.

How Is Eating And Drinking Foods That Contain Marijuana (Edibles) Different From Smoking Marijuana?

Because marijuana contains THC, there are health risks associated with using marijuana regardless of the how it is used. Some of these negative effects include having difficulty thinking and problem-solving, having problems with memory, learning and maintaining attention and demonstrating impaired coordination. Additionally, frequent use can lead to becoming addicted to marijuana. However, some risks may differ by the way it is used.

Smoke from marijuana contains many of the same toxins, irritants, and carcinogens as tobacco smoke. Smoking marijuana can lead to a greater risk of bronchitis, cough, and phlegm production. Whereas, edibles, which take longer to digest, take longer to produce an effect. Therefore, people may consume more to feel the effects faster. This may lead to people consuming very high doses and result in negative effects like anxiety, paranoia and, in rare cases, an extreme psychotic reaction (e.g., delusions, hallucinations, talking incoherently, and agitation).

It's Legal In Many States, So Doesn't That Mean Marijuana Is Safe?

The fact that it's legal does not mean that it is safe. Using marijuana at an early age can lead to negative health consequences.

- Heavy marijuana use (daily or near-daily) can do damage to memory, learning, and attention, which can last a week or more after the last time someone used.

- Using marijuana during pregnancy or while breastfeeding may harm the baby, just like alcohol or tobacco.

- Marijuana use has been linked to anxiety, depression, and schizophrenia, but scientists don't yet know whether it directly causes these diseases.

- Smoking any product, including marijuana, can damage your lungs and cardiovascular system.

Chapter 24

Marijuana Abuse Among U.S. Teens

The teen years are a time of rapid growth, exploration, and onset of risk taking. Taking risks with new behaviors provides kids and teens the opportunity to test their skills and abilities and discover who they are. But, some risk behaviors—such as using marijuana—can have harmful and long-lasting effects on a teen's health and well-being.

Marijuana And The Teen Brain

Unlike adults, the teen brain is actively developing and often will not be fully developed until the mid-20s. Marijuana use during this period may harm the developing teen brain.

Negative effects include:

- Difficulty thinking and problem solving

- Problems with memory and learning

- Impaired coordination

- Difficulty maintaining attention

Negative Effects On School And Social Life

Marijuana use in adolescence or early adulthood can have a serious impact on a teen's life.

About This Chapter: Text in this chapter begins with excerpts from "Marijuana And Public Health—What You Need To Know About Marijuana Use In Teens," Centers for Disease Control and Prevention (CDC), April 13, 2017; Text under the heading "How Many Teens Use Marijuana?" is excerpted from "Marijuana," National Institute on Drug Abuse (NIDA) for Teens, May 2017.

- **Decline in school performance.** Students who smoke marijuana may get lower grades and may more likely to drop out of high school than their peers who do not use.

- **Increased risk of mental health issues.** Marijuana use has been linked to a range of mental health problems in teens such as depression or anxiety. Psychosis has also been seen in teens at higher risk like those with a family history.

- **Impaired driving.** Driving while impaired by any substance, including marijuana, is dangerous. Marijuana negatively affects a number of skills required for safe driving, such as reaction time, coordination, and concentration.

- **Potential for addiction.** Research shows that about one in six teens who repeatedly use marijuana can become addicted, which means that they may make unsuccessful efforts to quit using marijuana or may give up important activities with friends and family in favor of using marijuana.

Facts About Marijuana

- 38 percent of high school students report having used marijuana in their life

- Research shows that marijuana use can have permanent effects on brain function the developing brain when use begins in adolescence, especially with regular or heavy use

- Frequent or long-term marijuana graduation hat use is linked to school dropout and lower educational achievement

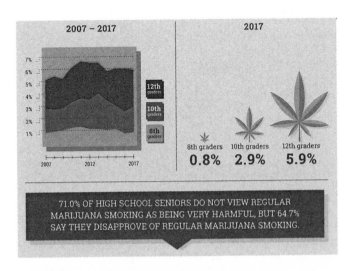

Figure 24.1. Daily Marijuana Use Mostly Steady

How Many Teens Use Marijuana?

Marijuana is the most commonly used illicit drug in the United States by teens as well as adults. The public discussions about medical marijuana and the public debate over the drug's legal status is leading to a reduced perception of harm among young people. In addition, some teens believe marijuana cannot be harmful because it is "natural." But not all natural plant substances are good for you—tobacco, cocaine, and heroin also come from plants.

Below is a table showing the percentage of teens who say they use marijuana.

Table 24.1. Trends In Prevalence Of Marijuana/Hashish For 8th Graders, 10th Graders, And 12th Graders; 2017 (In Percent)*

Drug	Time Period	8th Graders	10th Graders	12th Graders
Marijuana/ Hashish	Lifetime	13.50	30.70	45.00
	Past Year	10.10	25.50	37.10
	Past Month	5.50	(15.70)	22.90
	Daily	0.80	2.90	5.90

Data in brackets indicate a statistically significant downward trend from the previous year.

Marijuana use can lead to the development of problem use, known as a marijuana use disorder, which takes the form of addiction in severe cases. Data suggest that 30 percent of those who use marijuana may have some degree of marijuana use disorder. People who begin using marijuana before the age of 18 are four to seven times more likely to develop a marijuana use disorder than adults.

In 2015, about 4.0 million people in the United States met the diagnostic criteria for a marijuana use disorder; 138,000 voluntarily sought treatment for their marijuana use.

(Source: "Marijuana," National Institute on Drug Abuse (NIDA).)

Chapter 25

Health Effects Of Marijuana

How Does Marijuana Affect The Brain?

Marijuana has both short-and long-term effects on the brain.

Short-Term Effects

When a person smokes marijuana, tetrahydrocannabinol (THC) quickly passes from the lungs into the bloodstream. The blood carries the chemical to the brain and other organs throughout the body. The body absorbs THC more slowly when the person eats or drinks it. In that case, they generally feel the effects after 30 minutes to 1 hour. THC acts on specific brain cell receptors that ordinarily react to natural THC-like chemicals. These natural chemicals play a role in normal brain development and function.

Marijuana overactivates parts of the brain that contain the highest number of these receptors. This causes the "high" that people feel. Other effects include:

- Altered senses (for example, seeing brighter colors)

- Altered sense of time

- Changes in mood

- Impaired body movement

- Difficulty with thinking and problem solving

About This Chapter: Text beginning with the heading "How Does Marijuana Affect The Brain?" is excerpted from "Marijuana," National Institute on Drug Abuse (NIDA), February 2018; Text under the heading "Marijuana Use And Educational Outcomes" is excerpted from "Marijuana Use And Educational Outcomes," National Institute on Drug Abuse (NIDA), November 20, 2014. Reviewed July 2018.

- Impaired memory

- Hallucinations (when taken in high doses)

- Delusions (when taken in high doses)

- Psychosis (when taken in high doses)

Long-Term Effects

Marijuana also affects brain development. When people begin using marijuana as teenagers, the drug may impair thinking, memory, and learning functions and affect how the brain builds connections between the areas necessary for these functions. Researchers are still studying how long marijuana's effects last and whether some changes may be permanent.

For example, a study from New Zealand conducted in part by researchers at Duke University showed that people who started smoking marijuana heavily in their teens and had an ongoing marijuana use disorder lost an average of 8 IQ points between ages 13 and 38. The lost mental abilities didn't fully return to those who quit marijuana as adults. Those who started smoking marijuana as adults didn't show notable IQ declines.

In another study on twins, those who used marijuana showed a significant decline in general knowledge and in verbal ability (equivalent to 4 IQ points) between the preteen years and early adulthood, but no predictable difference was found between twins when one used marijuana and the other didn't. This suggests that the IQ decline in marijuana users may be caused by something other than marijuana, such as shared familial factors (e.g., genetics, family environment). National Institute on Drug Abuse's (NIDA) Adolescent Brain Cognitive Development (ABCD) study, a major longitudinal study, is tracking a large sample of young

When marijuana is smoked, THC and other chemicals in the plant pass from the lungs into the bloodstream, which rapidly carries them throughout the body to the brain. The person begins to experience effects almost immediately. Many people experience a pleasant euphoria and sense of relaxation. Other common effects, which may vary dramatically among different people, include heightened sensory perception (e.g., brighter colors), laughter, altered perception of time, and increased appetite.

Although detectable amounts of THC may remain in the body for days or even weeks after use, the noticeable effects of smoked marijuana generally last from one to two hours, and those of marijuana consumed in food or drink may last for many hours.

(Source: "Marijuana," National Institute on Drug Abuse (NIDA).)

Americans from late childhood to early adulthood to help clarify how and to what extent marijuana and other substances, alone and in combination, affect adolescent brain development.

What Are The Other Health Effects Of Marijuana?

Marijuana use may have a wide range of effects, both physical and mental.

Physical Effects

- **Breathing problems.** Marijuana smoke irritates the lungs, and people who smoke marijuana frequently can have the same breathing problems as those who smoke tobacco. These problems include daily cough and phlegm, more frequent lung illness, and a higher risk of lung infections. Researchers so far haven't found a higher risk for lung cancer in people who smoke marijuana.

- **Increased heart rate.** Marijuana raises heart rate for up to 3 hours after smoking. This effect may increase the chance of heart attack. Older people and those with heart problems may be at higher risk.

- **Problems with child development during and after pregnancy.** One study found that about 20 percent of pregnant women 24-years-old and younger screened positive for marijuana. However, this study also found that women were about twice as likely to screen positive for marijuana use via a drug test than they state in self-reported measures. This suggests that self-reported rates of marijuana use in pregnant females is not an accurate measure of marijuana use and may be underreporting their use. This concerns medical experts because marijuana use during pregnancy is linked to lower birth weight and increased risk of both brain and behavioral problems in babies. If a pregnant woman uses marijuana, the drug may affect certain developing parts of the fetus's brain. Children exposed to marijuana in the womb have an increased risk of problems with attention, memory, and problem-solving compared to unexposed children. Some research also suggests that moderate amounts of THC are excreted into the breast milk of nursing mothers. With regular use, THC can reach amounts in breast milk that could affect the baby's developing brain. More research is needed.

- **Intense nausea and vomiting.** Regular, long-term marijuana use can lead to some people to develop Cannabinoid Hyperemesis Syndrome. This causes users to experience regular cycles of severe nausea, vomiting, and dehydration, sometimes requiring emergency medical attention.

Mental Effects

Long-term marijuana use has been linked to mental illness in some people, such as:

- Temporary hallucinations

- Temporary paranoia

- Worsening symptoms in patients with schizophrenia—a severe mental disorder with symptoms such as hallucinations, paranoia, and disorganized thinking

Marijuana use has also been linked to other mental health problems, such as depression, anxiety, and suicidal thoughts among teens. However, study findings have been mixed.

Are There Effects Of Inhaling Secondhand Marijuana Smoke?

Can I Fail A Drug Test?

While it's possible to fail a drug test after inhaling secondhand marijuana smoke, it's unlikely. Studies show that very little THC is released into the air when a person exhales. Research findings suggest that, unless people are in an enclosed room, breathing in lots of smoke for hours at close range, they aren't likely to fail a drug test. Even if some THC was found in the blood, it wouldn't be enough to fail a test.

Can I Get High From Passive Exposure?

Similarly, it's unlikely that secondhand marijuana smoke would give nonsmoking people in a confined space a high from passive exposure. Studies have shown that people who don't use marijuana report only mild effects of the drug from a nearby smoker, under extreme conditions (breathing in lots of marijuana smoke for hours in an enclosed room).

Other Health Effects?

More research is needed to know if secondhand marijuana smoke has similar health risks as secondhand tobacco smoke. A study on rats suggests that secondhand marijuana smoke can do as much damage to the heart and blood vessels as secondhand tobacco smoke. But researchers haven't fully explored the effect of secondhand marijuana smoke on humans. What they do know is that the toxins and tar found in marijuana smoke could affect vulnerable people, such as children or people with asthma.

Marijuana Use And Educational Outcomes

Studies show that marijuana interferes with attention, motivation, memory, and learning. Students who use marijuana regularly tend to get lower grades and are more likely to drop out of high school than those who don't use. Those who use it regularly may be functioning at a reduced intellectual level most or all of the time.

Facts About Marijuana Use In Adolescence

- As the perception of harm decreases teen marijuana use increases.
- Everyday, 3,287 teens use marijuana for the first time.
- Marijuana may hurt the developing teen brain.
- The teen brain is still developing and it is especially vulnerable to drug use.
- Regular heavy marijuana use by teens can lead to an IQ drop of up to 8 points.

Heavy marijuana use by teens is linked to:

Educational Outcomes

- Lower grades and exam scores
- Less likely to enroll in college
- Less likely to graduate from high school or college

Life Outcomes

- Lower satisfaction with life
- More likely to earn a lower income
- More likely to be unemployed

Chapter 26

Marijuana Smoking And Respiratory Disorders

Like tobacco smoke, marijuana smoke is an irritant to the throat and lungs and can cause a heavy cough during use. It also contains levels of volatile chemicals and tar that are similar to tobacco smoke, raising concerns about risk for cancer and lung disease.

Marijuana smoking is associated with large airway inflammation, increased airway resistance, and lung hyperinflation, and those who smoke marijuana regularly report more symptoms of chronic bronchitis than those who do not smoke. One study found that people who frequently smoke marijuana had more outpatient medical visits for respiratory problems than those who do not smoke. Some case studies have suggested that, because of delta-9-tetrahydrocannabinol's (THC) immune-suppressing effects, smoking marijuana might increase susceptibility to lung infections, such as pneumonia, in people with immune deficiencies; however, a large acquired immunodeficiency syndrome (AIDS) cohort study did not confirm such an association. Smoking marijuana may also reduce the respiratory system's immune response, increasing the likelihood of the person acquiring respiratory infections, including pneumonia. Animal and human studies have not found that marijuana increases risk for emphysema.

Whether smoking marijuana causes lung cancer, as cigarette smoking does, remains an open question. Marijuana smoke contains carcinogenic combustion products, including about 50 percent more benzopyrene and 75 percent more benzanthracene (and more phenols, vinyl chlorides, nitrosamines, reactive oxygen species) than cigarette smoke. Because of how it is typically smoked (deeper inhale, held for longer), marijuana smoking leads to four times the

About This Chapter: Text in this chapter begins with excerpts from "What Are Marijuana's Effects On Lung Health?" National Institute on Drug Abuse (NIDA), June 2018; Text beginning with the heading "Marijuana Smoking Is Associated With A Spectrum Of Respiratory Disorders" is excerpted from "Marijuana Smoking Is Associated With A Spectrum Of Respiratory Disorders," National Institute on Drug Abuse (NIDA), October 1, 2006. Reviewed July 2018.

deposition of tar compared to cigarette smoking. However, while a few small, uncontrolled studies have suggested that heavy, regular marijuana smoking could increase risk for respiratory cancers, well-designed population studies have failed to find an increased risk of lung cancer associated with marijuana use.

One complexity in comparing the lung-health risks of marijuana and tobacco concerns the very different ways the two substances are used. While people who smoke marijuana often inhale more deeply and hold the smoke in their lungs for a longer duration than is typical with cigarettes, marijuana's effects last longer, so people who use marijuana may smoke less frequently than those who smoke cigarettes.

Additionally, the fact that many people use both marijuana and tobacco makes determining marijuana's precise contribution to lung cancer risk, if any, difficult to establish. Cell culture and animal studies have also suggested THC and cannabidiol (CBD) may have antitumor effects, and this has been proposed as one reason why stronger expected associations are not seen between marijuana use and lung cancer, but more research is needed on this question.

Marijuana Smoking Is Associated With A Spectrum Of Respiratory Disorders

A large epidemiological study suggests that marijuana smoke can cause the same types of respiratory damage as tobacco smoke. Significant associations between marijuana smoking and a variety of respiratory diseases also have been confirmed by an extensive review of clinical literature.

Within a few minutes after inhaling marijuana smoke, a person's heart rate speeds up, the breathing passages relax and become enlarged, and blood vessels in the eyes expand, making the eyes look bloodshot. The heart rate—normally 70–80 beats per minute—may increase by 20–50 beats per minute or may even double in some cases. Taking other drugs with marijuana can amplify this effect.

(Source: "Marijuana," National Institute on Drug Abuse (NIDA).)

Monitoring The Effects Of Tobacco And Marijuana

Dr. Brent Moore and colleagues at Yale University, the National Cancer Institute (NCI), and the University of Vermont (UVM) evaluated data from a nationally representative sample of 6,728 adults. Their analysis indicated that a history of more than 100 lifetime episodes of smoking marijuana, with at least one episode in the past month, increased an individual's risk of chronic bronchitis, coughing on most days, wheezing, chest sounds without a cold, and increased phlegm.

"The most significant difference between tobacco smoke and marijuana smoke is their principal active ingredients—nicotine in tobacco and THC in marijuana. Beyond that, marijuana contains at least as much tar and half again as many carcinogens as smoke from conventional tobacco," says Dr. Moore. "Quitting marijuana smoking may benefit respiratory health as much as quitting cigarettes, in addition to the clear and considerable health, psychological, and social benefits of no longer abusing an illicit drug."

The information Dr. Moore and his colleagues analyzed was gathered through the third National Health and Nutrition Examination Survey (NHANES III), conducted between 1988 and 1994. Participants included 4,789 nonsmokers of either tobacco or marijuana; 1,525 smokers of tobacco but not marijuana; 320 smokers of both marijuana and tobacco; and 94 who smoked marijuana only. On average, marijuana abusers had smoked the drug on 10 of the preceding 30 days, with 16 percent reporting daily or almost daily smoking. Tobacco smokers consumed roughly the same number of cigarettes—averaging 19.2 per day—whether or not they also smoked marijuana. Survey participants answered questions about their experiences of a range of respiratory symptoms and were examined for signs of respiratory abnormalities.

The researchers concluded that tobacco smokers who also smoked marijuana had a higher prevalence of most respiratory symptoms than tobacco-only smokers. Compared with tobacco-only smokers, however, those who also smoked marijuana were less likely to have had pneumonia during the previous year or to show spirometric evidence of obstructive pulmonary disorder. Commenting on this finding, Dr. Moore says that it is important to note that the marijuana smokers in the sample were significantly younger (average age 31.2 years) than the tobacco smokers (average age 41.5 years). "The marijuana-related respiratory effects correspond to a relatively young population, and NHANES III did not ask participants older than age 59 about drug use," he adds. "It is likely that respiratory effects will be higher in older marijuana smokers, and, because of the high prevalence of tobacco use among marijuana smokers, there appears to be an increased risk for illness due to cumulative effects of smoking both drugs."

Marijuana's Long-Term Pulmonary Effects

Further evidence of marijuana's respiratory toxicity emerged from a study conducted by Dr. Donald Tashkin at the University of California, Los Angeles. Dr. Tashkin conducted an extensive review of clinical and epidemiological research to determine the extent to which chronic marijuana smoking might lead to long-term pulmonary effects and diseases similar to those caused by tobacco. Unlike the NHANES III data examined by Dr. Moore, the studies evaluated by Dr. Tashkin made it possible to assess a possible association between marijuana smoking and respiratory cancers.

The results of animal and cell culture studies are mixed with respect to the carcinogenic effects of THC, some studies showing that THC promotes lung cancer growth and others showing an antitumoral effect on a variety of malignancies. Although the results of epidemiological studies are also mixed, a case-control study has failed to find a direct link between marijuana use (including heavy use) and lung, throat, or other head and neck cancers. "Nevertheless, there is evidence that suggests precarcinogenic effects in respiratory tissue," Dr. Tashkin says. "Biopsies of bronchial tissue provide evidence that regular marijuana smoking injures airway epithelial cells, leading to dysregulation of bronchial epithelial cell growth and eventually to possible malignant changes." Moreover, he adds, because marijuana smokers typically hold their breath four times as long as tobacco smokers after inhaling, marijuana smoking deposits significantly more tar and known carcinogens within the tar, such as polycyclic aromatic hydrocarbons (PAHs), in the airways. In addition to precancerous changes, Dr. Tashkin found that marijuana smoking is associated with a range of damaging pulmonary effects, including inhibition of the tumor-killing and bactericidal activity of alveolar macrophages, the primary immune cells within the lung.

Taken together, Dr. Tashkin's survey of clinical and epidemiological studies and Dr. Moore's assessment of self-reported and clinically observed effects provide an extensive catalog of respiratory and pulmonary damage associated with marijuana smoking. Smokers are subject to:

- Coughing and phlegm production on most days;

- Wheezing and other chest sounds;

- Acute and chronic bronchitis;

- Injury to airway tissue, including edema (swelling), increased vascularity, and increased mucus secretion; and

- Impaired function of immune system components (alveolar macrophages) in the lungs.

Chapter 27

Marijuana Smoking And Psychiatric Disorders

You may know that smoking marijuana can pose risks for a person's physical health and brain development, especially for teens. But did you know that, for some people, it carries risks for their mental health, too?

It doesn't just mean short-term memory problems or poor judgment—those can happen for anybody who smokes marijuana. It's about serious mental illness.

Researchers have found that some marijuana users have an increased risk for psychosis, a serious mental disorder where people have false thoughts (delusions) or see or hear things that aren't there (hallucinations). But there is still a lot to learn about whether marijuana use may lead to this loss of touch with reality, or if having a mental illness makes people more likely to use marijuana. And as with other drugs, things like the age of users, how early they started smoking pot, the amount of the drug they used, and their genetics all could make a difference in whether or not long-term problems develop.

It's Not Your Jeans That Matter—It's Your Genes

Regular marijuana users with a specific version of a particular gene, *AKT1*, are at a greater risk of developing psychosis than those who smoke it less often or not at all. How much greater? For people who smoke marijuana daily, the risk is up to seven times greater.

About This Chapter: Text in this chapter begins with excerpts from "Marijuana And Psychosis," National Institute on Drug Abuse (NIDA) for Teens, June 2, 2015; Text beginning with the heading "Marijuana Use And Psychiatric Disorders" is excerpted from "Marijuana—Is There A Link Between Marijuana Use And Psychiatric Disorders," National Institute on Drug Abuse (NIDA), May 2018.

The reason is that the *AKT1* gene affects how much dopamine is released in your brain. Dopamine is one of our brain's "feel-good" chemicals; it affects important brain functions such as behavior, motivation, and reward. When your brain releases dopamine (for example, after a beautiful bike ride or when you eat a delicious piece of chocolate), the release "teaches" your brain to seek out the same experience (reward) again. Some researchers believe that changes in dopamine levels are linked to psychosis.

Another study found that adults who used marijuana when they were teenagers and who carried a specific form of another gene for the enzyme catechol-O-methyltransferase (COMT) (which also impacts dopamine signaling) were at a higher risk of becoming psychotic.

Are You At Risk?

Right now, unless you've had your deoxyribonucleic acid (DNA) tested for those specific genes, you don't know. Many health professionals believe that in the future most of us will know much more about our genetic makeup, but for now and for regular marijuana users, it's an unknown risk—and you won't know until you've developed an addiction.

Even If You Don't Have Those Specific Genes, There's Still A Risk

A psychotic event can even happen to pot smokers without these specific genes that put them at risk for long-term serious mental illness. Although rare, marijuana-induced psychosis is becoming more common as people use higher potency forms, including edibles and oil extracts. The bottom line? It's important to know all the risks that can come with using marijuana.

Marijuana Use And Psychiatric Disorders

Several studies have linked marijuana use to increased risk for psychiatric disorders, including psychosis (schizophrenia), depression, anxiety, and substance use disorders, but whether and to what extent it actually causes these conditions is not always easy to determine. The amount of drug used, the age at first use, and genetic vulnerability have all been shown to influence this relationship. The strongest evidence to date concerns links between marijuana use and substance use disorders and between marijuana use and psychiatric disorders in those with a preexisting genetic or other vulnerability.

Research using longitudinal data from the National Epidemiological Survey on Alcohol and Related Conditions (NESARC) examined associations between marijuana use, mood and anxiety disorders, and substance use disorders. After adjusting for various confounding factors, no association between marijuana use and mood and anxiety disorders was found. The only significant associations were increased risk of alcohol use disorders, nicotine dependence, marijuana use disorder, and other drug use disorders.

Adverse Consequences Of Marijuana Use

Acute (present during intoxication)

- Impaired short-term memory
- Impaired attention, judgment, and other cognitive functions
- Impaired coordination and balance
- Increased heart rate
- Anxiety, paranoia
- Psychosis (uncommon)

Persistent (lasting longer than intoxication, but may not be permanent)

- Impaired learning and coordination
- Sleep problems

Long-Term (cumulative effects of repeated use)

- Potential for marijuana addiction
- Impairments in learning and memory with potential loss of IQ*
- Increased risk of chronic cough, bronchitis
- Increased risk of other drug and alcohol use disorders
- Increased risk of schizophrenia in people with genetic vulnerability**

*Loss of IQ among individuals with persistent marijuana use disorder who began using heavily during adolescence.

**These are often reported co-occurring symptoms/disorders with chronic marijuana use. However, research has not yet determined whether marijuana is causal or just associated with these mental problems.

A research has found that people who use marijuana and carry a specific variant of the *AKT1* gene, which codes for an enzyme that affects dopamine signaling in the striatum, are at increased risk of developing psychosis. The striatum is an area of the brain that becomes activated and flooded with dopamine when certain stimuli are present. One study found that the risk of psychosis among those with this variant was seven times higher for those who used marijuana daily compared with those who used it infrequently or used none at all.

Another study found an increased risk of psychosis among adults who had used marijuana in adolescence and also carried a specific variant of the gene for COMT, an enzyme that degrades neurotransmitters such as dopamine and norepinephrine. Marijuana use has also been shown to worsen the course of illness in patients who already have schizophrenia. As mentioned previously, marijuana can produce an acute psychotic reaction in nonschizophrenic people who use marijuana, especially at high doses, although this fades as the drug wears off.

Inconsistent and modest associations have been reported between marijuana use and suicidal thoughts and attempted suicide among teens. Marijuana has also been associated with an amotivational syndrome, defined as a diminished or absent drive to engage in typically rewarding activities. Because of the role of the endocannabinoid system in regulating mood and reward, it has been hypothesized that brain changes resulting from early use of marijuana may underlie these associations, but more research is needed to verify that such links exist and better understand them.

Chapter 28

Marijuana As Medicine

What Is Medical Marijuana?

The term medical marijuana refers to using the whole, unprocessed marijuana plant or its basic extracts to treat symptoms of illness and other conditions. The U.S. Food and Drug Administration (FDA) has not recognized or approved the marijuana plant as medicine. However, scientific study of the chemicals in marijuana, called cannabinoids, has led to two FDA-approved medications that contain cannabinoid chemicals in pill form. Continued research may lead to more medications. Because the marijuana plant contains chemicals that may help treat a range of illnesses and symptoms, many people argue that it should be legal for medical purposes. In fact, a growing number of states have legalized marijuana for medical use.

Why Isn't The Marijuana Plant An FDA-Approved Medicine?

The FDA requires carefully conducted studies (clinical trials) in hundreds to thousands of human subjects to determine the benefits and risks of a possible medication. So far, researchers haven't conducted enough large-scale clinical trials that show that the benefits of the marijuana plant (as opposed to its cannabinoid ingredients) outweigh its risks in patients it's meant to treat.

About This Chapter: This chapter includes text excerpted from "Marijuana As Medicine," National Institute on Drug Abuse (NIDA), May 2018.

Can Medical Marijuana Legalization Decrease Prescription Opioid Problems?

Some studies have suggested that medical marijuana legalization might be associated with decreased prescription opioid use and overdose deaths, but researchers don't have enough evidence yet to confirm this finding. For example, one study found that Medicare Part D prescriptions filled for all opioids decreased in states with medical marijuana laws. Another study examined Medicaid prescription data and found that medical marijuana laws and adult-use marijuana laws were associated with lower opioid prescribing rates (5.88% and 6.88% lower, respectively).

Additionally, one National Institute on Drug Abuse (NIDA)-funded study suggested a link between medical marijuana legalization and fewer overdose deaths from prescription opioids. These studies, however, are population-based and can't show that medical marijuana legalization caused the decrease in deaths or that pain patients changed their drug-taking behavior. A more detailed NIDA-funded analysis showed that legally protected medical marijuana dispensaries, not just medical marijuana laws, were also associated with a decrease in the following:

- Opioid prescribing
- Self-reports of opioid misuse
- Treatment admissions for opioid addiction

Additionally, some data suggests that medical marijuana treatment may reduce the opioid dose prescribed for pain patients, while another National Institutes of Health (NIH)-funded study suggests that cannabis use appears to increase the risk of developing and opioid use disorder. NIDA is funding additional studies to determine the link between medical marijuana use and the use or misuse of opioids for specific types of pain, and also its possible role for treatment of opioid use disorder.

What Are Cannabinoids?

Cannabinoids are chemicals related to delta-9-tetrahydrocannabinol (THC), marijuana's main mind-altering ingredient that makes people "high." The marijuana plant contains more than 100 cannabinoids. Scientists, as well as illegal manufacturers, have produced many cannabinoids in the lab. Some of these cannabinoids are extremely powerful and have led to serious health effects when misused.

The body also produces its own cannabinoid chemicals. They play a role in regulating pleasure, memory, thinking, concentration, body movement, awareness of time, appetite, pain, and the senses (taste, touch, smell, hearing, and sight).

Chemical Cannabidiol (CBD) And Childhood Epilepsy

There is growing interest in the marijuana chemical cannabidiol (CBD) to treat certain conditions such as childhood epilepsy, a disorder that causes a child to have violent seizures. Therefore, scientists have been specially breeding marijuana plants and making CBD in oil form for treatment purposes. These drugs aren't popular for recreational use because they aren't intoxicating.

How Might Cannabinoids Be Useful As Medicine?

The two main cannabinoids from the marijuana plant that are of medical interest are THC and CBD. THC can increase appetite and reduce nausea. THC may also decrease pain, inflammation (swelling and redness), and muscle control problems. Unlike THC, CBD is a cannabinoid that doesn't make people "high." It may be useful in reducing pain and inflammation, controlling epileptic seizures, and possibly even treating mental illness and addictions.

Many researchers, including those funded by the NIH, are continuing to explore the possible uses of THC, CBD, and other cannabinoids for medical treatment.

For instance, some animal studies have shown that marijuana extracts may help kill certain cancer cells and reduce the size of others. Evidence from one cell culture study with rodents suggests that purified extracts from whole-plant marijuana can slow the growth of cancer cells from one of the most serious types of brain tumors. Research in mice showed that treatment with purified extracts of THC and CBD, when used with radiation, increased the cancer-killing effects of the radiation.

Scientists are also conducting preclinical and clinical trials with marijuana and its extracts to treat symptoms of illness and other conditions, such as:

- Diseases that affect the immune system, including:

  - Human immunodeficiency virus (HIV) and acquired immunodeficiency syndrome (AIDS)

  - Multiple sclerosis (MS), which causes gradual loss of muscle control

- Inflammation

- Pain

- Seizures

- Substance use disorders (SUDs)

- Mental disorders

What Medications Contain Cannabinoids?

Two FDA-approved drugs, dronabinol and nabilone, contain THC. They treat nausea caused by chemotherapy and increase appetite in patients with extreme weight loss caused by AIDS. Continued research might lead to more medications. The United Kingdom, Canada, and several European countries have approved nabiximols (Sativex®), a mouth spray containing THC and CBD. It treats muscle control problems caused by MS, but it isn't FDA-approved. Epidiolex, a CBD-based liquid drug to treat certain forms of childhood epilepsy, is being tested in clinical trials but isn't yet FDA-approved.

Chapter 29

The U.S. Drug Enforcement Administration Position On Marijuana

The campaign to legitimize what is called "medical" marijuana is based on two propositions: first, that science views marijuana as medicine; and second, that the U.S. Drug Enforcement Administration (DEA) targets sick and dying people using the drug. Neither proposition is true. Specifically, smoked marijuana has not withstood the rigors of science—it is not medicine, and it is not safe. Moreover, the DEA targets criminals engaged in the cultivation and trafficking of marijuana, not the sick and dying. This is true even in the District of Columbia (DC) and the 19 states that have approved the use of "medical" marijuana.

Smoked Marijuana Is Not Medicine

In 1970, Congress enacted laws against marijuana based in part on its conclusion that marijuana has no scientifically proven medical value. Likewise, the U.S. Food and Drug Administration (FDA), which is responsible for approving drugs as safe and effective medicine, has thus far declined to approve smoked marijuana for any condition or disease. Indeed, the FDA has noted that "there is currently sound evidence that smoked marijuana is harmful," and "that no sound scientific studies support medical use of marijuana for treatment in the United States, and no animal or human data support the safety or efficacy of marijuana for general medical use."

About This Chapter: This chapter includes text excerpted from "The DEA Position On Marijuana," U.S. Drug Enforcement Administration (DEA), April 2013. Reviewed July 2018.

The United States Supreme Court has also declined to carve out an exception for marijuana under a theory of medical viability. In 2001, for example, the Supreme Court decided that a 'medical necessity' defense against prosecution was unavailable to defendants because Congress had purposely placed marijuana into Schedule I, which enumerates those controlled substances without any medical benefits.

The DEA and the federal government are not alone in viewing smoked marijuana as having no documented medical value. Voices in the medical community likewise do not accept smoked marijuana as medicine:

- The American Medical Association (AMA) has always endorsed "well-controlled studies of marijuana and related cannabinoids in patients with serious conditions for which preclinical, anecdotal, or controlled evidence suggests possible efficacy and the application of such results to the understanding and treatment of disease." In November 2009, the AMA amended its policy, urging that marijuana's status as a Schedule I controlled substance be reviewed "with the goal of facilitating the conduct of clinical research and development of cannabinoid-based medicines, and alternate delivery methods." The AMA also stated that "this should not be viewed as an endorsement of state-based medical cannabis programs, the legalization of marijuana, or that scientific evidence on the therapeutic use of cannabis meets the current standards for prescription drug product."

- The American Society of Addiction Medicine's (ASAM) public policy statement on "Medical Marijuana," clearly rejects smoking as a means of drug delivery. ASAM further recommends that "all cannabis, cannabis-based products and cannabis delivery devices should be subject to the same standards applicable to all other prescription medication and medical devices, and should not be distributed or otherwise provided to patients …" without FDA approval. ASAM also "discourages state interference in the federal medication approval process." ASAM continues to support these policies, and has also stated that they do not "support proposals to legalize marijuana anywhere in the United States."

- The American Cancer Society (ACS) "is supportive of more research into the benefits of cannabinoids. Better and more effective treatments are needed to overcome the side effects of cancer and its treatment. However, the ACS does not advocate the use of inhaled marijuana or the legalization of marijuana."

- The American Glaucoma Society (AGS) has stated that "although marijuana can lower the intraocular pressure, the side effects and short duration of action, coupled with the lack of evidence that its use alters the course of glaucoma, preclude recommending this drug in any form for the treatment of glaucoma at the present time."

- The Glaucoma Research Foundation (GRF) states that "the high dose of marijuana necessary to produce a clinically relevant effect on intraocular pressure in people with glaucoma in the short term requires constant inhalation, as much as every three hours. The number of significant side effects generated by long-term use of marijuana or long-term inhalation of marijuana smoke makes marijuana a poor choice in the treatment of glaucoma. To date, no studies have shown that marijuana—or any of its approximately 400 chemical components—can safely and effectively lower intraocular pressure better than the variety of drugs currently on the market."

- The American Academy of Pediatrics (AAP) believes that "any change in the legal status of marijuana, even if limited to adults, could affect the prevalence of use among adolescents." While it supports scientific research on the possible medical use of cannabinoids as opposed to smoked marijuana, it opposes the legalization of marijuana.

- The American Academy of Child and Adolescent Psychiatry (AACAP) "is concerned about the negative impact of medical marijuana on youth. Adolescents are especially vulnerable to the many adverse developments, cognitive, medical, psychiatric, and addictive effects of marijuana." Of greater concern to the AACAP is that "adolescent marijuana users are more likely than adult users to develop marijuana dependence, and their heavy use is associated with increased incidence and worsened course of psychotic, mood, and anxiety disorders." "The "medicalization" of smoked marijuana has distorted the perception of the known risks and purposed benefits of this drug." Based upon these concerns, the "AACAP opposes medical marijuana dispensing to adolescents."

- The National Multiple Sclerosis Society (NMSS) has stated that "based on studies to date—and the fact that long-term use of marijuana may be associated with significant, serious side effects—it is the opinion of the National Multiple Sclerosis Society's Medical Advisory Board that there are currently insufficient data to recommend marijuana or its derivatives as a treatment for multiple sclerosis (MS) symptoms. Research is continuing to determine if there is a possible role for marijuana or its derivatives in the treatment of MS. In the meantime, other well tested, FDA approved drugs are available to reduce spasticity."

In 1999, the Institute of Medicine (IOM) released a landmark study reviewing the supposed medical properties of marijuana. The study is frequently cited by "medical" marijuana advocates, but in fact, severely undermines their arguments.

- After release of the IOM study, the principal investigators cautioned that the active compounds in marijuana may have medicinal potential, and therefore, should be researched further. However, the study concluded that "there is little future in smoked marijuana as a medically approved medication."

- For some ailments, the IOM found "potential therapeutic value of cannabinoid drugs, primarily tetrahydrocannabinol (THC), for pain relief, control of nausea and vomiting, and appetite stimulation." However, it pointed out that "the effects of cannabinoids on the symptoms studied are generally modest, and in most cases, there are more effective medications (than smoked marijuana)."

- The study concluded that, at best, there is only anecdotal information on the medical benefits of smoked marijuana for some ailments, such as muscle spasticity. For other ailments, such as epilepsy and glaucoma, the study found no evidence of medical value and did not endorse further research.

- The IOM study explained that "smoked marijuana is a crude THC delivery system that also delivers harmful substances." In addition, "plants contain a variable mixture of biologically active compounds and cannot be expected to provide a precisely defined drug effect." Therefore, the study concluded that "there is little future in smoked marijuana as a medically approved medication."

- The principal investigators explicitly stated that using smoked marijuana in clinical trials "should not be designed to develop it as a licensed drug, but should be a stepping stone to the development of new, safe delivery systems of cannabinoids."

Thus, even scientists and researchers who believe that certain active ingredients in marijuana may have potential medicinal value openly discount the notion that smoked marijuana is or can become "medicine."

The U.S. Drug Enforcement Administration (DEA) supports ongoing research into potential medicinal uses of marijuana's active ingredients. As of January 2013:

- There are 125 researchers registered with DEA to perform studies with marijuana, marijuana extracts, and nontetrahydrocannabinol marijuana derivatives that exist in the plant, such as cannabidiol and cannabinol.

- Studies include evaluation of abuse potential, physical/psychological effects, adverse effects, therapeutic potential, and detection.

- Eighteen of the researchers are approved to conduct research with smoked marijuana on human subjects.

However, the clear weight of the evidence is that smoked marijuana is harmful. No matter what medical condition has been studied, other drugs already approved by the FDA have been proven to be safer than smoked marijuana.

The only drug currently approved by the FDA that contains the synthetic form of THC is Marinol®. Available through prescription, Marinol® comes in pill form, and is used to relieve nausea and vomiting associated with chemotherapy for cancer patients and to assist with loss of appetite with acquired immunodeficiency syndrome (AIDS) patients.

Sativex®, an oromucosal spray for the treatment of spasticity due to multiple sclerosis is already approved for use in Canada, New Zealand, Spain, and the United Kingdom. The oral liquid spray contains two of the cannabinoids found in marijuana—THC and cannabidiol (CBD)—but unlike smoked marijuana, removes contaminants, reduces the intoxicating effects, is grown in a structured and scientific environment, administers a set dosage and meets criteria for pharmaceutical products. GW Pharmaceuticals plans to submit Sativex® to the FDA in 2014 as a treatment for cancer pain.

Organizers behind the "medical" marijuana movement have not dealt with ensuring that the product meets the standards of modern medicine: quality, safety, and efficacy. There is no standardized composition or dosage; no appropriate prescribing information; no quality control; no accountability for the product; no safety regulation; no way to measure its effectiveness (besides anecdotal stories); and no insurance coverage. Science, not popular vote, should determine what medicine is.

Marijuana Is Dangerous To The User And Others

Without a clear understanding of the mental and physical effects of marijuana, its use on our youth, our families, and our society, we will never understand the ramifications it will have on the lives of our younger generation, the impact on their future, and its costs to our society.

Legalization of marijuana, no matter how it begins, will come at the expense of our children and public safety. It will create dependency and treatment issues, and open the door to use of other drugs, impaired health, delinquent behavior, and drugged drivers.

This is not the marijuana of the 1970s; today's marijuana is far more powerful. On May 14, 2009, analysis from the National Institute on Drug Abuse (NIDA)-funded University of Mississippi's (UM) Potency Monitoring Project revealed that marijuana potency levels in the United States are the highest ever reported since the scientific analysis of the drug began. This trend continues.

- The average amount of THC in seized samples has reached 15.1 percent. This compares to an average of just under four percent reported in 1983 and represents more than a tripling of the potency of the drug since that time.

- "We are increasingly concerned that regular or daily use of marijuana is robbing many young people of their potential to achieve and excel in school or other aspects of life," said NIDA Director Nora D. Volkow, MD. "THC, a key ingredient in marijuana, alters the ability of the hippocampus, a brain area related to learning and memory, to communicate effectively with other brain regions. In addition, we know from research that marijuana use that begins during adolescence can lower IQ and impair other measures of mental function in adulthood."

- "We should also point out that marijuana use that begins in adolescence increases the risk they will become addicted to the drug," said Volkow. "The risk of addiction goes from about 1 in 11 overall to 1 in 6 for those who start using in their teens, and even higher among daily smokers."

The statistics on the use of marijuana in the United States shows that marijuana use continues to rise.

- In 2011, an estimated 22.5 million American's aged 12 and older were current (past month) illicit drug users. This represents 8.7 percent of the population 12 and older. Marijuana was the most commonly used illicit drug with 18.1 million past month users.

- The use of illicit drug use among young adults aged 18–25 increased from 19.7 percent in 2008 to 21.4 percent in 2011, driven largely by an increase in marijuana use (from 16.6% in 2008 to 19% in 2011).

- In 2011, an estimated 3.1 million persons aged 12 and older used an illicit drug for the first time within the past 12 months. That equals about 8,400 initiates per day. The largest number of new initiates (7,200) used marijuana (2.6 million).

- Among 12 and 13 year olds, 1.3 percent used marijuana; for 14 and 15 year olds, it was 6.7 percent; and for 16 and 17 year olds, it climbed to 15.1 percent.

- Nearly 23 percent of high school seniors say they smoked marijuana in the month prior to the survey, and just over 36 percent say they smoked within the previous year. More than 11 percent of eighth graders said they used marijuana during the past year.

- An estimated 16.7 percent of past year marijuana users aged 12 and older used marijuana on 300 or more days within the past 12 months. This means that almost 5 million persons used marijuana on a daily or almost daily basis over a 12 month period.

- An estimated 39.1 percent (7.1 million) of current marijuana users aged 12 and older used marijuana on 20 or more days in the past month.

- Among persons 12 or older, an estimated 1.5 million first-time past year marijuana users initiated use prior to age 18.

- According to 2012 Monitoring the Future (MTF) Survey, one in every 15 high school seniors (16.5%) is a daily or near-daily marijuana user.

- The 2011 Partnership Attitude Tracking Study (PATS) found that nine percent of teens (nearly 1.5 million) smoked marijuana heavily (at least 20 times) in the past month. Overall, past-month teen use was up 80 percent from 2008.

  - Nearly half of teens (47%) have ever used marijuana—a 21 percent increase from 2008.

  - Two out of every five teens (39%) have tried marijuana during the past year, an increase from 31 percent in 2008.

  - Past-month use increased 42 percent, from 19 percent in 2008 to 27 percent in 2011 (an increase of 4 million teens).

  - Past-year use is up 26 percent from 31 percent in 2008 to 39 percent in 2011 (an increase of 6 million teens).

  - Lifetime use is up 21 percent, from 39 percent in 2008 to 47 percent in 2011 (an increase of 8 million teens).

Increasingly, the international community is joining the United States in recognizing the fallacy of arguments claiming marijuana use is a harmless activity with no consequences to others.

- Antonio Maria Costa, then Executive Director of the United Nations Office on Drugs and Crime (UNODC), noted in an article published in *The Independent on Sunday* "The debate over the drug is no longer about liberty; it's about health." He continued, "Evidence of the damage to mental health caused by cannabis use—from loss of concentration to paranoia, aggressiveness and outright psychosis—is mounting and cannot be ignored. Emergency-room admissions involving cannabis is rising, as is demand for rehabilitation treatment. It is time to explode the myth of cannabis as a 'soft' drug."

- The President of the International Narcotics Control Board (INCB), Raymond Yars, voiced grave concern about the referenda in the United States that would allow the recreational use of cannabis by adults. "Legalization of cannabis within these states would send wrong and confusing signals to youth and society in general, giving a false impression that drug abuse might be considered normal and even, most disturbingly, safe. Such a development could result in the expansion of drug abuse, especially among young people, and we must remember that all young people have a right to be protected from drug abuse and drug dependency."

"The concern with marijuana is not born out of any culture war mentality, but out of what science tells us about the drug's effects."

Marijuana As A Precursor To Abuse Of Other Drugs

- Teens who experiment with marijuana may be making themselves more vulnerable to heroin addiction later in life, if the findings from experiments with rats are any indication. "Cannabis has very long-term, enduring effects on the brain," according to Dr. Yamin Hurd of the Mount Sinai School of Medicine in New York, the study's lead author.

- Long-term studies on patterns of drug usage among young people show that very few of them use other drugs without first starting with marijuana. For example, one study found that among adults (age 26 and older) who had used cocaine, 62 percent had initiated marijuana use before age 15. By contrast, less than one percent of adults who never tried marijuana went on to use cocaine.

- Marijuana use in early adolescence is particularly ominous. Adults who were early marijuana users were found to be five times more likely to become dependent on any drug, eight times more likely to use cocaine in the future, and fifteen times more likely to use heroin later in life.

- An estimated 3.1 million persons aged 12 or older—an average of approximately 8,400 per day—used a drug other than alcohol for the first time in the past year according to the 2011 National Survey on Drug Use and Health. More than two-thirds (68 percent) of these new users reported that marijuana was the first drug they tried.

Chapter 30

Legalization And Decriminalization Of Marijuana

The legalization and decriminalization of marijuana has received a great deal of media attention across the country, and many states are considering whether they should legalize marijuana for recreational or medical use. States need information about the impacts of laws that legalize or decriminalize the use of marijuana, including its impact on driving safety and the state's driving while impaired (DWI) system.

A total of 25 states, the District of Columbia, and Guam allow marijuana and cannabis programs for medical use. The approved efforts in 17 states allow use of "low tetrahydrocannabinol (THC), high cannabidiol (CBD)" products for medical reasons in limited situations or as a legal defense. Four states and the District of Columbia have legalized marijuana for recreational use. Nine states have ballot measures for recreational or legal marijuana and four States were either gathering ballot signatures or certifying initiatives.

The Federal Policy On Medical Marijuana

In 2009, the Obama Administration began to deviate from previous strict enforcement policies, despite the fact that medical marijuana remains illegal under federal law. The U.S. Department of Justice (DOJ) sent a memo to federal prosecutors, encouraging them to

---

About This Chapter: Text in this chapter begins with excerpts from "Impact Of The Legalization And Decriminalization Of Marijuana On The DWI System," National Highway Traffic Safety Administration (NHTSA), June 2017; Text beginning with the heading "The Federal Policy On Medical Marijuana" is excerpted from "The Path Forward: Rethinking Federal Marijuana Policy," U.S. House of Representatives, April 9, 2018; Text under the heading "As Some States Implement New Marijuana Laws, Science Should Guide Public Health Policy" is excerpted from "As Some States Implement New Marijuana Laws, Science Should Guide Public Health Policy," National Institute on Drug Abuse (NIDA), December 8, 2016.

deprioritize prosecuting individuals "whose actions are in clear and unambiguous compliance with existing state laws providing for the medical use of marijuana," and instead focus on providers who violate both state and federal law, and those who operate medical facilities as a front for criminal activity. This letter is commonly referred to as the "Ogden Memo." As a result, many states moved forward with enacting medical marijuana laws and establishing systems for regulating production and distribution.

Since 2011, however, the DOJ further clarified its policy with the "Cole Memo," stating that laissez-faire approval does not apply to large-scale commercial operations that cultivate, sell, or distribute marijuana, regardless of whether or not they are in compliance with state law. DOJ claims that many of these facilities were operating as fronts for criminal activity which state regulation has been insufficient to prevent. The federal government has since continued to enforce federal law relating to medical marijuana, and facilities across the country have been raided by the U.S. Drug Enforcement Administration (DEA) or otherwise targeted by the DOJ. At the time of the report, a national example was a California case on the front page of the New York Times on January 14, 2013. Also of note, in 1998, the District of Columbia approved a medical marijuana measure. However, Congress responded by passing the "Barr Amendment," which prohibited DC from implementing this measure, until the Barr Amendment was overturned in 2009.

Public Opinion Shifts On Marijuana

While the United States spends billions of dollars incarcerating citizens and damaging lives, nearly half of the American public believes that marijuana should be legalized. This figure has steadily risen over the last 30 years, and 2011 marked the first time when a majority of Americans believed marijuana should be legalized. Among young Americans the numbers are even more overwhelmingly in support of changing policy. The American public demonstrates even stronger support for the use of medical marijuana. When polled, 70 percent favor allowing doctors to prescribe marijuana for reducing pain and suffering.

Challenges

Enforcement

The federal government must choose the degree to which it will enforce federal law in states that have legalized marijuana under state law. Strict enforcement will become increasingly difficult and costly as more states legalize marijuana. Additionally, the current system creates uncertainty that is only likely to grow without major reform of marijuana laws in Congress.

The presence of a black market for marijuana poses additional challenges to the federal government as it seeks to enforce existing drug policies, raiding dispensaries and operations that the government claims are tied to trafficking but that also sell into the medical market. Such enforcement limits the accessibility of medical marijuana for legitimate customers, and creates barriers to entry for those who seek to grow and sell marijuana legally.

Tax And Regulate Marijuana

Considering the growing number of jurisdictions that legalize medical marijuana and the two jurisdictions that legalize recreational use, it is time that Congress end the federal prohibition on marijuana, removing it from the Controlled Substances Act (CSA) and creating a regulatory and taxation framework, similar to the frameworks in place for alcohol and tobacco.

A specific tax on marijuana grown for all purposes should be imposed to help fund substance abuse dependency treatment, law enforcement, and help reduce the federal debt. Revenue estimates from taxing marijuana vary due to uncertainties surrounding the existing marijuana market and how legalization and regulation would impact price and consumption habits. Assuming increased legal consumption and reduction in prices, a $50 per ounce tax, for example, would raise estimated revenue of $20 billion annually. Any study of the fiscal impact should also include the savings generated by reduced expenditures on marijuana interdiction and enforcement. This represents a unique opportunity to save ruined lives, wasted enforcement and prison costs, while simultaneously creating a new industry, with new jobs and revenues that will improve the federal budget outlook. Passing such legislation would represent a key part of a comprehensive approach to marijuana reform. However Congress should also consider additional legislation that would ease problems during this transitional period, such as exempting medical marijuana specifically to ensure patient access, and alleviating specific tax and business challenges.

States To Enact Existing Medical Marijuana Laws Without Federal Interference

The federal government needs to allow states to enforce their laws without fear of interference by removing barriers to medical marijuana distribution and research. Descheduling marijuana in the Controlled Substances Act will ensure that patients and providers that operate in compliance with state law remain immune from federal prosecution. Congress should pass legislation that will accomplish this by declaring that in a state where medical marijuana is legal, no provision of the Controlled Substance Act, or the Federal Food, Drug and Cosmetic Act (FD&C Act) shall prohibit or restrict:

- The prescription or recommendation of marijuana for medical use by a medical professional

- An individual from obtaining, manufacturing, possessing, or transporting within their state marijuana for medical purposes

- A pharmacy or other entity authorized to distribute medical marijuana

- An authorized entity from producing, processing, or distributing marijuana

Taking such action will help ensure patients have safe access to medical marijuana, and ensure that states are free to enact comprehensive regulatory oversight of their programs without fear that they will be putting business owners and patients at risk or breaking federal law.

Medical Marijuana Research

Following the 1996 legalization of medical marijuana in California, a National Institutes of Health (NIH) panel of experts called for additional studies to properly evaluate marijuana's medical potential.

Yet, because of marijuana's classification as a Schedule I substance, the research data collected on specific medicinal effects of marijuana remains very limited. Researchers wishing to obtain marijuana for medical research must obtain a special license from the Drug Enforcement Administration and apply for access to the supply overseen by the National Institutes of Drug Abuse (NIDA). NIDA's mission is "to lead the nation in bringing the power of science to bear on drug abuse and addiction," and is decidedly not focused on medical research. Permission to obtain marijuana for medical research has been quite difficult. Thus while opponents of medical marijuana research often point to the absence of peer-reviewed studies that establish the medical benefits of marijuana, the absence of such studies is more directly a result of the extreme legal and funding difficulties surrounding conducting such a scientific study.

Medical marijuana is used to treat nausea, loss of appetite, muscle tension or spasms, chronic pain, and insomnia. It has often been used to treat these symptoms in patients suffering from cancer and the side effects of chemotherapy, human immunodeficiency virus (HIV), and other serious conditions.

As Some States Implement New Marijuana Laws, Science Should Guide Public Health Policy

After the election on November 8, 2016, marijuana is now or will soon be legal for adult recreational use in eight states plus the District of Columbia (DC). These states, and those that may join them in the future, will have choices to make in how they enact and implement their policies. Careful thought should be given to creating regulatory frameworks that prioritize public health. Science needs to be the guide.

A 2015 report prepared by the RAND Corporation for the state of Vermont pointed out that marijuana policy need not be seen as a binary choice between maintaining the status quo (prohibition) or putting in place a for-profit commercial model, such as those that now exist in Colorado and Washington. The latter could create an industry that stands to profit from encouraging heavy drug use by aggressively marketing its product and lobbying for less regulation. Heavy users account for the majority of sales currently in both the alcohol and tobacco industry. But a broad spectrum of models exists, varying in terms of who can provide marijuana (the state versus private or not-for-profit entities), what regulations govern how they operate, what kinds of products can be produced and distributed, including potency of the products, and how they are priced.

The United States experience with other legal drugs provides useful lessons for states to consider. Alcohol is often seen as the most obvious comparison to marijuana, as it is a legal drug with wide range of health and safety risks but also a history of prohibition that is now viewed by most as having been a failure. There are definite policy lessons to be learned from the country's experience with alcohol; raising the legal drinking age to 21 in the 1980s, for example, was associated with significant reductions in alcohol use and car crashes in young adults. But alcohol remains widely misused in all age groups, is cheap and readily available in most locales, and numerous adverse health and safety outcomes are attributable to it.

The U.S. experience with tobacco offers a different set of important and useful lessons. NIDA have seen continuous reductions in cigarette smoking and corresponding gains in public health for decades thanks to a number of efforts aimed at reducing demand for tobacco products, including significant increases in tobacco taxes, comprehensive smoke-free laws, hard-hitting media campaigns, and offering help for smokers to quit. In an article in *PLOS Medicine*, University of California San Francisco (UCSF) tobacco policy researchers Rachel Ann Barry and Stanton Glantz argue that a framework for marijuana that restricts demand by making marijuana expensive and its use socially nonnormative, similar to current tobacco policies, would help prevent marijuana from playing the same deleterious role in Americans' health and safety that alcohol misuse now does.

The degree of marijuana's harms relative to alcohol and tobacco remains widely debated, but there is no doubt that harms exist. Marijuana raises car crash risk; in some studies it has been associated with neurodevelopmental problems in prenatally exposed children; and its use by adolescents has been linked to cognitive impairments and poor educational outcomes and well-being. Although it is still not known whether marijuana raises lung cancer risk, it can adversely affect lung and heart health, potentially even via secondhand exposure. It is also addictive. Thus the wide societal perception that marijuana is a safe drug is not accurate. Absent appropriate regulation focused on protecting public health, the marijuana industry will capitalize on this misperception to increase demand for their product.

Part Five
Abuse Of Legally Available Substances

Chapter 31

Facts About The Abuse Of Prescription And Over-The-Counter (OTC) Medications

What Are Prescription Drugs?

A drug is a substance intended for use in the diagnosis, cure, mitigation, treatment, or prevention of disease. Here are the main differences between over-the-counter (OTC) drugs and prescription drugs.

Prescription drugs are:

- Prescribed by a doctor

- Bought at a pharmacy

- Prescribed for and intended to be used by one person

- Regulated by U.S. Food and Drug Administration (FDA) through the New Drug Application (NDA) process

What Is Prescription Drug Misuse?

Prescription drug misuse has become a large public health problem, because misuse can lead to addiction, and even overdose deaths.

About This Chapter: Text under the heading "What Are Prescription Drugs?" is excerpted from "Prescription Drugs And Over-The-Counter (OTC) Drugs: Questions And Answers," U.S. Food and Drug Administration (FDA), November 13, 2017; Text beginning with the heading "What Is Prescription Drug Misuse?" is excerpted from "Prescription Drugs," National Institute on Drug Abuse (NIDA) for Teens, March 2017; Text beginning with the heading "What Are Over-The-Counter (OTC) Medicines?" is excerpted from "Over-The-Counter Medicines," National Institute on Drug Abuse (NIDA), December 2017.

For teens, it is a growing problem:

- After marijuana and alcohol, prescription drugs are the most commonly misused substances by Americans age 14 and older.

- Teens misuse prescription drugs for a number of reasons, such as to get high, to stop pain, or because they think it will help them with school work.

- Many teens get prescription drugs they misuse from friends and relatives, sometimes without the person knowing.

- Boys and girls tend to misuse some types of prescription drugs for different reasons. For example, boys are more likely to misuse prescription stimulants to get high, while girls tend to misuse them to stay alert or to lose weight.

Also known as:

Opioids: Happy Pills, Hillbilly Heroin, OC, Oxy, Oxycotton, Percs, and Vikes

Depressants: A-minus, Barbs, Candy, Downers, Phennies, Reds, Red Birds, Sleeping Pills, Tooies, Tranks, Yellow Jackets, Yellows, and Zombie Pills

Stimulants: Bennies, Black Beauties, Hearts, Roses, Skippy, The Smart Drug, Speed, and Vitamin R, and Uppers

What Makes Prescription Drugs Unsafe

Prescription drugs are often strong medications, which is why they require a prescription in the first place. Every medication has some risk for harmful effects, sometimes serious ones. Doctors consider the potential benefits and risks to each patient before prescribing medications and take into account a lot of different factors, described below. When they are misused, they can be just as dangerous as drugs that are made illegally.

- **Personal information.** Before prescribing a drug, health providers take into account a person's weight, how long they've been prescribed the medication, other medical conditions, and what other medications they are taking. Someone misusing prescription drugs may overload their system or put themselves at risk for dangerous drug interactions that can cause seizures, coma, or even death.

- **Form and dose.** Doctors know how long it takes for a pill or capsule to dissolve in the stomach, release drugs to the blood, and reach the brain. When misused, prescription drugs may be taken in larger amounts or in ways that change the way the drug works in the body and brain, putting the person at greater risk for an overdose. For example, when people who misuse OxyContin crush and inhale the pills, a dose that normally works over the course of 12 hours hits the central nervous system (CNS) all at once. This effect increases the risk for addiction and overdose.

- **Side effects.** Prescription drugs are designed to treat a specific illness or condition, but they often affect the body in other ways, some of which can be uncomfortable and in some cases, dangerous. These are called side effects. For example, opioid pain relievers can help with pain, but they can also cause constipation and sleepiness. Stimulants, such as Adderall, increase a person's ability to pay attention, but they also raise blood pressure and heart rate, making the heart work harder. These side effects can be worse when prescription drugs are not taken as prescribed or are used in combination with other substances.

How Prescription Drugs Are Misused

- **Taking someone else's prescription medication.** Even when someone takes another person's medication for its intended purposes (such as to relieve pain, to stay awake, or to fall asleep) it is considered misuse.

- **Taking a prescription medication in a way other than prescribed.** Taking your own prescription in a way that it is not meant to be taken is also misuse. This includes taking more of the medication than prescribed or changing its form—for example, breaking or crushing a pill or capsule and then snorting the powder.

- **Taking a prescription medication to get high.** Some types of prescription drugs also can produce pleasurable effects or "highs." Taking the medication only for the purpose of getting high is considered prescription drug misuse.

- **Mixing it with other drugs.** In some cases, if you mix your prescription drug with alcohol and certain other drugs, it is considered misuse and it can be dangerous.

Commonly Misused Prescription Drugs

There are three kinds of prescription drugs that are commonly misused.

- **Opioids**—used to relieve pain, such as Vicodin, OxyContin, or codeine

- **Depressants**—used to relieve anxiety or help a person sleep, such as Valium or Xanax

- **Stimulants**—used for treating attention deficit hyperactivity disorder (ADHD), such as Adderall and Ritalin

What Happens To Your Brain When You Use Prescription Drugs?

In the brain, neurotransmitters such as dopamine send messages by attaching to receptors on nearby cells. The actions of these neurotransmitters and receptors cause the effects from prescription drugs. Each class of prescription drugs works a bit differently in the brain:

- Prescription opioid pain medications bind to molecules on cells known as opioid receptors—the same receptors that respond to heroin. These receptors are found on nerve cells in many areas of the brain and body, especially in brain areas involved in the perception of pain and pleasure.

- Prescription stimulants, such as Ritalin, have similar effects to cocaine, by causing a buildup of the brain chemicals dopamine and norepinephrine.

- Prescription depressants make a person feel calm and relaxed in the same manner as the club drugs gamma-hydroxybutyrate (GHB) and Rohypnol.

What Happens To Your Body When You Use Prescription Drugs?

Prescription drugs can help with medical problems when used as directed. However, whether they are used properly or misused, there can be side effects:

- Using opioids like oxycodone and codeine can cause you to feel sleepy, sick to your stomach, and constipated. At higher doses, opioids can make it hard to breathe properly and can cause overdose and death.

- Using stimulants like Adderall or Ritalin can make you feel paranoid (feeling like someone is going to harm you even though they aren't). It also can cause your body temperature to get dangerously high and make your heart beat too fast. This is especially likely if stimulants are taken in large doses or in ways other than swallowing a pill.

- Using depressants like barbiturates can cause slurred speech, shallow breathing, sleepiness, disorientation, and lack of coordination. People who misuse depressants regularly and then stop suddenly may experience seizures. At higher doses depressants can also cause overdose and death, especially when combined with alcohol.

Can You Overdose Or Die If You Use Prescription Drugs?

Yes, more than half of the drug overdose deaths in the United States each year are caused by prescription drug misuse. Deaths from overdoses of prescription drugs have been increasing since the early 1990s, largely due to increases in the misuse of prescription opioid pain relievers. More than 29,700 people died from a prescription drug overdose in 2015, with alarming increases among young people ages 15–24. Mixing different types of prescription drugs can be particularly dangerous. For example, benzodiazepines interact with opioids and increase the risk of overdose. Also, combining opioids (pain relievers) with alcohol can make breathing problems worse and can lead to death.

Are Prescription Drugs Addictive?

Yes, prescription drugs that affect the brain, including opioid pain relievers, stimulants, and depressants, can cause physical dependence that could lead to addiction. Medications that affect the brain can change the way it works—especially when they are taken over an extended period of time or with escalating doses. They can change the reward system, making it harder for a person to feel good without the drug and possibly leading to intense cravings, which make it hard to stop using.

This dependence on the drug happens because the brain and body adapt to having drugs in the system for a while. A person may need larger doses of the drug to get the same initial effects. This is known as "tolerance." When drug use is stopped, uncomfortable withdrawal symptoms can occur. When people continue to use the drug despite a range of negative consequences, it is considered an addiction.

How Many Teens Use Prescription Drugs?

Prescription and OTC drugs are the most commonly misused substances by Americans age 14 and older, after marijuana and alcohol.

Below is a table showing the percentage of teens who misuse prescription drugs.

Table 31.1. Trends In Prevalence Of Any Prescription Drug For 12th Graders; 2014–2017 (In Percent)*

Drug	Time Period	12th Graders			
		2014	**2015**	**2016**	**2017**
Any Prescription Drug	Lifetime	(19.90)	18.30	18.00	16.50
	Past Year	(13.90)	12.90	12.00	10.90
	Past Month	6.40	5.90	5.40	4.90

*Data in brackets indicate statistically significant change from the previous year.

What Should I Do If Someone I Know Needs Help?

If you or a friend are in crisis and need to speak with someone now, please call:

- National Suicide Prevention Lifeline (NSPL) at 800-273-TALK (800-273-8255) (they don't just talk about suicide—they cover a lot of issues and will help put you in touch with someone close by).

If you need information on treatment and where you can find it, you can call:

- Substance Abuse Treatment Facility Locator at 800-662-HELP (800-662-4357) or visit www.findtreatment.samhsa.gov.

Prevention Of Prescription Drug Misuse

Patients can take steps to ensure that they use prescription medications appropriately by:

- Following the directions as explained on the label or by the pharmacist.
- Being aware of potential interactions with other drugs as well as alcohol.
- Never stopping or changing a dosing regimen without first discussing it with the doctor.
- Never using another person's prescription, and never giving their prescription medications to others.
- Storing prescription stimulants, sedatives, and opioids safely.

(Source: "How Can Prescription Drug Misuse Be Prevented?" National Institute on Drug Abuse (NIDA).)

What Are Over-The-Counter (OTC) Medicines?

Over-the-counter (OTC) medicines are those that can be sold directly to people without a prescription. OTC medicines treat a variety of illnesses and their symptoms including pain, coughs and colds, diarrhea, constipation, acne, and others. Some OTC medicines have active ingredients with the potential for misuse at higher-than-recommended dosages.

How Do People Use And Misuse OTC Medicines?

Misuse of an OTC medicine means:

- Taking medicine in a way or dose other than directed on the package

- Taking medicine for the effect it causes—for example, to get high

- Mixing OTC medicines together to create new products

"Behind-The-Counter"

Pseudoephedrine, a nasal decongestant found in many OTC cold medicines, can be used to make methamphetamine. For this reason, products containing pseudoephedrine are sold "behind the counter" nationwide. A prescription is not needed in most states, but in states that do require a prescription, there are limits on how much a person can buy each month. In some states, only people 18 years of age or older can buy pseudoephedrine.

What Are Some Of The Commonly Misused OTC Medicines?

There are two OTC medicines that are most commonly misused.

Dextromethorphan (DXM) is a cough suppressant found in many OTC cold medicines. The most common sources of abused DXM are "extra-strength" cough syrup, tablets and gel capsules. OTC medications that contain DXM often also contain antihistamines and decongestants. DXM may be swallowed in its original form or may be mixed with soda for flavor, called "robo-tripping" or "skittling." Users sometimes inject it. These medicines are often misused in combination with other drugs, such as alcohol and marijuana.

Loperamide is an antidiarrheal that is available in tablet, capsule, or liquid form. When misusing loperamide, people swallow large quantities of the medicine. It is unclear how often this drug is misused.

How Do These OTC Medicines Affect The Brain?

DXM is an opioid without effects on pain reduction and does not act on the opioid receptors. When taken in large doses, DXM causes a depressant effect and sometimes a hallucinogenic effect, similar to phencyclidine (PCP) and ketamine. Repeatedly seeking to experience that feeling can lead to addiction-a chronic relapsing brain condition characterized by the inability to stop using a drug despite damaging consequences to a person's life and health.

Loperamide is an opioid designed not to enter the brain. However, when taken in large amounts and combined with other substances, it may cause the drug to act in a similar way to other opioids. Other opioids, such as certain prescription pain relievers and heroin, bind to and activate opioid receptors in many areas of the brain, especially those involved in feelings of pain and pleasure. Opioid receptors are also located in the brainstem, which controls important processes, such as blood pressure, arousal, and breathing.

What Are The Health Effects Of These OTC Medicines?

Dextromethorphan (DXM)

Short-term effects of DXM misuse can range from mild stimulation to alcohol- or marijuana-like intoxication. At high doses, a person may have hallucinations or feelings of physical distortion, extreme panic, paranoia, anxiety, and aggression.

Other health effects from DXM misuse can include the following:

- Hyperexcitability
- Poor motor control
- Lack of energy
- Stomach pain
- Vision changes
- Slurred speech
- Increased blood pressure
- Sweating

Misuse of DXM products containing acetaminophen can cause liver damage.

Loperamide

In the short term, loperamide is sometimes misused to lessen cravings and withdrawal symptoms; however, it can cause euphoria, similar to other opioids.

Loperamide misuse can also lead to fainting, stomach pain, constipation, eye changes, and loss of consciousness. It can cause the heart to beat erratically or rapidly, or cause kidney problems. These effects may increase if taken with other medicines that interact with loperamide. Other effects have not been well studied and reports are mixed, but the physical consequences of loperamide misuse can be severe.

Opioid Withdrawal Symptoms

These symptoms include:

- Muscle and bone pain
- Sleep problems
- Diarrhea and vomiting
- Cold flashes with goosebumps
- Uncontrollable leg movements
- Severe cravings

Can A Person Overdose On These OTC Medicines?

Yes, a person can overdose on cold medicines containing DXM or loperamide. An overdose occurs when a person uses enough of the drug to produce a life-threatening reaction or death. As with other opioids, when people overdose on DXM or loperamide, their breathing often slows or stops. This can decrease the amount of oxygen that reaches the brain, a condition called hypoxia. Hypoxia can have short- and long-term mental effects and effects on the nervous system, including coma and permanent brain damage and death.

How Can These OTC Medicine Overdoses Be Treated?

A person who has overdosed needs immediate medical attention. Call 911. If the person has stopped breathing or if breathing is weak, begin cardiopulmonary resuscitation (CPR).

DXM overdoses can also be treated with naloxone. Certain medications can be used to treat heart rhythm problems caused by loperamide overdose. If the heart stops, healthcare providers will perform CPR and other cardiac support therapies.

Can Misuse Of These OTC Medicines Lead To Addiction?

Yes, misuse of DXM or loperamide can lead to addiction. An addiction develops when continued use of the drug causes issues, such as health problems and failure to meet responsibilities at work, school, or home. The symptoms of withdrawal from DXM and loperamide have not been well studied.

How Can People Get Treatment For Addiction To These OTC Medicines?

There are no medications approved specifically to treat DXM or loperamide addiction. Behavioral therapies, such as cognitive behavioral therapy (CBT) and contingency management, may be helpful. CBT helps to modify the patient's drug-use expectations and behaviors, and effectively manage triggers and stress. Contingency management provides vouchers or small cash rewards for positive behaviors such as staying drug-free.

Chapter 32

Trends In The Abuse Of Prescription And OTC Medications Among U.S. Teens

Opioids

Opioids are a class of drugs that include the illegal drug heroin, synthetic opioids such as fentanyl, and pain relievers available legally by prescription, such as oxycodone (OxyContin®), hydrocodone (Vicodin®), codeine, morphine, and many others.

Statistics And Trends

Table 32.1. Trends In Prevalence Of Various Drugs For 8th Graders, 10th Graders, And 12th Graders; 2017 (In Percent)*

Drug	Time Period	8th Graders	10th Graders	12th Graders
Heroin	Past Year	0.30	0.20	0.40
Narcotics other than Heroin	Past Year	–	–	4.20
OxyContin	Past Year	0.80	2.20	2.70
Vicodin	Past Year	0.70	1.50	[2.00]

*Data in brackets indicate statistically significant change from the previous year.

About This Chapter: This chapter includes text excerpted from "Opioids," National Institute on Drug Abuse (NIDA), June 7, 2018.

Table 32.2. Trends In Prevalence Of Various Drugs For Ages 12 Or Older, Ages 12–17, Ages 18–25, And Ages 26 Or Older; 2016 (In Percent)

Drug	Time Period	Ages 12 Or Older	Ages 12–17	Ages 18–25	Ages 26 Or Older
Heroin	Past Year	0.40	0.10	0.70	0.30
Pain Relievers	Past Year	4.30	3.50	7.10	3.90

Hydrocodone products are used for pain relief and cough suppression and produce effects comparable to oral morphine. Hydrocodone products are the most frequently prescribed opioids in the United States, and they are also the most abused narcotic in the United States.

(Source: "Prescription For Disaster—How Teens Abuse Medicine," U.S. Drug Enforcement Administration (DEA).)

Prescription Medicines

When used as prescribed by a doctor, prescription medicines can be helpful in treating many illnesses. Stimulants are helpful in managing attention deficit hyperactivity disorder (ADHD) and narcolepsy. Central nervous system (CNS) depressants treat anxiety, panic, and sleep disorders. Opioids are prescribed to treat pain, coughing, and diarrhea. But when these medicines are misused, they can have serious consequences.

Statistics And Trends

Table 32.3. Trends In Prevalence Of Various Drugs For 8th Graders, 10th Graders, And 12th Graders; 2017 (In Percent)*

Drug	Time Period	8th Graders	10th Graders	12th Graders
Any Prescription Drug	Past Year	–	–	10.90
Adderall	Past Year	1.30	4.00	5.50
Amphetamine	Past Year	3.50	5.60	5.90
Narcotics other than Heroin	Past Year	–	–	4.20
OxyContin	Past Year	0.80	2.20	2.70
Ritalin	Past Year	(0.40)	0.80	1.30
Tranquilizers	Past Year	2.00	4.10	4.70
Vicodin	Past Year	0.70	1.50	(2.00)

*Data in brackets indicate statistically significant change from the previous year.

Table 32.4. Trends In Prevalence Of Psychotherapeutics (Nonmedical Use) For Ages 12 Or Older, Ages 12–17, Ages 18–25, And Ages 26 Or Older; 2016 (In Percent)

Drug	Time Period	Ages 12 or Older	Ages 12–17	Ages 18–25	Ages 26 or Older
Psychotherapeutics (Nonmedical Use)	Lifetime	–	–	–	–
	Past Year	6.90	5.30	14.50	5.90
	Past Month	2.30	1.60	4.60	2.00

According to a national survey, 17.8 percent of high school students took a prescription drug without a doctor's prescription (such as OxyContin®, Percocet®, Vicodin®, codeine, Adderall®, Ritalin® or Xanax®), once or more in the past year. When looking at high school students' use by state, Arkansas had the highest use with 21.5 percent of students reporting they took a prescription drug without a doctor's prescription, while Utah had the lowest use with 8.7 percent of students reporting that they took a prescription drug without a doctor's prescription.

(Source: "Prescription For Disaster—How Teens Abuse Medicine," U.S. Drug Enforcement Administration (DEA).)

Steroids (Anabolic)

Anabolic steroids are synthetic variations of the male sex hormone testosterone. The proper term for these compounds is anabolic-androgenic steroids (AAS). "Anabolic" refers to muscle building, and "androgenic" refers to increased male sex characteristics. Some common names for anabolic steroids are Gear, Juice, Roids, and Stackers.

Statistics And Trends

Table 32.5. Trends In Prevalence Of Steroids For 8th Graders, 10th Graders, And 12th Graders; 2017 (In Percent)

Drug	Time Period	8th Graders	10th Graders	12th Graders
Steroids	Lifetime	1.10	1.10	0.60
	Past Year	0.60	0.70	1.10
	Past Month	0.30	0.30	0.80

There are over 100 different types of anabolic steroids. Steroids are taken orally, injected, taken under the tongue, or applied with topical creams that allow steroids to enter the bloodstream. There are different regimens for taking steroids to increase body mass; they are widely published and available on the Internet.

(Source: "Prescription For Disaster—How Teens Abuse Medicine," U.S. Drug Enforcement Administration (DEA).)

Over-The-Counter (OTC) Medicines

Over-the-counter (OTC) medicines are those that can be sold directly to people without a prescription. OTC medicines treat a variety of illnesses and their symptoms including pain, coughs and colds, diarrhea, constipation, acne, and others. Some OTC medicines have active ingredients with the potential for misuse at higher-than-recommended dosages.

Statistics And Trends

Table 32.6. Trends In Prevalence Of Cough Medicine (Nonprescription) For 8th Graders, 10th Graders, And 12th Graders; 2017 (In Percent)

Drug	Time Period	8th Graders	10th Graders	12th Graders
Cough Medicine (nonprescription)	Past Year	2.10	3.60	3.20

Chapter 33

Commonly Abused Pain Relievers

What Is Prescription Opioid Misuse?

Prescription opioids are medications that are chemically similar to endorphins—opioids that our body makes naturally to relieve pain—and also similar to the illegal drug heroin. In nature, opioids are found in the seed pod of the opium poppy plant. Opioid medications can be natural (made from the plant), semi-synthetic (modified in a lab from the plant), and fully synthetic (completely made by people).

Prescription opioids usually come in pill form and are given to treat severe pain—for example, pain from dental surgery, serious sports injuries, or cancer. Opioids are also commonly prescribed to treat other kinds of pain that lasts a long-time (chronic pain), but it is unclear if they are effective for long-term pain.

> Also known as: Happy Pills, Hillbilly Heroin, OC, Oxy, Percs, or Vikes

For most people, when opioids are taken as prescribed by a medical professional for a short time, they are relatively safe and can reduce pain effectively. However, dependence and addiction are still potential risks when taking prescription opioids. Dependence means you feel withdrawal symptoms when not taking the drug. Continued use can lead to addiction, where you continue to use despite negative consequences. These risks increase when these

---

About This Chapter: This chapter includes text excerpted from "Prescription Pain Medications (Opioids)," National Institute on Drug Abuse (NIDA) for Teens, March 2017.

medications are misused. Prescription medications are some of the most commonly misused drugs by teens, after tobacco, alcohol, and marijuana.

Common opioids and their medical uses are listed below.

Common Opioid Types

- Oxycodone (OxyContin, Percodan, Percocet)

- Hydrocodone (Vicodin, Lortab, Lorcet)

- Diphenoxylate (Lomotil)

- Morphine (Kadian, Avinza, MS Contin)

- Codeine fentanyl (Duragesic)

- Propoxyphene (Darvon)

- Hydromorphone (Dilaudid)

- Meperidine (Demerol)

- Methadone

Conditions They Treat

- Severe pain, often after surgery

- Acute (severe) pain

- Some forms of chronic pain (severe)

- Cough and diarrhea

Fentanyl is a powerful opioid prescribed for extreme pain that is 50–100 times more potent than morphine. It is extremely dangerous if misused, and is sometimes added to illicit drugs sold by drug dealers.

Table 33.1. Types Of Opioids

Type Of Opioid	How Are They Derived	Examples
Natural opioids (sometimes called opiates)	Nitrogen-containing base chemical compounds, called alkaloids, that occur in plants such as the opium poppy	Morphine, codeine, thebaine

Table 33.1. Continued

Type Of Opioid	How Are They Derived	Examples
Semi-synthetic/human-made opioids	Created in labs from natural opioids	Hydromorphone, hydrocodone, and oxycodone (the prescription drug OxyContin), heroin (which is made from morphine)
Fully synthetic/human-made opioids	Completely human-made	Fentanyl, pethidine, levorphanol, methadone, tramadol, dextropropoxyphene

How Prescription Opioids Are Misused

People misuse prescription opioid medications by taking them in a way that is not intended, such as:

- Taking someone else's prescription, even if it is for a legitimate medical purpose like relieving pain

- Taking an opioid medication in a way other than prescribed—for instance, taking more than your prescribed dose or taking it more often, or crushing pills into powder to snort or inject the drug

- Taking the opioid prescription to get high

- Mixing them with alcohol or certain other drugs. Your pharmacist can tell you what other drugs are safe to use with prescription pain relievers.

What Happens To Your Brain When You Use Prescription Opioids?

Opioids attach to specific proteins, called opioid receptors, on nerve cells in the brain, spinal cord, gut, and other organs. When these drugs attach to their receptors, they block pain messages sent from the body through the spinal cord to the brain. They can also reduce or stop other essential functions like breathing. Opioid receptors are also located in the brain's reward center, where they cause a large release of the neurotransmitter dopamine. This causes a strong feeling of relaxation and euphoria (extreme good feelings). Repeated surges of dopamine in the reward center from drug-taking can lead to addiction.

What Happens To Your Body When You Use Prescription Opioids?

In addition to pain relief and euphoria, other effects of opioids include:

- Sleepiness

- Confusion

- Nausea (feeling sick to the stomach)

- Constipation

- Slowed or stopped breathing

Can You Overdose Or Die If You Use Prescription Opioids?

Yes, you can overdose and die from prescription opioid misuse. In fact, taking just one large dose could cause the body to stop breathing. Deaths from overdoses of prescription drugs have been increasing since the early 1990s, largely due to the increase in misuse of prescription opioid pain relievers. Nearly 23,000 people died from an overdose of a prescription pain

Signs Of Overdose

Signs of a possible prescription opioid overdose are:

- Slow breathing
- Blue lips and fingernails
- Cold damp skin
- Shaking
- Vomiting or gurgling noise

People who are showing symptoms of overdose need urgent medical help (call 911 immediately). A drug called naloxone can be given to reverse the effects of an opioid overdose and prevent death—but only if it is given in time. Naloxone is available as an easy-to-use nasal spray or autoinjector. It is often carried by emergency first responders, including police officers and emergency medical services. In some states, doctors can now prescribe naloxone in advance to people who use prescription opioids or to their family members, so that in the event of an overdose, it can be given right away without waiting for emergency personnel (who may not arrive in time).

medication in 2015, with alarming increases among young people ages 15–24. The risk of overdose and death increase if you combine opioids with alcohol or other medications that also slow breathing, such as Benzodiazepines (e.g., Xanax).

What About Prescription Opioids And Heroin Use?

Prescription opioids are chemically closely related to heroin, and their effects, especially when misused, can be very similar. Because heroin may be cheaper to get, people who have become addicted to prescription pain medications sometimes switch to using heroin. Nearly 80 percent of people addicted to heroin started first with prescription opioids. However, the transition to heroin use from prescription opioids is still rare; only about four percent of people who misuse prescription opioids use heroin. Even so, because millions of people are using prescription opioids, this adds up to hundreds of thousands of heroin users.

Are Prescription Opioids Addictive?

Yes, prescription opioids can be addictive. People who misuse prescription opioids are at greater risk of becoming addicted to opioids than people who take them as prescribed by a doctor.

Opioid withdrawal can cause:

- Restlessness
- Muscle and bone pain
- Sleep problems
- Diarrhea
- Vomiting (throwing up)
- Cold flashes with goosebumps ("cold turkey")
- Involuntary leg movements

Carefully following the doctor's instructions for taking a medication can make it less likely that someone will develop dependence or addiction, because the medication is prescribed in amounts and forms that are considered appropriate for that person. Doctors should always weigh the risks of opioid dependence and addiction against the benefits of the medication, and patients should communicate any issues or concerns to their doctor as soon as they arise. The earlier a problem is identified, the better the chances are for long-term recovery.

How Many Teens Use Prescription Opioids?

Below table 33.2 showing the percentage of teens who misuse prescription opioid pain medicines.

Table 33.2. Trends In Prevalence Of Various Drugs For 8th Graders, 10th Graders, And 12th Graders; 2017 (In Percent)*

Drug	Time Period	8th Graders	10th Graders	12th Graders
Vicodin	Past Year	0.70	1.50	(2.00)
OxyContin	Past Year	0.80	2.20	2.70

Data in brackets indicate statistically significant change from the previous year.

More than one third of adults nationwide reported prescription opioid use in 2015, with substantial numbers reporting misuse and use disorders, according to a report compiled to estimate the prevalence of, and explore the motivations for, opioid use and misuse. The data showed that pain relief was most commonly cited as the reason for the misuse of opioids and that close to half of those who misused obtained them free from a family member or friend.

(Source: "Pain Relief Most Reported Reason For Misuse Of Opioid Pain Relievers," National Institute on Drug Abuse (NIDA).)

What Should I Do If Someone I Know Needs Help?

If you, or a friend, are in crisis and need to speak with someone now:

- Call National Suicide Prevention Lifeline (NSPL) at 800-273-TALK (800-273-8255) (they don't just talk about suicide—they cover a lot of issues and will help put you in touch with someone close by).

If you need information on drug treatment and where you can find it, the Substance Abuse and Mental Health Services Administration (SAMHSA) can help.

- Call Substance Abuse Treatment Facility Locator at 800-662-HELP (800-662-4357).

- Visit the locator online at www.findtreatment.samhsa.gov.

Chapter 34

Commonly Abused Sedatives And Tranquilizers

What Are Prescription Central Nervous System (CNS) Depressants?

Central nervous system (CNS) depressants are medicines that include sedatives, tranquilizers, and hypnotics. These drugs can slow brain activity, making them useful for treating anxiety, panic, acute stress reactions, and sleep disorders. CNS depressants cause drowsiness; sedatives are often prescribed to treat sleep disorders like insomnia and hypnotics can induce sleep, whereas tranquilizers are prescribed to treat anxiety or to relieve muscle spasms.

Some examples of CNS depressants grouped by their respective drug class are:

Benzodiazepines

- Diazepam (Valium®)

- Clonazepam (Klonopin®)

- Alprazolam (Xanax®)

- Triazolam (Halcion®)

- Estazolam (Prosom®)

About This Chapter: This chapter includes text excerpted from "Prescription CNS Depressants," National Institute on Drug Abuse (NIDA), March 2018.

Nonbenzodiazepine Sedative Hypnotics

- Zolpidem (Ambien®)

- Eszopiclone (Lunesta®)

- Zaleplon (Sonata®)

Barbiturates

- Mephobarbital (Mebaral®)

- Phenobarbital (Luminal®)

- Pentobarbital sodium (Nembutal®)

Main Reasons For Misusing Sedatives

Among people aged 12 or older in 2015 who misused prescription sedatives in the past year, the most common reason for the last misuse was to help with sleep (71.7%), which is the reason sedatives are prescribed. Even if people took sedatives to help them sleep, this use constituted misuse if people took them without a prescription, more often than prescribed, or at higher dosages than prescribed.

Other reasons for the last misuse among people who misused sedatives were to relax or relieve tension (12.0%) and to feel good or get high (5.9%). Less commonly reported reasons included to help with feelings or emotions (3.7%), to experiment to see what the drug was like (3.7%), and to increase or decrease the effects of some other drug (1.2%). In addition, 1.8 percent of past year misusers of sedatives reported that some other reason was their main reason for their last misuse.

(Source: "Prescription Drug Use And Misuse In The United States: Results From The 2015 National Survey On Drug Use And Health," Substance Abuse and Mental Health Services Administration (SAMHSA).)

How Do People Use And Misuse Prescription CNS Depressants?

Most prescription CNS depressants come in pill, capsule, or liquid form, which a person takes by mouth. Misuse of prescription CNS depressants means:

- Taking medicine in a way or dose other than prescribed

- Taking someone else's medicine

- Taking medicine for the effect it causes—to get high

When misusing a prescription CNS depressant, a person can swallow the medicine in its normal form or can crush pills or open capsules.

How Do CNS Depressants Affect The Brain?

Most CNS depressants act on the brain by increasing activity of *gamma-aminobutyric acid* (GABA), a chemical that inhibits brain activity. This action causes the drowsy and calming effects that make the medicine effective for anxiety and sleep disorders. People who start taking CNS depressants usually feel sleepy and uncoordinated for the first few days until the body adjusts to these side effects. Other effects from use and misuse can include:

- Slurred speech

- Poor concentration

- Confusion

- Headache

- Light-headedness

- Dizziness

- Dry mouth

- Problems with movement and memory

- Lowered blood pressure

- Slowed breathing

If a person takes CNS depressants long term, he or she might need larger doses to achieve therapeutic effects. Continued use can also lead to dependence and withdrawal when use is abruptly reduced or stopped. Suddenly stopping can also lead to harmful consequences like seizures.

Can A Person Overdose On CNS Depressants?

Yes, a person can overdose on CNS depressants. An overdose occurs when the person uses enough of a drug to produce life-threatening symptoms or death. When people overdose on a CNS depressant, their breathing often slows or stops. This can decrease the amount of oxygen that reaches the brain, a condition called hypoxia. Hypoxia can have short- and long-term mental effects and effects on the nervous system, including coma and permanent brain damage.

How Can A CNS Depressant Overdose Be Treated?

The most important step to take is to call 911, so a person who has overdosed can receive immediate medical attention. Flumazenil (Romazicon®) is a medication that medical personnel can use to treat benzodiazepine overdose and has also been shown effective in treating overdose from sleep medicines. The drug might not completely reverse slowed breathing and can lead to seizures in some patients who are taking certain antidepressants. Flumazenil is short-acting, and the patient may need more of it every 20 minutes until he or she recovers. For barbiturates and nonbenzodiazepines, body temperature, pulse, breathing, and blood pressure should be monitored while waiting for the drug to be eliminated.

Can Prescription CNS Depressant Use Lead To Addiction And Substance Use Disorder (SUD)?

Yes, use or misuse of prescription CNS depressants can lead to problem use, known as a substance use disorder (SUD), which takes the form of addiction in severe cases. Long-term use of prescription CNS depressants, even as prescribed by a doctor, can cause some people to develop a tolerance, which means that they need higher and/or more frequent doses of the drug to get the desired effects. A SUD develops when continued use of the drug leads to negative consequences such as health problems or failure to meet responsibilities at work, school, or home, but despite all that the drug use continues.

Those who have become addicted to a prescription CNS depressant and stop using the drug abruptly may experience a withdrawal. Withdrawal symptoms—which can begin as early as a few hours after the drug was last taken—include:

- Seizures

- Shakiness

- Anxiety

- Agitation

- Insomnia

- Overactive reflexes

- Increased heart rate, blood pressure, and temperature with sweating

- Hallucinations

- Severe cravings

People addicted to prescription CNS depressants should not attempt to stop taking them on their own. Withdrawal symptoms from these drugs can be severe and—in the case of certain medications-potentially life-threatening.

How Can People Get Treatment For Prescription CNS Depressant Addiction?

There isn't a lot of research on treating people for addiction to prescription CNS depressants. However, people addicted to these medications should undergo medically supervised detoxification because the dosage they take should be tapered gradually. Counseling, either in an outpatient or inpatient program, can help people through this process. One type of counseling, cognitive behavioral therapy (CBT), focuses on modifying the person's thinking, expectations, and behaviors while improving ways to cope with life's stresses. CBT has helped people successfully adapt to stop using benzodiazepines. Often prescription CNS depressant misuse occurs along with the use of other drugs, such as alcohol or opioids. In those cases, the person should seek treatment that addresses the multiple addictions.

Chapter 35

Commonly Abused Prescription Stimulants

What Are Prescription Stimulants?

Prescription stimulants are medicines generally used to treat attention deficit hyperactivity disorder (ADHD) and narcolepsy—uncontrollable episodes of deep sleep. They increase alertness, attention, and energy.

What Are Common Prescription Stimulants?

- Dextroamphetamine (Dexedrine®)

- Dextroamphetamine/amphetamine combination product (Adderall®)

- Methylphenidate (Ritalin®, Concerta®)

Popular slang terms for prescription stimulants include Speed, Uppers, and Vitamin R.

How Do People Use And Misuse Prescription Stimulants?

Most prescription stimulants come in tablet, capsule, or liquid form, which a person takes by mouth.

About This Chapter: Text beginning with the heading "What Are Prescription Stimulants?" is excerpted from "Prescription Stimulants," National Institute on Drug Abuse (NIDA), June 2018; Text under the heading "Five Myths About ADHD Drugs" is excerpted from "5 Myths About ADHD Drugs," National Institute on Drug Abuse (NIDA) for Teens, December 12, 2013. Reviewed July 2018.

Misuse of a prescription stimulant means:

- Taking medicine in a way or dose other than prescribed

- Taking someone else's medicine

- Taking medicine only for the effect it causes—to get high

When misusing a prescription stimulant, people can swallow the medicine in its normal form. Alternatively, they can crush tablets or open the capsules, dissolve the powder in water, and inject the liquid into a vein. Some can also snort or smoke the powder.

Do Prescription Stimulants Make You Smarter?

Some people take prescription stimulants to try to improve mental performance. Teens and college students sometimes misuse them to try to get better grades, and older adults misuse them to try to improve their memory. Taking prescription stimulants for reasons other than treating ADHD or narcolepsy could lead to harmful health effects, such as addiction, heart problems, or psychosis.

How Do Prescription Stimulants Affect The Brain And Body?

Prescription stimulants increase the activity of the brain chemicals dopamine and norepinephrine. Dopamine is involved in the reinforcement of rewarding behaviors. Norepinephrine affects blood vessels, blood pressure and heart rate, blood sugar, and breathing.

Short-Term Effects

People who use prescription stimulants report feeling a "rush" (euphoria) along with the following:

- Increased blood pressure and heart rate

- Increased breathing

- Decreased blood flow

- Increased blood sugar

- Opened-up breathing passages

At high doses, prescription stimulants can lead to a dangerously high body temperature, an irregular heartbeat, heart failure, and seizures.

What Are The Other Health Effects Of Prescription Stimulants?

Repeated misuse of prescription stimulants, even within a short period, can cause psychosis, anger, or paranoia. If the drug is injected, it is important to note that sharing drug injection equipment and having an impaired judgment from drug misuse can increase the risk of contracting infectious diseases such as human immunodeficiency virus (HIV) and hepatitis.

Can A Person Overdose On Prescription Stimulants?

Yes, a person can overdose on prescription stimulants. An overdose occurs when the person uses enough of the drug to produce a life-threatening reaction or death.

Risk Of Later Substance Use

Some people may be concerned about later substance misuse in children and teens who've been prescribed stimulant drugs to treat ADHD. Studies so far have not shown a difference in later substance use in young people with ADHD treated with prescription stimulants compared with those who didn't receive such treatment. This suggests that treatment with ADHD medication does not positively or negatively affect a person's risk of developing problem use.

When people overdose on a prescription stimulant, they most commonly experience several different symptoms, including restlessness, tremors, overactive reflexes, rapid breathing, confusion, aggression, hallucinations, panic states, abnormally increased fever, muscle pains and weakness.

They also may have heart problems, including an irregular heartbeat leading to a heart attack, nerve problems that can lead to a seizure, abnormally high or low blood pressure, and circulation failure. Stomach issues may include nausea, vomiting, diarrhea, and abdominal cramps. In addition, an overdose can result in convulsions, coma, and fatal poisoning.

How Can A Prescription Stimulant Overdose Be Treated?

Because prescription stimulant overdose often leads to a heart attack or seizure, the most important step to take is to call 911 so a person who has overdosed can receive immediate medical attention. First responders and emergency room doctors try to treat the overdose with the intent of restoring blood flow to the heart and stopping the seizure with care or with medications if necessary.

Can Prescription Stimulant Use Lead To Substance Use Disorder And Addiction?

Yes, misuse of prescription stimulants can lead to a substance use disorder (SUD), which takes the form of addiction in severe cases. Long-term use of stimulants, even as prescribed by a doctor, can cause a person to develop a tolerance, which means that he or she needs higher and/or more frequent doses of the drug to get the desired effects. An SUD develops when continued use of the drug causes issues, such as health problems and failure to meet responsibilities at work, school, or home. Concerns about use should be discussed with a healthcare provider.

If a person develops an SUD and stops the use of the prescription stimulant, he or she can experience withdrawal. Withdrawal symptoms can include:

- Fatigue
- Depression
- Sleep problems

How Can People Get Treatment For Prescription Stimulant Addiction?

Behavioral therapies, including cognitive behavioral therapy (CBT) and contingency management (motivational incentives), can be effective in helping to treat people with prescription stimulant addiction. Cognitive behavioral therapy helps to modify the patient's drug-use expectations and behaviors, and it can effectively manage triggers and stress. Contingency management provides vouchers or small cash rewards for positive behaviors such as staying drug-free.

Prescription stimulants—like Adderall and Ritalin—have been in the news because some high school and college students say they take these drugs to help them study better or party longer.

Five Myths About ADHD Drugs

Let's look at five myths about prescription stimulants.

Myth #1: Drugs like Ritalin and Adderall can make you smarter.

Fact: While these drugs may help you focus, they don't help you learn better, and they won't improve your grades.

Being "smart" is about improving your ability to master new skills, concepts, and ideas. Like a muscle, the brain gets stronger through exercise. Learning strengthens brain connections through repetition and practice to enhance cognition—"smartness"—over a lifetime. Short-cuts, like abusing prescription stimulants, do not "exercise" the brain.

Research has shown that students who abuse prescription stimulants actually have lower grade point average (GPA) in high school and college than those who don't.

Myth #2: Prescription stimulants are just "brain vitamins."

Fact: Unlike vitamins, these drugs contain ingredients that can change brain chemistry and may have serious side effects.

Also, unlike vitamins, they require a doctor's prescription. If you take these drugs more often than directed, in too high a dose, or in some way other than by mouth, you are abusing the drug, which can lead to addiction.

Myth #3: These drugs can't hurt you.

Fact: Prescription stimulants like Adderall or Ritalin are safe and effective when prescribed for people with ADHD and used properly. But the same drugs, when used by someone without ADHD, can be dangerous.

Stimulants taken without a medical reason can disrupt brain communication. When used improperly or in excess, they can cause mood swings and loss of sleep, and can increase your blood pressure, heart rate, and body temperature.

Myth #4: Taking someone else's prescription—just once in a while—is okay.

Fact: Doctors prescribe medicine based on your weight, symptoms, and body chemistry. Doctors may adjust how much you take or change to a different medication to better treat symptoms or respond to side effects.

When you take a stimulant prescribed for a friend or family member, you haven't been looked at by a doctor. The possible side effects can make you sick. Side effects include elevated heart rate, dizziness, and fainting—or, even worse, heart attacks and stroke. Side effects may also include depression and exhaustion.

Myth #5: If your doctor prescribed the drug, it doesn't matter how you take it.

Fact: If you are diagnosed with ADHD, stimulants the doctor prescribes for you can help. But always be sure to take the medication exactly as directed—no more, no less.

Also, be sure to tell your doctor everything that's going on at home and at school. Combining prescription stimulants with other drugs or alcohol can be dangerous.

And don't help your friends or family members abuse prescription drugs by sharing your pills with them.

Chapter 36

What You Should Know About The Abuse Of Cold And Cough Medicines

What Are Cough And Cold Medicines?

Millions of Americans take cough and cold medicines each year to help with symptoms of colds, and when taken as instructed, these medicines can be safe and effective. However, several cough and cold medicines contain ingredients that are psychoactive (mind-altering) when taken in higher-than-recommended dosages, and some people misuse them. These products also contain other ingredients that can add to the risks. Many of these medicines are bought "over-the-counter" (OTC), meaning you do not need a prescription to have them.

> Also known as: Candy, Dex, Drank, Lean, Robo, Robotripping, Skittles, Triple C, Tussin, or Velvet

Two commonly misused cough and cold medicines are:

- **Cough syrups and capsules containing dextromethorphan (DXM).** These OTC cough medicines are safe for stopping coughs during a cold if you take them as directed. Taking more than the recommended amount can produce euphoria (a relaxed pleasurable feeling) but also dissociative effects (like you are detached from your body).

About This Chapter: This chapter includes text excerpted from "Cough And Cold Medicine (DXM And Codeine Syrup)," National Institute on Drug Abuse (NIDA) for Teens, May 2017.

- **Promethazine-codeine cough syrup.** These prescription medications contain an opioid drug called codeine, which stops coughs, but when taken in higher doses produces a "buzz" or "high."

How Cough And Cold Medicines Are Misused

Cough and cold medicines are usually sold in liquid syrup, capsule, or pill form. They may also come in a powder. Drinking promethazine-codeine cough syrup mixed with soda (a combination called syrup, sizzurp, purple drank, barre, or lean) was referenced frequently in some popular music beginning in the late 1990s and has become increasingly popular among youth in several areas of the country. Young people are often more likely to misuse cough and cold medicines containing DXM than some other drugs because these medicines can be purchased without a prescription.

What Happens To Your Brain When You Misuse Cough Or Cold Medicines?

When cough and cold medicines are taken as directed, they safely treat symptoms caused by colds and flu. But when taken in higher quantities or when such symptoms aren't present, they may affect the brain in ways very similar to illegal drugs, and can even lead to addiction.

DXM acts on the same brain cell receptors as drugs like ketamine or phencyclidine (PCP). A single high dose of DXM can cause hallucinations (imagined experiences that seem real). Ketamine and PCP are called "dissociative" drugs, which means they make you feel separated from your body or your environment, and they twist the way you think or feel about something or someone.

Codeine attaches to the same cell receptors as opioids like heroin. High doses of promethazine-codeine cough syrup can produce euphoria similar to that produced by other opioid drugs. Also, both codeine and promethazine depress activities in the central nervous system (CNS) (brain and spinal cord), which produces calming effects.

Both codeine and DXM cause an increase in the amount of dopamine in the brain's reward pathway. Extra amounts of dopamine increase the feeling of pleasure and at the same time cause important messages to get lost, causing a range of effects from lack of motivation to serious health problems. Repeatedly seeking to experience that feeling can lead to addiction.

Cough and cold medicines are usually consumed orally in tablet, capsule, or syrup form. They may be mixed with soda for flavor and are often abused in combination with other drugs, such as alcohol or marijuana.

To avoid nausea produced by high doses of the expectorant guaifenesin commonly found in DXM-containing syrups, young people may instead abuse Coricidin® HBP cough and cold capsules (street name C-C-C or triple-C), which contain DXM but lack guaifenesin.

Drinking promethazine-codeine cough syrup mixed with soda (a combination called syrup, sizzurp, purple drank, barre, or lean) was referenced frequently in some popular music beginning in the late 1990s and has become increasingly popular among youth in several areas of the country. A variation of "purple drank" is promethazine-codeine cough syrup mixed with alcohol. Users may also flavor the mixture with the addition of hard candies.

(Source: "Cough And Cold Medicine Abuse," National Institute on Drug Abuse (NIDA).)

What Happens To Your Body When You Misuse Cough Or Cold Medicines?

DXM misuse can cause:

- Loss of coordination

- Numbness

- Feeling sick to the stomach

- Increased blood pressure

- Faster heartbeat

- In rare instances, lack of oxygen to the brain, creating lasting brain damage, when DXM is taken with decongestants

Promethazine-codeine cough syrup misuse can cause:

- Slowed heart rate

- Slowed breathing (high doses can lead to overdose and death)

Cough and cold medicines are even more dangerous when taken with alcohol or other drugs.

Are Cough And Cold Medicines Addictive?

Yes, high doses and repeated misuse of cough and cold medicines can lead to addiction. That's when a person seeks out and takes the drug over and over again, even though it is causing health or other problems.

Can You Overdose Or Die If You Use Cough And Cold Medicines?

Yes. Misuse of promethazine-codeine cough syrup slows down the CNS, which can slow or stop the heart and lungs. Mixing it with alcohol greatly increases this risk. Promethazine-codeine cough syrup has been linked to the overdose deaths of a few prominent musicians.

How Many Teens Misuse Cough And Cold Medicines?

Below is a table showing the percentage of teens who misuse cough and cold medicines.

Table 36.1. Trends In Prevalence Of Cough Medicine (Nonprescription) For 8th Graders, 10th Graders, And 12th Graders, 2017 (In Percent)

Drug	Time Period	8th Graders	10th Graders	12th Graders
Cough Medicine (Nonprescription)	Past Year	2.1	3.6	3.2

What Should I Do If Someone I Know Needs Help?

If you, or a friend, are in crisis and need to speak with someone now:

- Call National Suicide Prevention Lifeline (NSPL) at 800-273-TALK (800-273-8255) (they don't just talk about suicide—they cover a lot of issues and will help put you in touch with someone close by).

If you need information on drug treatment and where you can find it, the Substance Abuse and Mental Health Services Administration (SAMHSA) can help.

- Call Substance Abuse Treatment Facility Locator at 800-662-HELP (800-662-4357).

- Visit the locator online at www.findtreatment.samhsa.gov.

Chapter 37

Anabolic Steroids: Risks And Health Consequences

What Are Anabolic Steroids?

Anabolic steroids are human-made medications related to testosterone (male sex hormone). Doctors use anabolic steroids to treat hormone problems in men, delayed puberty, and muscle loss from some diseases. Bodybuilders and athletes may misuse anabolic steroids to build muscles and improve athletic performance, often taking doses much higher than would be prescribed for a medical condition. Using them this way is not legal—or safe, and can have long-term consequences.

Anabolic steroids are only one type of steroid. Other types of steroids include cortisol, estrogen, and progesterone. These are different chemicals and do not have the same effects.

Also known as: Anabolic-androgenic Steroids, Juice, or Roids

Common brand names: Androsterone, Deca-durabolin, Dianabol, Equipoise, Oxandrin, and Winstrol

How Anabolic Steroids Are Misused

When people take steroids without a doctor's prescription or in ways other than as prescribed, they are abusing steroids. Some people who abuse steroids take pills; others use needles to inject steroids into their muscles.

About This Chapter: This chapter includes text excerpted from "Anabolic Steroids," National Institute on Drug Abuse (NIDA) for Teens, March 2017.

What Happens To Your Brain When You Misuse Anabolic Steroids?

Anabolic steroids affect a part of the brain called the limbic system, which controls mood. Long-term steroid abuse can lead to aggressive behavior and extreme mood swings. This is sometimes referred to as "roid rage." Steroids can also lead to feeling paranoid (like someone or something is out to get you), jealousy, delusions (belief in something that is not true), and feeling invincible (like nothing can hurt you).

What Happens To Your Body When You Misuse Anabolic Steroids?

Abuse of anabolic steroids has been linked with serious health problems. They include:

- High blood pressure
- Changes in blood cholesterol (increases in "bad" cholesterol or low-density lipoproteins (LDL), decreases in "good" cholesterol or high-density lipoproteins (HDL))
- Enlarged heart
- Heart attack or stroke (even in young people)
- Liver disease, including cancer
- Kidney problems or failure
- Severe acne

Males

- Breast growth and shrinking of testicles
- Low sperm count/infertility (unable to have children)
- Increased risk for prostate cancer

Females

- Voice deepening
- Growth of facial hair
- Male-pattern baldness

- Changes in or end of menstrual cycle/getting your period

- Enlargement of clitoris

In addition, if teens abuse anabolic steroids, they may never achieve their full height because anabolic steroids can stop growth in the middle of puberty.

Can You Overdose Or Die If You Misuse Anabolic Steroids?

Yes. Although it is rare, there are a few ways steroid use can cause death.

- **Heart attacks and strokes.** Steroid misuse can lead to a condition called atherosclerosis, in which fat builds up inside arteries and makes it hard for blood to flow. When blood flow to the heart is blocked, a heart attack can occur. If blood flow to the brain is blocked, a stroke can occur.

- **Human immunodeficiency virus (HIV).** People who inject anabolic steroids using needles may share dirty drug injection equipment that can spread serious viral infections such as human immunodeficiency virus (HIV) / acquired immunodeficiency syndrome (AIDS) or hepatitis (a liver disease).

- **Depression.** Steroid misuse can lead to depression, especially during withdrawal. In rare cases, this can contribute to destructive behaviors, including suicide.

- **Cancer.** There is some scientific evidence that repeated use of anabolic steroids can contribute to the development of liver and prostate cancer.

Are Anabolic Steroids Addictive?

They can be. Addiction to steroids is different compared to other drugs of misuse, because users don't become high when using; however, they can experience withdrawal symptoms. People who do become addicted keep using steroids despite bad effects on their bodies and lives. Also, people who misuse steroids typically spend a large amount of time and money obtaining the drugs, another sign they could be addicted.

When they stop using steroids, people can experience uncomfortable symptoms such as feeling depressed, mood swings, feeling tired or restless, loss of appetite, being unable to sleep (insomnia), and the desire to take more steroids. Depression can be very dangerous, because it sometimes leads people to think of or attempt suicide (killing themselves). If not treated, some symptoms of depression that are linked with anabolic steroid withdrawal have lasted for a year or more after the person stops taking the drugs.

How Many Teens Misuse Anabolic Steroids?

Below is a table showing the percentage of teens who misuse steroids.

Table 37.1. Trends In Prevalence Of Steroids For 8th Graders, 10th Graders, And 12th Graders; 2017 (In Percent)

Drug	Time Period	8th Graders	10th Graders	12th Graders
Steroids	Lifetime	1.1	1.1	0.6
	Past Year	0.6	0.7	1.1
	Past Month	0.3	0.3	0.8

Commonly Misused Steroids

Oral Steroids

- Anadrol (Oxymetholone)
- Anavar (Oxandrolone)
- Dianabol (Methandienone)
- Winstrol (Stanozolol)
- Restandol (Testosterone undecanoate)

Injectable Steroids

- Deca-Durabolin (Nandrolone decanoate)
- Durabolin (Nandrolone phenpropionate)
- Depo-Testosterone (Testosterone cypionate)
- Agovirin (Testosterone propionate)
- Retandrol (Testosterone phenylpropionate)
- Equipoise (Boldenone undecylenate)

(Source: "Steroids And Other Appearance And Performance Enhancing Drugs (APEDs)," National Institute on Drug Abuse (NIDA).)

What Should I Do If Someone I Know Needs Help?

If you, or a friend, are in crisis and need to speak with someone now:

- Call National Suicide Prevention Lifeline at 800-273-TALK (800-273-8255) (they don't just talk about suicide—they cover a lot of issues and will help put you in touch with someone close by).

If you need information on drug treatment and where you can find it, the Substance Abuse and Mental Health Services Administration (SAMHSA) can help.

- Call Substance Abuse Treatment Facility Locator at 800-662-HELP (800-662-4357).

- Visit the locator online at www.findtreatment.samhsa.gov.

Chapter 38

Sports Supplements

Dietary supplements to enhance exercise and athletic performance come in a variety of forms, including tablets, capsules, liquids, powders, and bars. Many of these products contain numerous ingredients in varied combinations and amounts. Among the more common ingredients are amino acids, protein, creatine, and caffeine. According to one estimate, retail sales of the category of "sports nutrition supplements" totaled $5.67 billion in 2016, or 13.8 percent of $41.16 billion total sales for dietary supplements and related nutrition products for that year.

It is difficult to make generalizations about the extent of dietary supplement use by athletes because the studies on this topic are heterogeneous. But the data suggest that:

- A larger proportion of athletes than the general U.S. population takes dietary supplements.

- Elite athletes (e.g., professional athletes and those who compete on a national or international level) use dietary supplements more often than their nonelite counterparts.

- The supplements used by male and female athletes are similar, except that a larger proportion of women use iron and a larger proportion of men take vitamin E, protein, and creatine.

For any individual to physically perform at his or her best, a nutritionally adequate diet and sufficient hydration are critical. The *Dietary Guidelines for Americans* (DGA) and MyPlate recommend such an eating plan for everyone. Athletes require adequate daily amounts of calories, fluids, carbohydrates (to maintain blood glucose levels and replace muscle glycogen;

About This Chapter: Text in this chapter begins with excerpts from "Dietary Supplements For Exercise And Athletic Performance," Office of Dietary Supplements (ODS), National Institutes of Health (NIH), June 30, 2017; Text under the heading "Sports Supplements: Not A Safe 'Quick Fix'" is excerpted from "Sports Supplements: Not A Safe 'Quick Fix,'" National Institute on Drug Abuse (NIDA) for Teens, September 24, 2013. Reviewed July 2018.

typically 1.4–4.5 g/lb body weight (3–10 g/kg body weight)), protein (0.55–0.9 g/lb body weight (1.2–2.0 g/kg body weight)), fat (20–35% of total calories), and vitamins and minerals.

A few dietary supplements might enhance performance only when they add to, but do not substitute for, this dietary foundation. Athletes engaging in endurance activities lasting more than an hour or performed in extreme environments (e.g., hot temperatures or high altitudes) might need to replace lost fluids and electrolytes and consume additional carbohydrates for energy. Even with proper nutritional preparation, the results of taking any dietary supplement(s) for exercise and athletic performance vary by level of training; the nature, intensity, and duration of the activity; and the environmental conditions.

Sellers claim that dozens of ingredients in dietary supplements can enhance exercise and athletic performance. Well-trained elite and recreational athletes might use products containing one or more of these ingredients to train harder, improve performance, and achieve a competitive edge. However, the National Athletic Trainers' Association (NATA) acknowledges in a position statement that because the outcomes of studies of various performance-enhancing substances are often equivocal, using these substances can be "controversial and confusing."

> A survey of 1,248 students aged 16 years or older in five U.S. colleges and universities in 2009–2010 found that 66 percent reported use of any supplement. The reasons for use included enhanced muscle strength (20% of users), performance enhancement (19% of users), and increased endurance (7% of users). Products taken for these purposes included protein, amino acids, herbal supplements, caffeine, creatine, and combination products.
>
> In a national survey of about 21,000 U.S. college athletes, respondents reported taking protein products (41.7%), energy drinks and shots (28.6%), creatine (14.0%), amino acids (12.1%), multivitamins with caffeine (5.7%), beta-hydroxy-beta-methylbutyrate (HMB; 0.2%), dehydroepiandrosterone (DHEA; 0.1%), and an unspecified mix of "testosterone boosters" (1.6%). Men were much more likely to take performance-enhancing products than women, except for energy drinks and shots. Among the sports with the highest percentage of users of performance-enhancing products were ice hockey, wrestling, and baseball among the men and volleyball, swimming, and ice hockey among the women.

Sports Supplements: Not A Safe "Quick Fix"

When working out or playing sports, you may feel like you want to up your game. There are lots of sports products out there that claim to help you run faster, be stronger, or play longer—but be careful. It's important to make sure any sports supplement or "vitamin" you want to take is safe. The ingredients in sports products are not required to meet the same high standards as medications. This means it's up to you to find out what's in any pills, drinks, or powders before you take them.

Know What You Put In Your Body

In July 2013, USPlabs, a maker of several sports products, destroyed $8 million worth of its sports supplements Jack3d and OxyElite Pro, after the government said the two products might be dangerous. These two products had the stimulant dimethylamylamine (DMAA), which the government warns can cause heart problems like shortness of breath and heart attacks. Stimulants are drugs that increase your energy and speed up your body. In 2011, two U.S. soldiers may have died after using Jack3d. The government is still trying to find out if that is true. The military has removed all products with DMAA from military bases to be safe.

But that's not all.

- Companies claim DMAA is a natural ingredient, but researchers believe it is made in chemistry labs and added to supplements.

- In 2010, the World Anti-Doping Agency (WADA) banned DMAA.

- As of April 2013, the government had 86 reports of illness and death related to DMAA.

Do Your Research

If you are thinking about taking a sports product, do more than just read the label. Look into the ingredients and all the effects they may have on your body. Ask your coach if he or she knows anything about the product. A healthy body is the best body, so make sure you know what you are taking and that it is right for you.

Chapter 39

Caffeine

What Is Caffeine?

Caffeine is a bitter substance that occurs naturally in more than 60 plants including:

- Coffee beans

- Tea leaves

- Kola nuts, which are used to flavor soft drink colas

- Cacao pods, which are used to make chocolate products

There is also synthetic (human-made) caffeine, which is added to some medicines, foods, and drinks. For example, some pain relievers, cold medicines, and over-the-counter (OTC) medicines for alertness contain synthetic caffeine. So do energy drinks and "energy-boosting" gums and snacks.

Most people consume caffeine from drinks. The amounts of caffeine in different drinks can vary a lot, but it is generally:

- An 8-ounce cup of coffee: 95–200 mg

- A 12-ounce can of cola: 35–45 mg

- An 8-ounce energy drink: 70–100 mg

- An 8-ounce cup of tea: 14–60 mg

About This Chapter: Text beginning with the heading "What Is Caffeine?" is excerpted from "Caffeine," MedlinePlus, National Institutes of Health (NIH), April 2, 2015; Text beginning with the heading "Caffeine: Breaking Down The Buzz" is excerpted from "The Buzz on Caffeine," National Institute on Drug Abuse (NIDA) for Teens, June 25, 2014. Reviewed July 2018.

> **Question:** What's the most widely used drug?
>
> It's not marijuana—and no, it's not tobacco or alcohol either. 9 out of 10 Americans take it in some form every day, and it's not limited to adults.
>
> **Hint:** According to a recent study published by the American Academy of Pediatrics (AAP), nearly three-fourths (75%) of children, teens, and young adults use it daily too—in the form of soda, coffee, and energy drinks.
>
> **Answer:** Caffeine!
>
> That's right, caffeine is a drug—a stimulant drug, to be exact. It's even possible to be physically dependent on it—which means that a person who is used to drinking lots of caffeinated beverages can experience withdrawal symptoms if they quit.
>
> *(Source: "The Buzz On Caffeine," National Institute on Drug Abuse (NIDA) for Teens.)*

What Are Caffeine's Effects On The Body?

Caffeine has many effects on your body's metabolism. It:

- stimulates your central nervous system, which can make you feel more awake and give you a boost of energy

- is a diuretic, meaning that it helps your body get rid of extra salt and water by urinating more

- increases the release of acid in your stomach, sometimes leading to an upset stomach or heartburn

- may interfere with the absorption of calcium in the body

- increases your blood pressure

Within one hour of eating or drinking caffeine, it reaches its peak level in your blood. You may continue to feel the effects of caffeine for 4–6 hours.

What Are The Side Effects From Too Much Caffeine?

For most people, it is not harmful to consume up to 400 mg of caffeine a day. If you do eat or drink too much caffeine, it can cause health problems, such as:

- Restlessness and shakiness

- Insomnia

- Headaches

- Dizziness

- Rapid or abnormal heart rhythm

- Dehydration

- Anxiety

- Dependency, so you need to take more of it to get the same results

Some people are more sensitive to the effects of caffeine than others.

What Are Energy Drinks, And Why Can They Be A Problem?

Energy drinks are beverages that have added caffeine. The amount of caffeine in energy drinks can vary widely, and sometimes the labels on the drinks do not give you the actual amount of caffeine in them. Energy drinks may also contain sugars, vitamins, herbs, and supplements. Companies that make energy drinks claim that the drinks can increase alertness and improve physical and mental performance. This has helped make the drinks popular with American teens and young adults. There's limited data showing that energy drinks might temporarily improve alertness and physical endurance. There is not enough evidence to show that they enhance strength or power. But what we do know is that energy drinks can be dangerous because they have large amounts of caffeine. And since they have lots of sugar, they can contribute to weight gain and worsen diabetes. Sometimes young people mix their energy drinks with alcohol. It is dangerous to combine alcohol and caffeine. Caffeine can interfere with your ability to recognize how drunk you are, which can lead you to drink more. This also makes you more likely to make bad decisions.

Who Should Avoid Or Limit Caffeine?

You should check with your healthcare provider about whether you should limit or avoid caffeine if you:

- Are pregnant, since caffeine passes through the placenta to your baby

- Are breastfeeding, since a small amount of caffeine that you consume is passed along to your baby

- Have sleep disorders, including insomnia

- Have migraines or other chronic headaches

- Have anxiety

- Have gastroesophageal reflux disease (GERD) or ulcers

- Have fast or irregular heart rhythms

- Have high blood pressure

- Take certain medicines or supplements, including stimulants, certain antibiotics, asthma medicines, and heart medicines. Check with your healthcare provider about whether there might be interactions between caffeine and any medicines and supplements that you take.

- Are a child or teen. Neither should have as much caffeine as adults. Children can be especially sensitive to the effects of caffeine.

Caffeine is the most widely used stimulant in the world and use by adolescents has more than doubled since 1980. Chronic caffeine use produces greater tolerance in adolescents compared with adults, suggesting that caffeine may cause greater brain changes in young people. Caffeine consumption is also known to be correlated with increased risk for illicit drug use and substance use disorders."

(Source: "Adolescent Caffeine Use And Cocaine Sensitivity," National Institute on Drug Abuse (NIDA).)

Caffeine: Breaking Down The Buzz

Caffeine has a perk-up effect because it blocks a brain chemical, adenosine, which causes sleepiness. On its own, moderate amounts of caffeine rarely cause harmful long-term health effects, although it is definitely possible to take too much caffeine and get sick as a result.

Consuming too much caffeine can make you feel jittery or jumpy—your heart may race and your palms may sweat, kind of like a panic attack. It may also interfere with your sleep, which is especially important while your brain is still developing.

Some caffeine drinks and foods will affect you more than others, because they contain very different amounts.

Table 39.1. Amounts Of Caffeine

Caffeine Source	Caffeine Content
8 oz black tea	14–70 milligrams (mg)
12 oz cola	23–35 mg
8.4 oz Red Bull	75–80 mg
8 oz regular coffee	95–200 mg
1 cup semi-sweet chocolate chips	104 mg
2 oz 5-Hour Energy Shot	200–207 mg

But it's more than just how much caffeine a beverage has that can make it harmful. Even though energy drinks don't necessarily have more caffeine than other popular beverages (that is, unless you take 8 ounces of 5-hour Energy Shot, which has 400 milligrams!), it's the way they are sometimes used that worries health experts.

In 2011, of the 20,783 emergency room visits because of energy drinks, 42 percent were because the user combined them with other drugs (e.g., prescription drugs, alcohol, or marijuana).

Caffeine + Alcohol = Danger

Mixing alcohol and caffeine is serious business. As a stimulant, caffeine sort of has the opposite effect on the brain as alcohol, which is a depressant. But don't think the effects of each are canceled out! In fact, drinking caffeine doesn't reduce the intoxication effect of alcohol (that is, how drunk you become) or reduce its cognitive impairments (that is, your ability to walk or drive or think clearly). But it does reduce alcohol's sedation effects, so you feel more awake and probably drink for longer periods of time, and you may think you are less drunk than you really are.

That can be super dangerous. People who consume alcohol mixed with energy drinks are 3 times more likely to binge drink than people who do not report mixing alcohol with energy drinks.

Stay Away From Caffeine?

Drinking a cup of coffee, or eating a bar of chocolate, is usually not a big deal. But there are alternatives to caffeine if you're looking for an energy burst but don't want to get that jittery feeling caffeine sometimes causes. Here are a few alternatives you can try to feel energized without overdoing the caffeine:

- **Sleep.** This may sound obvious, but getting enough sleep is important. Teens need 9 hours of sleep a night.

- **Eat regularly.** When you don't eat, your glucose (sugar) levels drop, making you feel drained. Some people find it helpful to eat four or five smaller meals throughout the day instead of fewer big meals.

- **Drink enough water.** Since our bodies are more than two-thirds H_2O, we need at least 64 ounces of water a day.

- **Take a walk.** If you're feeling drained in the middle of the day, it helps to move around. Do sit-ups or jumping jacks. Go outside for a brisk walk or ride your bike.

What Is Caffeine Withdrawal?

If you have been consuming caffeine on a regular basis and then suddenly stop, you may have caffeine withdrawal. Symptoms can include:

- Headaches
- Drowsiness
- Irritability
- Nausea
- Difficulty concentrating

These symptoms usually go away after a couple of days.

(Source: "Caffeine," MedlinePlus, National Institutes of Health (NIH).)

Chapter 40

Inhalant Abuse

What Are Inhalants?

Inhalants are chemicals found in ordinary household or workplace products that people inhale on purpose to get "high." Because many inhalants can be found around the house, people often don't realize that inhaling their fumes, even just once, can be very harmful to the brain and body and can lead to death. In fact, the chemicals found in these products can change the way the brain works and cause other problems in the body.

> Also known as: Bold (nitrites), Laughing gas (nitrous oxide), Poppers (amyl nitrite and butyl nitrite), Rush (nitrites), Snappers (amyl nitrite), Whippets (fluorinated hydrocarbons)

Although different inhalants cause different effects, they generally fall into one of four categories.

Volatile solvents are liquids that become a gas at room temperature. They are found in:

- Paint thinner, nail polish remover, degreaser, dry-cleaning fluid, gasoline, and contact cement

- Some art or office supplies, such as correction fluid, felt-tip marker fluid, and electronic contact cleaner

Aerosols are sprays that contain propellants and solvents. They include:

About This Chapter: This chapter includes text excerpted from "Inhalants," National Institute on Drug Abuse (NIDA) for Teens, March 2017.

- Spray paint, hair spray, deodorant spray, vegetable oil sprays, and fabric protector spray

Gases may be in household or commercial products, or used in the medical field to provide pain relief. They are found in:

- Butane lighters, propane tanks, whipped cream dispensers, and refrigerant gases

- Anesthesia, including ether, chloroform, halothane, and nitrous oxide (commonly called "laughing gas")

Nitrites are a class of inhalants used mainly to enhance sexual experiences. Organic nitrites include amyl, butyl, and cyclohexyl nitrites and other related compounds. Amyl nitrite was used in the past by doctors to help with chest pain and is sometimes used today to diagnose heart problems. Nitrites are now banned (prohibited by the Consumer Product Safety Commission (CPSC)) but can still be found, sold in small bottles labeled as "video head cleaner," "room odorizer," "leather cleaner," or "liquid aroma."

How Inhalants Are Used

People who use inhalants breathe in the fumes through their nose or mouth, usually by "sniffing," "snorting," "bagging," or "huffing." It's called different names depending on the substance and equipment used.

What Happens To Your Brain When You Use Inhalants?

The lungs absorb inhaled chemicals into the bloodstream very quickly, sending them throughout the brain and body. Nearly all inhalants (except nitrites) produce a pleasurable effect by slowing down brain activity. Nitrites, in contrast, expand and relax blood vessels.

Short-Term Effects

Within seconds, users feel intoxicated and experience effects similar to those of alcohol, such as slurred speech, lack of coordination, euphoria (a feeling of intense happiness), and dizziness. Some users also experience lightheadedness, hallucinations (seeing things that are not really there), and delusions (believing something that is not true). If enough of the chemical is inhaled, nearly all solvents and gases produce anesthesia—a loss of sensation—and can lead to unconsciousness.

The high usually lasts only a few minutes, causing people to continue the high by inhaling repeatedly, which is very dangerous. Repeated use in one session can cause a person to lose consciousness and possibly even die.

With repeated inhaling, many users feel less inhibited and less in control. Some may feel drowsy for several hours and have a headache that lasts a while.

Long-Term Effects

Inhalants often contain more than one chemical. Some chemicals leave the body quickly, but others stay for a long time and get absorbed by fatty tissues in the brain and central nervous system (CNS). Over the long term, the chemicals can cause serious problems:

- **Damage to nerve fibers.** Long-term inhalant use can break down the protective sheath around certain nerve fibers in the brain and elsewhere in the body. This hurts the ability of nerve cells to send messages, which can cause muscle spasms and tremors or even permanent trouble with basic actions like walking, bending, and talking. These effects are similar to what happens to people with the disease multiple sclerosis (MS).

- **Damage to brain cells.** Inhalants also can damage brain cells by preventing them from getting enough oxygen. The effects of this condition, also known as brain hypoxia, depend on the area of the brain that gets damaged. The hippocampus, for example, is responsible for memory, so someone who repeatedly uses inhalants may be unable to learn new things or may have a hard time carrying on simple conversations. If the cerebral cortex is damaged, it will affect a person's ability to solve complex problems and plan ahead. And, if the cerebellum is affected, it can cause a person to move slowly or be clumsy.

What Happens To Your Body When You Use Inhalants?

Regular use of inhalants can cause serious harm to vital organs and systems besides the brain. Inhalants can cause:

- Heart damage

- Liver failure

- Muscle weakness

- Aplastic anemia—the body produces fewer blood cells

- Nerve damage, which can lead to chronic pain

Damage to these organs is not reversible even when the person stops abusing inhalants.

Signs Of Inhalant Use

Sometimes you can see signs that tell you a person is using inhalants, such as:

- Chemical odors on breath or clothing
- Paint or other stains on the face, hands, or clothing
- Hidden empty spray paint or solvent containers, or rags or clothing soaked with chemicals
- Drunk or disoriented actions
- Slurred speech
- Nausea (feeling sick) or loss of appetite and weight loss
- Confusion, inattentiveness, lack of coordination, irritability, and depression
- Purchase of excessive amounts of products used as inhalants

---

Effects Of Specific Chemicals

Depending on the type of inhalant used, the harmful health effects will differ. The table below lists some of the harmful effects of inhalants.

Table 40.1. Effects Of Specific Chemicals

Inhalant	Examples	Possible Effects
Amyl nitrite, butyl nitrite	Poppers, video head cleaner	• Sudden sniffing death • Weakened immune system • Damage to red blood cells (interfering with oxygen supply to vital tissues)
Benzene	Gasoline	• Bone marrow damage • Weakened immune system • Increased risk of leukemia (a form of cancer) • Reproductive system complications

Table 40.1. Continued

Inhalant	Examples	Possible Effects
Butane, propane	Lighter fluid, hair and pain sprays	• Sudden sniffing death from heart effects
		• Serious burn injuries
Freon (difluoroethane substitutes)	Refrigerant and aerosol propellant	• Sudden sniffing death
		• Breathing problems and death (from sudden cooling of airways)
		• Liver damage
Methylene chloride	Paint thinners and removers, degreasers	• Reduced ability of blood to carry oxygen to the brain and body
		• Changes to heart muscle and heartbeat
Nitrous oxide, hexane	"Laughing gas"	• Death from lack of oxygen to the brain
		• Altered perception and motor coordination
		• Loss of sensation
		• Spasms
		• Blackouts caused by blood pressure changes
		• Depression of heart muscle functioning
Toluene	Gasoline, paint thinners and removers, correction fluid	• Brain damage (loss of brain tissue, impaired thinking, loss of coordination, limb spasms, hearing and vision loss)
		• Liver and kidney damage
Trichloroethylene	Spot removers, degreasers	• Sudden sniffing death
		• Liver disease
		• Reproductive problems
		• Hearing and vision loss

Can You Overdose Or Die If You Use Inhalants?

Yes, using inhalants can cause death, even after just one use, by:

- **Sudden sniffing death**—heart beats quickly and irregularly, and then suddenly stops (cardiac arrest)

- **Asphyxiation**—toxic fumes replace oxygen in the lungs so that a person stops breathing

- **Suffocation**—air is blocked from entering the lungs when inhaling fumes from a plastic bag placed over the head

- **Convulsions or seizures**—abnormal electrical discharges in the brain

- **Coma**—the brain shuts down all but the most vital functions

- **Choking**—inhaling vomit after inhalant use

- **Injuries**—accidents, including driving, while intoxicated

How Can An Inhalant Overdose Be Treated?

Because inhalant overdose can lead to seizures or cause the heart to stop, first responders and emergency room doctors try to treat the overdose by treating these conditions. They will try to stop the seizure or restart the heart.

(Source: "Inhalants," National Institute on Drug Abuse (NIDA).)

Are Inhalants Addictive?

It isn't common, but addiction can happen. Some people, particularly those who use inhalants a lot and for a long time, report a strong need to continue using inhalants. Using inhalants over and over again can cause mild withdrawal when stopped. In fact, research in animal models shows that toluene can affect the brain in a way that is similar to other drugs of use (e.g., amphetamines). Toluene increases dopamine activity in reward areas of the brain, and the long-term disruption of the dopamine system is one of the key factors leading to addiction.

How Many Teens Use Inhalants?

Inhalants are often among the first drugs that young adolescents use. In fact, they are one of the few classes of drugs that are used more by younger adolescents than older ones. Inhalant use can become chronic and continue into adulthood.

Below is a table showing the percentage of teens who use inhalants.

Table 40.2. Trends In Prevalence Of Inhalants For 8th Graders, 10th Graders, And 12th Graders, 2017 (In Percent)*

Drug	Time Period	8th Graders	10th Graders	12th Graders
Inhalants	Lifetime	(8.90)	6.10	4.90
	Past Year	(4.70)	2.30	1.50
	Past Month	2.10	1.10	0.80

Data in brackets indicate a statistically significant change from the previous year.

What Should I Do If Someone I Know Needs Help?

If you, or a friend, are in crisis and need to speak with someone now:

- Call National Suicide Prevention Lifeline (NSPL) at 800-273-TALK (800-273-8255) (they don't just talk about suicide—they cover a lot of issues and will help put you in touch with someone close by).

If you need information on drug treatment and where you can find it, the Substance Abuse and Mental Health Services Administration (SAMHSA) can help.

- Call Substance Abuse Treatment Facility Locator at 800-662-HELP (800-662-4357)

- Visit the locator online at www.findtreatment.samhsa.gov

Part Six
Abuse Of Illegal Substances

Chapter 41

Club Drugs And Raves

What Are Club Drugs?

Club drugs are a pharmacologically heterogeneous group of psychoactive compounds that tend to be abused by teens and young adults at a nightclub, bar, rave, or trance scene. Gamma-hydroxybutyrate (GHB), Rohypnol, and ketamine are some of the drugs in this group; so are 3,4-methylenedioxymethamphetamine (MDMA) (ecstasy) and methamphetamine.

Gamma-Hydroxybutyric Acid (GHB)*

What Is It?

Prescribed as Xyrem, it is also known as the "date rape drug." It comes in a liquid or as a white powder that is dissolved in water, juice, or alcohol. In liquid form, GHB is clear and colorless and slightly salty in taste.

Street Names

- G
- Georgia Home Boy
- Goop
- Grievous Bodily Harm
- Liquid X
- Scoop
- Liquid Ecstasy

About This Chapter: Text beginning with the heading "What Are Club Drugs?" is excerpted from "Club Drugs (GHB, Ketamine, And Rohypnol)," National Institute on Drug Abuse (NIDA), December 2014. Reviewed July 2018; Text under the heading "Statistics And Trends" is excerpted from "Club Drugs," National Institute on Drug Abuse (NIDA), June 11, 2018; Text under the heading "What Should I Do If Someone I Know Needs Help?" is excerpted from "MDMA (Ecstasy Or Molly)," National Institute on Drug Abuse (NIDA) for Teens, May 2017.

How Is It Used?

- Usually, a liquid, mixed in a beverage

- White powder normally dissolved in a liquid

How Does It Affect The Body?

- Hallucinations

- Euphoria, drowsiness, decreased anxiety, excited and aggressive behavior

- Overdose symptoms: unconsciousness, seizures, slowed heart rate, greatly slowed breathing, lower body temperature, vomiting, nausea, coma, death

- Addictive. Withdrawal symptoms: insomnia, anxiety, tremors, increased heart rate and blood pressure, psychotic thoughts.

Text excerpted from "GHB—Gamma-Hydroxybutyric Acid," Get Smart About Drugs, U.S. Drug Enforcement Administration (DEA)

Rohypnol*

What Is It?

Depressant and benzodiazepine with generic name Flunitrazepam. It is not approved for medical use in the United States. Used by cocaine abusers to relieve side effects, and also used as a "date rape" drug.

> ## Street Names
>
> - Circles
> - Forget Me Pill
> - La Rocha
> - Lunch Money Drug
> - Mexican Valium
> - Pingus
> - R2
> - Roach 2
> - Ruffies
> - Rophies
> - Wolfies

How Is It Used?

- Oblong olive green tablet, swallowed, crushed and snorted

- Can be dissolved in liquids
- When placed in a light-colored drink, will dye it blue

How Does It Affect The Body?

- Muscle relaxant
- Decreased anxiety
- Drowsiness, amnesia, sleep
- Slurred speech, loss of coordination
- Impaired mental function, confusion
- Addictive

Text excerpted from "Rohypnol," Get Smart About Drugs, U.S. Drug Enforcement Administration (DEA)

Ketamine*

What Is It?

General, short-acting anesthetic with hallucinogenic effects. Sometimes used to facilitate sexual assault crimes.

Street Names

- Special K
- Cat Valium
- Kit Kat
- K
- Super Acid

- Super K
- Purple
- Special LA Coke
- Jet
- Vitamin K

How Is It Used?

- Injected
- Liquid mixed with liquids
- Powder that is snorted mixed in drinks, or smoked

How Does It Affect The Body?

- Hallucinatory effects last 30-60 minutes

- Distorts sights and sounds

- Induces feelings of calmness and relaxation, relief from pain

- Immobility and amnesia

- Body feels out of control

- Agitation, depression, unconsciousness

- Hallucinations

- Flashbacks

Text excerpted from "Ketamine," Get Smart About Drugs, U.S. Drug Enforcement Administration (DEA)

How Are Club Drugs Abused?

Raves and trance events are generally night-long dances, often held in warehouses. Many who attend raves and trances do not use club drugs, but those who do may be attracted to their generally low cost and the intoxicating highs that are said to deepen the rave or trance experience.

- Rohypnol is usually taken orally, although there are reports that it can be ground up and snorted.

- GHB and Rohypnol have both been used to facilitate date rape (also known as "drug rape," "acquaintance rape," or "drug-assisted" assault). They can be colorless, tasteless, and odorless, and can be added to beverages and ingested unbeknownst to the victim. When mixed with alcohol, Rohypnol can incapacitate victims and prevent them from resisting sexual assault.

- GHB also has anabolic effects (it stimulates protein synthesis) and has been sought by bodybuilders to aid in fat reduction and muscle building.

- Ketamine is usually snorted or injected intramuscularly.

How Do Club Drugs Affect The Brain?

- GHB acts on at least two sites in the brain: the $GABA_B$ receptor and a specific GHB binding site. At high doses, GHB's sedative effects may result in sleep, coma, or death.

Before You Risk It...

- **Know the law.** It is illegal to buy or sell club drugs. It is also a federal crime to use any controlled substance to aid in a sexual assault.

- **Get the facts.** Despite what you may have heard, club drugs can be addictive.

- **Stay informed.** The club drug scene is constantly changing. New drugs and new variations of drugs appear all of the time.

- **Know the risks.** Mixing club drugs together or with alcohol is extremely dangerous. The effects of one drug can magnify the effects and risks of another. In fact, mixing substances can be lethal.

- **Look around you.** The vast majority of teens are not using club drugs. While Ecstasy is considered to be the most frequently used club drug, less than 1 percent of 12- to 17-year-olds use it on a regular basis. In fact, 98 percent of people this age have never even tried Ecstasy.

(Source: "The Truth About Club Drugs," Substance Abuse and Mental Health Services Administration (SAMHSA).)

Rohypnol, like other benzodiazepines, acts at the $GABA_A$ receptor. It can produce anterograde amnesia, in which individuals may not remember events they experienced while under the influence of the drug.

- Ketamine is a dissociative anesthetic, so called because it distorts perceptions of sight and sound and produces feelings of detachment from the environment and self. Ketamine acts on a type of glutamate receptor N-methyl-D-aspartate (NMDA) receptor to produce its effects, similar to those of the drug phencyclidine (PCP). Low-dose intoxication results in impaired attention, learning ability, and memory. At higher doses, ketamine can cause dreamlike states and hallucinations; and at higher doses still, ketamine can cause delirium and amnesia.

Addictive Potential

- Repeated use of GHB may lead to withdrawal effects, including insomnia, anxiety, tremors, and sweating. Severe withdrawal reactions have been reported among patients presenting from an overdose of GHB or related compounds, especially if other drugs or alcohol are involved.

- Like other benzodiazepines, chronic use of Rohypnol can produce tolerance and dependence.

- There have been reports of people binging on ketamine, a behavior that is similar to that seen in some cocaine- or amphetamine-dependent individuals. Ketamine users can develop signs of tolerance and cravings for the drug.

What Other Adverse Effects Do Club Drugs Have On Health?

Uncertainties about the sources, chemicals, and possible contaminants used to manufacture many club drugs make it extremely difficult to determine toxicity and associated medical consequences.

- Coma and seizures can occur following use of GHB. Combined use with other drugs such as alcohol can result in nausea and breathing difficulties. GHB and two of its precursors, gamma-butyrolactone (GBL) and butanediol (BD), have been involved in poisonings, overdoses, date rapes, and deaths.

- Rohypnol may be lethal when mixed with alcohol and/or other CNS depressants.

- Ketamine, in high doses, can cause impaired motor function, high blood pressure, and potentially fatal respiratory problems.

What Treatment Options Exist?

There is very little information in scientific literature about treatment for persons who abuse or are dependent upon club drugs.

- There are no GHB detection tests for use in emergency rooms, and as many clinicians are unfamiliar with the drug, many GHB incidents likely go undetected. According to case reports, however, patients who abuse GHB appear to present both a mixed picture of severe problems upon admission and good response to treatment, which often involves residential services.

- Treatment for Rohypnol follows accepted protocols for any benzodiazepine, which may consist of a 3- to 5-day inpatient detoxification program with 24-hour intensive medical monitoring and management of withdrawal symptoms, since withdrawal from benzodiazepines can be life threatening.

- Patients with a Ketamine overdose are managed through supportive care for acute symptoms, with special attention to cardiac and respiratory functions.

Statistics And Trends

Below are the tables showing the percentage of teens who use various club drugs.

Table 41.1. Trends In Prevalence Of Various Drugs For 8th Graders, 10th Graders, And 12th Graders (In Percent)

Drug	Time Period	8th Graders	10th Graders	12th Graders
GHB	Past Year	–	–	0.40
Ketamine	Past Year	–	–	1.20
LSD	Lifetime	1.30	3.00	5.00
	Past Year	0.90	2.10	3.30
MDMA	Lifetime	1.50	2.80	4.90
	Past Year	0.90	1.70	2.60
Methamphetamine	Lifetime	0.70	0.90	1.10
	Past Year	0.50	0.40	0.60
Rohypnol	Lifetime	0.60	0.70	–
	Past Year	0.40	0.30	0.80

Table 41.2. Trends In Prevalence Of Various Drugs For Ages 12 Or Older, Ages 12–17, And Ages 18–25 (In Percent)

Drug	Time Period	Ages 12 Or Older	Ages 12–17	Ages 18–25
LSD	Lifetime	9.60	1.20	8.30
	Past Year	0.70	0.80	3.40
MDMA	Lifetime	6.90	1.20	11.60
	Past Year	0.90	0.70	3.50
Methamphetamine	Lifetime	5.40	0.30	2.40
	Past Year	0.50	0.10	0.80
Psychotherapeutics (Nonmedical Use)	Lifetime	–	–	–
	Past Year	6.90	5.30	14.50

What Should I Do If Someone I Know Needs Help?

If you, or a friend, are in crisis and need to speak with someone now:

- Call National Suicide Prevention Lifeline (NSPL) at 800-273-TALK (800-273-8255) (they don't just talk about suicide—they cover a lot of issues and will help put you in touch with someone close by)

If you need information on drug treatment and where you can find it, the Substance Abuse and Mental Health Services Administration (SAMHSA) can help.

- Call Substance Abuse Treatment Facility Locator at 800-662-HELP (800-662-4357)

- Visit the locator online at www.findtreatment.samhsa.gov

Chapter 42

MDMA (Ecstasy Or Molly)

What Is MDMA (Ecstasy Or Molly)?

MDMA, short for 3,4-methylenedioxymethamphetamine, is most commonly known as Ecstasy or Molly. It is a man-made drug that produces energizing effects similar to the stimulants called amphetamines, as well as psychedelic effects, similar to the hallucinogens mescaline and lysergic acid diethylamide (LSD). MDMA is known as a "club drug" because of its popularity in the nightclub scene, at "raves" (all-night dance parties), and music festivals or concerts. MDMA's effects generally last from three to six hours.

MDMA is a Schedule I substance, which means that the U.S. government has determined that it has no medical benefit and a high potential for abuse. Researchers, however, continue to investigate the possible medical benefits, for example, with patients that have posttraumatic stress disorder (PTSD) and terminal cancer patients with anxiety. However, those patients are under strict medical supervision.

> Also known as: Adam, Beans, Clarity, E, Ecstasy, Hug, Love drug, Lover's speed, Molly, X, or XTC

How MDMA Is Used

Most people who use MDMA take it in a pill, tablet, or capsule. The pills can be different colors and sometimes have cartoon-like images on them. Some people take more than one pill at a time, called "bumping." The popular term "Molly" (slang for molecular) refers to the pure

About This Chapter: This chapter includes text excerpted from "MDMA (Ecstasy Or Molly)," National Institute on Drug Abuse (NIDA) for Teens, May 2017.

crystalline powder form of MDMA, usually sold in capsules. But this is mostly a marketing gimmick—testing on "Molly" seized by police shows a variety of other ingredients.

In fact, researchers and law enforcement have found that much of the Ecstasy sold today contains other harmful and possibly deadly drugs in addition to MDMA. In some recent cases, drugs sold as MDMA actually contain no MDMA at all. Frequently, MDMA is mixed with or replaced by synthetic cathinones, the chemicals in "bath salts. Some MDMA pills, tablets, and capsules have also been found to contain caffeine, dextromethorphan (found in some cough syrups), amphetamines, phencyclidine (PCP), or cocaine.

What Happens To Your Brain When You Use MDMA?

Once an MDMA pill or capsule is swallowed, it takes about 15 minutes for the drug to enter the bloodstream and reach the brain. MDMA produces its effects by increasing the activity of three neurotransmitters (the chemical messengers of brain cells): serotonin, dopamine, and norepinephrine. Let's take a look at the importance of these chemicals:

- **Serotonin**—Plays a role in controlling our mood, aggression, sexual activity, sleep, and feelings of pain. The extra serotonin that is released by MDMA likely causes mood-lifting effects in users. People who use MDMA might feel very alert, or "hyper," at first. Some experience altered sense of time and other changes in perception, such as a more intense sense of touch. Serotonin also triggers the release of the hormones oxytocin and vasopressin, which play a role in feelings of love, sexual arousal, and trust. This may be why users report feeling a heightened sense of emotional closeness and empathy.

- **Dopamine**—Helps to control movement, motivation, emotions, and sensations like pleasure. The extra dopamine causes a surge of feelings of joy and increased energy.

- **Norepinephrine**—Increases heart rate and blood pressure, which are particularly risky for people who have problems with their heart and blood circulation

Because MDMA increases the activity of these chemicals, some users experience negative effects. They may become anxious and agitated, become sweaty, have chills, or feel faint or dizzy. Even those who don't feel negative effects during use can experience negative aftereffects. These are caused by the brain no longer having enough serotonin after the surge that was triggered by using MDMA. Days or even weeks after use, people can experience confusion, depression, sleep problems, drug craving, and anxiety, because the surge of serotonin caused by MDMA reduces the brain's supply of this important chemical.

Effects Of Long-Term Use

Researchers are not sure if MDMA causes long-term brain changes or if such effects are reversible when someone stops using the drug. However, studies have shown that some heavy MDMA users experience problems that are long lasting, including confusion, depression, and problems with memory and attention.

What Happens To Your Body When You Use MDMA?

The changes that take place in the brain with MDMA use affect the user in other ways as well. These include:

- Increases in heart rate and blood pressure

- Muscle tension

- Teeth clenching

- Nausea (feeling sick) and possible vomiting

- Blurred vision

- Faintness

- Chills or sweating

- Higher body temperature (can lead to serious heart, liver, or kidney problems)

- Increased risk for unsafe sex

Because MDMA does not always break down in the body, it can interfere with its own metabolism. This can cause harmful levels of the drug to build up in the body if it is taken repeatedly within short periods of time. High levels of the drug in the bloodstream can increase the risk for seizures and affect the heart's ability to beat normally.

Can You Overdose Or Die If You Use MDMA?

Yes, you can die from MDMA use. MDMA can cause problems with the body's ability to control temperature, especially when it is used in active, hot settings (like dance parties or concerts). On rare occasions, this can lead to a sharp rise in body temperature (known as hyperthermia), which can cause liver, kidney, or heart failure or even death.

Is MDMA Addictive?

Researchers don't yet know. What is known is that MDMA targets the same neurotransmitters that are targeted by other addictive drugs. Researchers are still working to understand MDMA's addictive properties. But, some users experience unpleasant withdrawal symptoms after regular (daily or almost daily) use of the drug is reduced or stopped, such as:

- Fatigue

- Loss of appetite

- Depression

- Trouble concentrating

How Can MDMA Use Be Prevented?

Providing accurate scientific information regarding the effects of MDMA is important for reducing the negative health effects associated with use of this drug. Young adults who use MDMA report that friends, substance use disorder treatment programs, and physicians are their most trusted sources of information about MDMA. Many also report that the internet is an important source of information, suggesting that prevention websites should be designed to be responsive to the needs of this population. In addition, the use of peer-led advocacy and drug prevention programs may be a promising approach to reduce MDMA use among adolescents and young adults.

New technologies could also help in delivering messages to high school and college students about the effects of MDMA use. For example, one study showed that an online school-based prevention program reduced students' intentions to use MDMA and other drugs.

(Source: "MDMA (Ecstasy) Abuse," National Institute on Drug Abuse (NIDA).)

How Many Teens Use MDMA?

Below is a table showing the percentage of teens who use MDMA.

Table 42.1. Trends In Prevalence Of MDMA For 8th Graders, 10th Graders, And 12th Graders (In Percent)

Drug	Time Period	8th Graders	10th Graders	12th Graders
MDMA	Lifetime	1.5	2.8	4.9
	Past Year	0.9	1.7	2.6
	Past Month	0.4	0.5	0.9

What Should I Do If Someone I Know Needs Help?

If you, or a friend, are in crisis and need to speak with someone now:

- Call National Suicide Prevention Lifeline (NSPL) at 800-273-TALK (800-273-8255) (they don't just talk about suicide—they cover a lot of issues and will help put you in touch with someone close by)

If you need information on drug treatment and where you can find it, the Substance Abuse and Mental Health Services Administration (SAMHSA) can help.

- Call Substance Abuse Treatment Facility Locator at 800-662-HELP (800-662-4357)

- Visit the locator online at www.findtreatment.samhsa.gov

Chapter 43

Hallucinogens: LSD, Psilocybin, And PCP

What Are Hallucinogens?

Hallucinogens are a diverse group of drugs that alter perception (awareness of surrounding objects and conditions), thoughts, and feelings. They cause hallucinations, or sensations and images that seem real though they are not. Hallucinogens can be found in some plants and mushrooms (or their extracts) or can be human-made. People have used hallucinogens for centuries, mostly for religious rituals. Common hallucinogens include the following:

- **Ayahuasca** is a tea made from one of several Amazonian plants containing dimethyltryptamine (DMT), the primary mind-altering ingredient. Ayahuasca is also known as Hoasca, Aya, and Yagé.

- **Dimethyltryptamine (DMT)** is a powerful chemical found in some Amazonian plants. Manufacturers can also make DMT in a lab. The drug is usually a white crystalline powder. A popular name for DMT is Dimitri.

About This Chapter: Text beginning with the heading "What Are Hallucinogens?" is excerpted from "Hallucinogens," National Institute on Drug Abuse (NIDA), January 2016; Text under the heading "What Is Lysergic Acid Diethylamide (LSD)?" is excerpted from "Drugs Of Abuse," U.S. Drug Enforcement Administration (DEA), January 23, 2018; Text under the heading "What Is Phencyclidine (PCP)?" is excerpted from "PCP (Phencyclidine)," Get Smart About Drugs, U.S. Drug Enforcement Administration (DEA), July 10, 2017; Text under the heading "Statistics And Trends" is excerpted from "Hallucinogens," National Institute on Drug Abuse (NIDA), June 11, 2018; Text under the heading "What Should I Do If Someone I Know Needs Help?" is excerpted from "MDMA (Ecstasy Or Molly)," National Institute on Drug Abuse (NIDA) for Teens, May 2017.

- **D-lysergic acid diethylamide (LSD)** is one of the most powerful mood-changing chemicals. It is a clear or white odorless material made from lysergic acid, which is found in a fungus that grows on rye and other grains. LSD has many other names, including Acid, Blotter, Dots, and Yellow Sunshine.

- **Peyote (mescaline)** is a small, spineless cactus with mescaline as its main ingredient. Peyote can also be synthetic. Buttons, Cactus, and Mesc are common names for peyote.

- **4-phosphoryloxy-N,N-dimethyltryptamine (psilocybin)** comes from certain types of mushrooms found in tropical and subtropical regions of South America, Mexico, and the United States. Other names for psilocybin include Little Smoke, Magic Mushrooms, Purple Passion, and Shrooms.

Some hallucinogens also cause users to feel out of control or disconnected from their body and environment. Common examples include the following:

- **Dextromethorphan (DXM)** is a cough suppressant and mucus-clearing ingredient in some over-the-counter (OTC) cold and cough medicines (syrups, tablets, and gel capsules). Robo is another popular name for DXM.

- **Ketamine** is used as a surgery anesthetic for humans and animals. Much of the ketamine sold on the streets comes from veterinary offices. While available as an injectable liquid, manufacturers mostly sell it as a powder or as pills. Other names for ketamine include K, Special K, or Cat Valium.

- **Phencyclidine (PCP)** was developed in the 1950s as a general anesthetic for surgery. It's no longer used for this purpose due to serious side effects. While PCP can be found in a variety of forms, including tablets or capsules, liquid and white crystal powder are the most common forms. PCP has various other names, such as Angel Dust, Hog, Love Boat, and Peace Pill.

- **Salvia divinorum (salvia)** is a plant common to southern Mexico and Central and South America. Other names for salvia are Diviner's Sage, Maria Pastora, Sally-D, and Magic Mint.

How Do People Use Hallucinogens?

People use hallucinogens in a wide variety of ways, as shown in the following figure:

	Ayahuasca	DMT	LSD	Peyote	Psilocybin	DXM	Ketamine	PCP	Salvia
Swallowing as tablets or pills		✓	✓				✓	✓	
Swallowing as liquid		✓	✓	✓					
Consuming raw or dried	✓			✓	✓				✓
Brewing into tea	✓			✓	✓				✓
Snorting							✓	✓	
Injecting							✓	✓	
Inhaling, vaporizing, or smoking		✓						✓	✓
Absorbing through the lining in the mouth using drug-soaked paper pieces			✓						

Figure 43.1. Hallucinogens Usage

Hallucinogenic and dissociative drugs have been used for a variety of reasons. Historically, hallucinogenic plants have been used for religious rituals to induce states of detachment from reality and precipitate "visions" thought to provide mystical insight or enable contact with a spirit world or "higher power." More recently, people report using hallucinogenic drugs for more social or recreational purposes, including to have fun, help them deal with stress, or enable them to enter into what they perceive as a more enlightened sense of thinking or being. Hallucinogens have also been investigated as therapeutic agents to treat diseases associated with perceptual distortions, such as schizophrenia, obsessive-compulsive disorder (OCD), bipolar disorder, and dementia. Anecdotal reports and small studies have suggested that ayahuasca may be a potential treatment for substance use disorders and other mental health issues, but no large-scale research has verified its efficacy.

(Source: "Hallucinogens And Dissociative Drugs," National Institute on Drug Abuse (NIDA).)

How Do Hallucinogens Affect The Brain?

Research suggests that hallucinogens work at least partially by temporarily disrupting communication between brain chemical systems throughout the brain and spinal cord. Some hallucinogens interfere with the action of the brain chemical serotonin, which regulates:

- Mood

- Sensory perception

- Sleep

- Hunger

- Body temperature

- Sexual behavior

- Muscle control

Other hallucinogens interfere with the action of the brain chemical glutamate, which regulates:

- Pain perception

- Responses to the environment

- Emotion

- Learning and memory

Short-Term Effects

The effects of hallucinogens can begin within 20–90 minutes and can last as long as 6–12 hours. Salvia's effects are more short-lived, appearing in less than 1 minute and lasting less than 30 minutes. Hallucinogen users refer to the experiences brought on by these drugs as "trips," calling the unpleasant experiences "bad trips."

Along with hallucinations, other short-term general effects include:

- Increased heart rate

- Nausea

- Intensified feelings and sensory experiences

- Changes in sense of time (for example, time passing by slowly)

Specific short-term effects of some hallucinogens include:

- Increased blood pressure, breathing rate, or body temperature

- Loss of appetite

- Dry mouth

- Sleep problems

- Mixed senses (such as "seeing" sounds or "hearing" colors)

- Spiritual experiences

- Feelings of relaxation or detachment from self/environment

- Uncoordinated movements

- Excessive sweating

- Panic

- Paranoia—extreme and unreasonable distrust of others

- Psychosis—disordered thinking detached from reality

Long-Term Effects

Little is known about the long-term effects of hallucinogens. Researchers do know that ketamine users may develop symptoms that include ulcers in the bladder, kidney problems, and poor memory. Repeated use of PCP can result in long-term effects that may continue for a year or more after use stops, such as:

- Speech problems

- Memory loss

- Weight loss

- Anxiety

- Depression and suicidal thoughts

Though rare, long-term effects of some hallucinogens include the following:

- **Persistent psychosis**—a series of continuing mental problems, including:

  - Visual disturbances

  - Disorganized thinking

- Paranoia

- Mood changes

- **Flashbacks**—recurrences of certain drug experiences. They often happen without warning and may occur within a few days or more than a year after drug use. In some users, flashbacks can persist and affect daily functioning, a condition known as hallucinogen persisting perceptual disorder (HPPD). These people continue to have hallucinations and other visual disturbances, such as seeing trails attached to moving objects.

- Symptoms that are sometimes mistaken for other disorders, such as stroke or a brain tumor

What Are Other Risks Of Hallucinogens?

Other risks or health effects of many hallucinogens remain unclear and need more research. Known risks include the following:

- Some psilocybin users risk poisoning and possibly death from using a poisonous mushroom by mistake.

- High doses of PCP can cause seizures, coma, and death, though death more often results from accidental injury or suicide during PCP intoxication. Interactions between PCP and depressants such as alcohol and benzodiazepines (prescribed to relieve anxiety or promote sleep—alprazolam (Xanax®), for instance) can also lead to coma.

- Some bizarre behaviors resulting from hallucinogens that users display in public places may prompt public health or law enforcement personnel intervention.

- While hallucinogens' effects on the developing fetus are unknown, researchers do know that mescaline in peyote may affect the fetus of a pregnant woman using the drug.

Are Hallucinogens Addictive?

Evidence indicates that certain hallucinogens can be addictive or that people can develop a tolerance to them. Use of some hallucinogens also produces tolerance to other similar drugs. For example, LSD is not considered an addictive drug because it doesn't cause uncontrollable drug-seeking behavior. However, LSD does produce tolerance, so some users who take the drug repeatedly must take higher doses to achieve the same effect. This is an extremely dangerous practice, given the unpredictability of the drug. In addition, LSD produces tolerance to other hallucinogens, including psilocybin. On the other hand, PCP is a hallucinogen that can be addictive. People who stop repeated use of PCP experience drug cravings, headaches, and sweating as common withdrawal symptoms. Scientists need more research into the tolerance or addiction potential of hallucinogens.

How Can People Get Treatment For Addiction To Hallucinogens?

There are no government-approved medications to treat addiction to hallucinogens. While inpatient and/or behavioral treatments can be helpful for patients with a variety of addictions, scientists need more research to find out if behavioral therapies are effective for addiction to hallucinogens.

What Is Lysergic Acid Diethylamide (LSD)?

Lysergic acid diethylamide (LSD) is a potent hallucinogen that has a high potential for abuse and currently has no accepted medical use in treatment in the United States.

What Is Its Origin?

LSD is produced in clandestine laboratories in the United States.

What Are Common Street Names?

Common names for LSD include:

- Acid
- Blotter Acid
- Dots
- Mellow Yellow
- Windowpane

What Does It Look Like?

LSD is sold on the street in tablets, capsules, and occasionally in liquid form. It is an odorless and colorless substance with a slightly bitter taste. LSD is often added to absorbent paper, such as blotter paper, and divided into small decorated squares, with each square representing one dose.

How Is It Abused?

LSD is abused orally.

What Is Its Effect On The Mind?

During the first hour after ingestion, users may experience visual changes with extreme changes in mood. While hallucinating, the user may suffer impaired depth and time perception accompanied by distorted perception of the shape and size of objects, movements, colors, soundtouch, and the user's own body image. The ability to make sound judgments and see common dangers is impaired, making the user susceptible to personal injury. It is possible for users to suffer acute anxiety and depression after an LSD "trip" and flashbacks have been reported days, and even months, after taking the last dose.

What Is Its Effect On The Body?

The physical effects include:

- Dilated pupils
- Higher body temperature
- Increased heart rate and blood pressure
- Sweating
- Loss of appetite
- Sleeplessness
- Dry mouth
- Tremors

What Are Its Overdose Effects?

Longer, more intense "trip" episodes, psychosis, and possible death.

Which Drugs Cause Similar Effects?

LSD's effects are similar to other hallucinogens, such as PCP, mescaline, and peyote.

What Is Its Legal Status In The United States?

LSD is a Schedule I substance under the Controlled Substances Act (CSA). Schedule I substances have a high potential for abuse, no currently accepted medical use in treatment in the United States, and a lack of accepted safety for use under medical supervision.

What Is Psilocybin?

Psilocybin is a chemical obtained from certain types of fresh or dried mushrooms.

What Is Its Origin?

Psilocybin mushrooms are found in Mexico, Central America, and the United States.

What Are Common Street Names?

Common street names include:

- Magic Mushrooms
- Mushrooms
- Shrooms

What Does It Look Like?

Mushrooms containing psilocybin are available fresh or dried and have long, slender stems topped by caps with dark gills on the underside. Fresh mushrooms have white or whitish-gray stems; the caps are dark brown around the edges and light brown or white in the center. Dried mushrooms are usually rusty brown with isolated areas of off-white.

How Is It Abused?

Psilocybin mushrooms are ingested orally. They may also be brewed as a tea or added to other foods to mask their bitter flavor.

What Is Its Effect On The Mind?

The psychological consequences of psilocybin use include hallucinations and an inability to discern fantasy from reality. Panic reactions and psychosis also may occur, particularly if a user ingests a large dose.

What Is Its Effect On The Body?

The physical effects include:

- Nausea
- Vomiting
- Muscle weakness
- Lack of coordination

What Are Its Overdose Effects?

Effects of overdose include:

- Longer
- More intense "trip" episodes
- Psychosis
- Possible death

Abuse of psilocybin mushrooms could also lead to poisoning if one of the many varieties of poisonous mushrooms is incorrectly identified as a psilocybin mushroom.

Which Drugs Cause Similar Effects?

Psilocybin effects are similar to other hallucinogens, such as mescaline and peyote.

What Is Its Legal Status In The United States?

Psilocybin is a Schedule I substance under the Controlled Substances Act, meaning that it has a high potential for abuse, no currently accepted medical use in treatment in the United States, and a lack of accepted safety for use under medical supervision.

What Is Phencyclidine (PCP)?

PCP is a synthetically produced hallucinogen.

What Are Common Street Names?

- Angel Dust
- Boat
- Crystal
- Embalming Fluid
- Hog
- Ozone
- Rocket Fuel
- Shermans

- Supergrass
- Tic Tac
- Wack
- Zoom

How Is It Used?

- Tablets, capsules are swallowed
- In powder form, snorted
- Leafy material sprayed or dipped in liquid and smoked

How Does It Affect The Body?

- Dissociative drug, induces distortion of sight and sound and produces feelings of detachment
- Disorientation, delirium
- Sedation, immobility, amnesia
- Numbness, slurred speech, loss of coordination
- Feeling of strength, power, and invulnerability
- Increased blood pressure, rapid and shallow breathing, elevated heart rate and temperature
- Addictive

Statistics And Trends

Below are the tables showing the percentage of teens who use hallucinogens.

Table 43.1. Monitoring The Future Study: Trends In Prevalence Of Various Drugs For 8th Graders, 10th Graders, And 12th Graders; 2017 (In Percent)

Drug	Time Period	Graders	10th Graders	12th Graders
Hallucinogens	Lifetime	1.90	4.20	6.70
	Past Year	1.10	2.80	4.40
	Past Month	0.50	1.10	1.60
LSD	Lifetime	1.30	3.00	5.00
	Past Year	0.90	2.10	3.30
	Past Month	0.30	0.80	1.20
PCP	Past Year	–	–	1.00

Table 43.2. National Survey On Drug Use And Health: Trends In Prevalence Of Various Drugs For Ages 12 Or Older, Ages 12–17, And Ages 18–25; 2016 (In Percent)

Drug	Time Period	Ages 12 Or Older	Ages 12–17	Ages 18–25
Hallucinogens	Lifetime	15.40	2.70	17.20
	Past Year	1.80	1.80	6.90
	Past Month	0.50	0.50	1.90
LSD	Lifetime	9.60	1.20	8.30
	Past Year	0.70	0.80	3.40
	Past Month	0.10	0.20	0.60
PCP	Lifetime	2.40	0.20	0.70
	Past Year	0.00	0.10	0.00
	Past Month	0.00	0.00	^

^indicate low precision; no estimate reported.

What Should I Do If Someone I Know Needs Help?

If you, or a friend, are in crisis and need to speak with someone now:

- Call National Suicide Prevention Lifeline (NSPL) at 800-273-TALK (800-273-8255) (they don't just talk about suicide—they cover a lot of issues and will help put you in touch with someone close by)

If you need information on drug treatment and where you can find it, the Substance Abuse and Mental Health Services Administration (SAMHSA) can help.

- Call Substance Abuse Treatment Facility Locator at 800-662-HELP (800-662-4357)

- Visit the locator online at www.findtreatment.samhsa.gov

Chapter 44

Stimulants: An Overview

What Are Stimulants?

Stimulants speed up the body's systems. This class of drugs includes prescription drugs such as amphetamines (Adderall and Dexedrine), methylphenidate (Concerta and Ritalin), diet aids (such as Didrex, Bontril, Preludin, Fastin, Adipex P, Ionamin, and Meridia), and illicitly produced drugs such as methamphetamine, cocaine, and methcathinone.

What Is Their Origin?

Stimulants are diverted from legitimate channels and clandestinely manufactured exclusively for the illicit market.

What Are Common Street Names?

Common street names for stimulants include:

- Bennies
- Black Beauties
- Cat
- Coke

- Crank
- Crystal
- Flake
- Ice

About This Chapter: Text beginning with the heading "What Are Stimulants?" is excerpted from "Drugs Of Abuse," U.S. Drug Enforcement Administration (DEA), January 23, 2018; Text under the heading "What Should I Do If Someone I Know Needs Help?" is excerpted from "MDMA (Ecstasy Or Molly)," National Institute on Drug Abuse (NIDA) for Teens, May 2017.

- Pellets
- R-Ball
- Skippy
- Snow
- Speed
- Uppers
- Vitamin R

What Do They Look Like?

Stimulants come in the form of:

- Pills
- Powder
- Rocks
- Injectable liquids

How Are They Abused?

Stimulants can be pills or capsules that are swallowed. Smoking, snorting, or injecting stimulants produces a sudden sensation known as a "rush" or a "flash." Abuse is often associated with a pattern of binge use—sporadically consuming large doses of stimulants over a short period of time. Heavy users may inject themselves every few hours, continuing until they have depleted their drug supply or reached a point of delirium, psychosis, and physical exhaustion. During heavy use, all other interests become secondary to recreating the initial euphoric rush.

How Do People Use And Misuse Prescription Stimulants?

Most prescription stimulants come in tablet, capsule, or liquid form, which a person takes by mouth. Misuse of a prescription stimulant means:

Taking medicine in a way or dose other than prescribed

- Taking someone else's medicine
- Taking medicine only for the effect it causes—to get high

When misusing a prescription stimulant, people can swallow the medicine in its normal form. Alternatively, they can crush tablets or open the capsules, dissolve the powder in water, and inject the liquid into a vein. Some can also snort or smoke the powder.

(Source: "Prescription Stimulants," National Institute on Drug Abuse (NIDA).)

What Is Their Effect On The Mind?

When used as drugs of abuse and not under a doctor's supervision, stimulants are frequently taken to:

- Produce a sense of exhilaration, enhance self-esteem, improve mental and physical performance, increase activity, reduce appetite, extend wakefulness for prolonged period, and "get high." Chronic, high-dose use is frequently associated with agitation, hostility, panic, aggression, and suicidal or homicidal tendencies. Paranoia, sometimes accompanied by both auditory and visual hallucinations, may also occur. Tolerance, in which more and more drug is needed to produce the usual effects, can develop rapidly, and psychological dependence occurs. In fact, the strongest psychological dependence observed occurs with the more potent stimulants, such as amphetamine, methylphenidate, methamphetamine, cocaine, and methcathinone. Abrupt cessation is commonly followed by depression, anxiety, drug craving, and extreme fatigue, known as a "crash."

Do Prescription Stimulants Make You Smarter?

Some people take prescription stimulants to try to improve mental performance. Teens and college students sometimes misuse them to try to get better grades, and older adults misuse them to try to improve their memory. Taking prescription stimulants for reasons other than treating attention deficit hyperactivity disorder (ADHD) or narcolepsy could lead to harmful health effects, such as addiction, heart problems, or psychosis.

(Source: "Prescription Stimulants," National Institute on Drug Abuse (NIDA).)

What Is Their Effect On The Body?

Stimulants are sometimes referred to as uppers and reverse the effects of fatigue on both mental and physical tasks. Therapeutic levels of stimulants can produce exhilaration, extended wakefulness, and loss of appetite. These effects are greatly intensified when large doses of stimulants are taken. Taking too large a dose at one time or taking large doses over an extended period of time may cause such physical side effects as:

- Dizziness
- Tremors
- Headache
- Flushed skin

- Chest pain with palpitations

- Excessive sweating

- Vomiting

- Abdominal cramps

What Are Their Overdose Effects?

In overdose, unless there is medical intervention, high fever, convulsions, and cardiovascular collapse may precede death. Because accidental death is partially due to the effects of stimulants on the body's cardiovascular and temperature regulating systems, physical exertion increases the hazards of stimulant use.

Which Drugs Cause Similar Effects?

Some hallucinogenic substances, such as ecstasy, have a stimulant component to their activity.

What Is Their Legal Status In The United States?

A number of stimulants have no medical use in the United States but have a high potential for abuse. These stimulants are controlled in Schedule I. Some prescription stimulants are not controlled, and some stimulants like tobacco and caffeine don't require a prescription—though society's recognition of their adverse effects has resulted in a proliferation of caffeine-free products and efforts to discourage cigarette smoking. Stimulant chemicals in over-the-counter products, such as ephedrine and pseudoephedrine, can be found in allergy and cold medicine. As required by The Combat Methamphetamine Epidemic Act of 2005 (CMEA), a retail outlet must store these products out of reach of customers, either behind the counter or in a locked cabinet. Regulated sellers are required to maintain a written or electronic form of a logbook to record sales of these products. In order to purchase these products, customers must now show a photo identification issued by a state or federal government. They are also required to write or enter into the logbook: their name, signature, address, date, and time of sale. In addition to the above, there are daily and monthly sales limits set for customers.

What Should I Do If Someone I Know Needs Help?

If you, or a friend, are in crisis and need to speak with someone now:

• Call National Suicide Prevention Lifeline (NSPL) at 800-273-TALK (800-273-8255) (they don't just talk about suicide—they cover a lot of issues and will help put you in touch with someone close by)

If you need information on drug treatment and where you can find it, the Substance Abuse and Mental Health Services Administration (SAMHSA) can help.

• Call Substance Abuse Treatment Facility Locator at 800-662-HELP (800-662-4357)

• Visit the locator online at www.findtreatment.samhsa.gov

Chapter 45

Cocaine, Crack, And Khat

What Is Cocaine?

Cocaine is a powerfully addictive stimulant drug made from the leaves of the coca plant native to South America. Although healthcare providers can use it for valid medical purposes, such as local anesthesia for some surgeries, cocaine is an illegal drug. As a street drug, cocaine looks like a fine, white, crystal powder. Street dealers often mix it with things like cornstarch, talcum powder, or flour to increase profits. They may also mix it with other drugs such as the stimulant amphetamine.

Popular nicknames for cocaine include:

- Blow
- Coke
- Crack
- Rock
- Snow

About This Chapter: Text under the heading "What Is Cocaine?" is excerpted from "DrugFacts: Cocaine," National Institute on Drug Abuse (NIDA), June 2016; Text under the heading "What Is Crack Cocaine?" is excerpted from "Crack Cocaine Fast Facts," U.S. Department of Justice (DOJ), April 2003. Reviewed July 2018; Text under the heading "What Is Khat?" is excerpted from "Drugs Of Abuse," U.S. Drug Enforcement Administration (DEA), January 23, 2018; Text under the heading "Statistics And Trends" is excerpted from "Cocaine," National Institute on Drug Abuse (NIDA), June 11, 2018; Text under the heading "What Should I Do If Someone I Know Needs Help?" is excerpted from "MDMA (Ecstasy Or Molly)," National Institute on Drug Abuse (NIDA) for Teens, May 2017.

How Do People Use Cocaine?

People snort cocaine powder through the nose, or they rub it into their gums. Others dissolve the powder in water and inject it into the bloodstream. Some people inject a combination of cocaine and heroin, called a Speedball. Another popular method of use is to smoke cocaine that has been processed to make a rock crystal (also called "freebase cocaine"). The crystal is heated to produce vapors that are inhaled into the lungs. This form of cocaine is called Crack, which refers to the crackling sound of the rock as it's heated. People who use cocaine often take it in binges—taking the drug repeatedly within a short time, at increasingly higher doses—to maintain their high.

How Does Cocaine Affect The Brain?

Cocaine increases levels of the natural chemical messenger dopamine in brain circuits controlling pleasure and movement. Normally, the brain releases dopamine in these circuits in response to potential rewards, like the smell of good food. It then recycles back into the cell that released it, shutting off the signal between nerve cells. Cocaine prevents dopamine from recycling, causing excessive amounts to build up between nerve cells. This flood of dopamine ultimately disrupts normal brain communication and causes cocaine's high.

Short-Term Effects

Short-term health effects of cocaine include:

- Extreme happiness and energy
- Mental alertness
- Hypersensitivity to sight, sound, and touch
- Irritability
- Paranoia—extreme and unreasonable distrust of others

Some people find that cocaine helps them perform simple physical and mental tasks more quickly, although others experience the opposite effect. Large amounts of cocaine can lead to bizarre, unpredictable, and violent behavior.

Cocaine's effects appear almost immediately and disappear within a few minutes to an hour. How long the effects last and how intense they are depend on the method of use. Injecting or smoking cocaine produces a quicker and stronger but shorter-lasting high than snorting. The high from snorting cocaine may last 15–30 minutes. The high from smoking may last 5–10 minutes.

What Are The Other Health Effects Of Cocaine Use?

Other health effects of cocaine use include:

- Constricted blood vessels

- Dilated pupils

- Nausea

- Raised body temperature and blood pressure

- Faster heartbeat

- Tremors and muscle twitches

- Restlessness

Long-Term Effects

Some long-term health effects of cocaine depend on the method of use and include the following:

- **Snorting:** Loss of sense of smell, nosebleeds, frequent runny nose, and problems with swallowing.

- **Consuming by mouth:** Severe bowel decay from reduced blood flow.

- **Needle injection:** Higher risk for contracting human immunodeficiency virus (HIV), hepatitis C, and other bloodborne diseases. However, even people involved with non-needle cocaine use place themselves at a risk for HIV because cocaine impairs judgment, which can lead to risky sexual behavior with infected partners.

Other long-term effects of cocaine use include being malnourished, because cocaine decreases appetite, and movement disorders, including Parkinson's disease, which may occur after many years of use. In addition, people report irritability and restlessness resulting from cocaine binges, and some also experience severe paranoia, in which they lose touch with reality and have auditory hallucinations—hearing noises that aren't real.

Can A Person Overdose On Cocaine?

Yes, a person can overdose on cocaine. An overdose occurs when the person uses too much of a drug and has a toxic reaction that results in serious, harmful symptoms or death. An overdose can be intentional or unintentional. Death from overdose can occur on the first use of cocaine or unexpectedly thereafter. Many people who use cocaine also drink alcohol at the same time, which is particularly risky and can lead to overdose. Others mix cocaine with heroin, another dangerous—and deadly—combination. Some of the most frequent and severe health consequences leading to overdose involve the heart and blood vessels, including irregular heart rhythm and heart attacks, and the nerves, including seizures and strokes.

Cocaine Tightens Blood Vessels

Cocaine causes the body's blood vessels to become narrow, constricting the flow of blood. This is a problem. It forces the heart to work harder to pump blood through the body. (If you've ever tried squeezing into a tight pair of pants, then you know how hard it is for the heart to pump blood through narrowed blood vessels.)

When the heart works harder, it beats faster. It may work so hard that it temporarily loses its natural rhythm. This is called fibrillation, and it can be very dangerous because it stops the flow of blood through the body.

Many of cocaine's effects on the heart are actually caused by cocaine's impact on the brain—the body's control center.

(Source: "Mind Over Matter: Cocaine," National Institute on Drug Abuse (NIDA).)

How Can A Cocaine Overdose Be Treated?

Because cocaine overdose often leads to a heart attack, stroke, or seizure, first responders and emergency room doctors try to treat the overdose by treating these conditions, with the intent of:

- Restoring blood flow to the heart (heart attack)

- Restoring oxygen-rich blood supply to the affected part of the brain (stroke)

- Stopping the seizure

How Does Cocaine Use Lead To Addiction?

As with other drugs, repeated use of cocaine can cause long-term changes in the brain's reward circuit and other brain systems, which may lead to addiction. The reward circuit eventually adapts to the excess dopamine brought on by the drug. As a result, people take stronger and more frequent doses to achieve the same high and feel relief from initial withdrawal. Withdrawal symptoms include:

- Depression

- Fatigue

- Increased appetite

- Unpleasant dreams and insomnia

- Slowed thinking

How Can People Get Treatment For Cocaine Addiction?

Behavioral therapy may be used to treat cocaine addiction. Examples include:

- Cognitive behavioral therapy (CBT)

- Contingency management, or motivational incentives—providing rewards to patients who remain substance free

- Therapeutic communities—drug-free residences in which people in recovery from substance use disorders help each other to understand and change their behaviors

While no government-approved medicines are currently available to treat cocaine addiction, researchers are testing some treatments, including:

- Disulfiram (used to treat alcoholism)

- Modanifil (used to treat narcolepsy—a disorder characterized by uncontrollable episodes of deep sleep)

- Lorcaserin (used to treat obesity)

What Is Crack Cocaine?

Crack cocaine is a highly addictive and powerful stimulant that is derived from powdered cocaine using a simple conversion process. Crack emerged as a drug of abuse in the mid-1980s. It is abused because it produces an immediate high and because it is easy and inexpensive to produce—rendering it readily available and affordable.

How Is It Produced?

Crack is produced by dissolving powdered cocaine in a mixture of water and ammonia or sodium bicarbonate (baking soda). The mixture is boiled until a solid substance forms. The solid is removed from the liquid, dried, and then broken into the chunks (rocks) that are sold as crack cocaine.

What Does It Look Like?

Crack typically is available as rocks. Crack rocks are white (or off-white) and vary in size and shape.

How Is Crack Abused?

Crack is nearly always smoked. Smoking crack cocaine delivers large quantities of the drug to the lungs, producing an immediate and intense euphoric effect.

Who Uses Crack?

Individuals of all ages use crack cocaine—data reported in the National Household Survey on Drug Abuse indicate that an estimated 6,222,000 U.S. residents aged 12 and older used crack at least once in their lifetime. The survey also revealed that hundreds of thousands of teenagers and young adults use crack cocaine—150,000 individuals aged 12–17 and 1,003,000 individuals aged 18–25 used the drug at least once.

Crack cocaine use among high school students is a particular problem. Nearly 4 percent of high school seniors in the United States used the drug at least once in their lifetime, and more than 1 percent used the drug in the past month, according to the University of Michigan's Monitoring the Future Survey.

What Are The Risks?

Cocaine, in any form, is a powerfully addictive drug, and addiction seems to develop more quickly when the drug is smoked—as crack is—than snorted—as powdered cocaine typically is. In addition to the usual risks associated with cocaine use (constricted blood vessels; increased temperature, heart rate, and blood pressure; and risk of cardiac arrest and seizure), crack users may experience acute respiratory problems, including coughing, shortness of breath, and lung trauma and bleeding. Crack cocaine smoking also can cause aggressive and paranoid behavior.

What Is It Called?

Street terms for crack cocaine include:

- 24-7
- Badrock
- Beat
- Candy
- Chemical
- Cloud

- Cookies
- Crumbs
- Crunch and munch
- Devil drug
- Dice
- Electric kool-aid

- Fat bags
- French fries
- Glo
- Gravel
- Grit
- Hail
- Hard ball
- Hard rock
- Hotcakes
- Ice cube
- Jelly beans
- Nuggets

- Paste
- Piece
- Prime time
- Product
- Raw
- Rock(s)
- Scrabble
- Sleet
- Snow coke
- Tornado
- Troop

Is Crack Cocaine Illegal?

Yes, crack cocaine is illegal. Crack cocaine is a Schedule II substance under the Controlled Substances Act (CSA). Schedule II drugs, which include phencyclidine (PCP) and methamphetamine, have a high potential for abuse. Abuse of these drugs may lead to severe psychological or physical dependence.

What Is Khat?

Khat is a flowering evergreen shrub that is abused for its stimulant-like effect. Khat has two active ingredients, cathine and cathinone.

What Is Its Origin?

Khat is native to East Africa and the Arabian Peninsula, where the use of it is an established cultural tradition for many social situations.

What Are Common Street Names?

Common street names for Khat include:

- Abyssinian Tea

- African Salad

- Catha
- Chat

- Kat
- Oat

What Does It Look Like?

Khat is a flowering evergreen shrub. Khat that is sold and abused is usually just the leaves, twigs, and shoots of the Khat shrub.

How Is It Abused?

Khat is typically chewed like tobacco, then retained in the cheek and chewed intermittently to release the active drug, which produces a stimulant-like effect. Dried Khat leaves can be made into tea or a chewable paste, and Khat can also be smoked and even sprinkled on food.

How Much Is Available In The United States?

The availability of khat in the United States has been increasing since 1995. According to the Federal-wide Drug Seizure System (FDSS), law enforcement seizures of khat increased from 14 metric tons in 1995 to over 37 metric tons in 2001. During the first six months of 2002, nearly 30 metric tons of khat was seized. El Paso Intelligence Center reported that law enforcement seized 32, 39, 37, 54, 47, and 32 metric tons of khat in 2000, 2001, 2002, 2003, 2004, and through September 2005, respectively.

How Much Does It Cost To Manufacture?

Khat is purchased from farmers in the horn of Africa region for about $1 per kilogram. Warlords operating in this area use their planes to ship the khat to countries in Europe, where khat is still legal. The khat is sold to middlemen for $200/kg, a profit of $199 per kilogram. The drugs are then shipped to the United States and elsewhere.

How Much Does Khat Sell For In The United States?

Khat generally sells for $300–$600 per kilogram or $30–$60 per bundle (which is 40 leafed twigs measuring 12–15 inches in length).

(Source: "Khat AKA: Catha Edulis," U.S. Drug Enforcement Administration (DEA).)

What Is Its Effect On The Mind?

Khat can induce manic behavior with:

- Grandiose delusions
- Paranoia

- Nightmares
- Hallucinations
- Hyperactivity

Chronic Khat abuse can result in violence and suicidal depression.

What Is Its Effect On The Body?

Khat causes an immediate increase in blood pressure and heart rate. Khat can also cause a brown staining of the teeth, insomnia, and gastric disorders. Chronic abuse of Khat can cause physical exhaustion.

What Are Its Overdose Effects?

The dose needed to constitute an overdose is not known, however, it has been historically associated with those who are long-term chewers of the leaves.

Symptoms of toxicity include:

- Delusions
- Loss of appetite
- Difficulty with breathing
- Increases in both blood pressure and heart rate

Additionally, there are reports of liver damage (chemical hepatitis) and of cardiac complications, specifically myocardial infarctions. This mostly occurs among long-term chewers of khat or those who have chewed too large a dose.

Which Drugs Cause Similar Effects?

Khat's effects are similar to other stimulants, such as cocaine, amphetamine, and methamphetamine.

What Is Its Legal Status In The United States?

The chemicals found in khat are controlled under the Controlled Substances Act (CSA). Cathine is a Schedule IV stimulant, and cathinone is a Schedule I stimulant under the CSA, meaning that it has a high potential for abuse, no currently accepted medical use in treatment in the United States, and a lack of accepted safety for use under medical supervision.

Statistics And Trends

Below are the tables showing the percentage of teens who use cocaine.

Table 45.1. Monitoring The Future Study: Trends In Prevalence Of Various Drugs For 8th Graders, 10th Graders, And 12th Graders; 2017 (In Percent)

Drug	Time Period	8th Graders	10th Graders	12th Graders
Cocaine	Lifetime	1.30	2.10	4.20
	Past Year	0.80	1.40	2.70
	Past Month	0.40	0.50	1.20
Crack Cocaine	Lifetime	0.80	0.80	1.70
	Past Year	0.50	0.60	1.00
	Past Month	0.30	0.30	0.60

Table 45.2. National Survey On Drug Use And Health: Trends In Prevalence Of Various Drugs For Ages 12 Or Older, Ages 12–17, And Ages 18–25; 2016 (In Percent)

Drug	Time Period	Ages 12 Or Older	Ages 12–17	Ages 18–25
Cocaine	Lifetime	14.40	0.90	11.30
	Past Year	1.90	0.50	5.60
	Past Month	0.70	0.10	1.60
Crack Cocaine	Lifetime	3.30	0.10	1.10
	Past Year	0.30	0.00	0.30
	Past Month	0.20	0.00	0.00

What Should I Do If Someone I Know Needs Help?

If you, or a friend, are in crisis and need to speak with someone now:

- Call National Suicide Prevention Lifeline (NSPL) at 800-273-TALK (800-273-8255) (they don't just talk about suicide—they cover a lot of issues and will help put you in touch with someone close by)

If you need information on drug treatment and where you can find it, the Substance Abuse and Mental Health Services Administration (SAMHSA) can help.

- Call Substance Abuse Treatment Facility Locator at 800-662-HELP (800-662-4357)

- Visit the locator online at www.findtreatment.samhsa.gov

Chapter 46

Methamphetamine And Yaba

What Is Methamphetamine?

Methamphetamine is a stimulant drug usually used as a white, bitter-tasting powder or a pill. Crystal methamphetamine is a form of the drug that looks like glass fragments or shiny, bluish-white rocks. It is chemically similar to amphetamine (a drug used to treat attention deficit hyperactivity disorder (ADHD) and narcolepsy, a sleep disorder). Other common names for methamphetamine include chalk, crank, crystal, ice, meth, and speed.

How Do People Use Methamphetamine?

People can take methamphetamine by:

- Inhaling/smoking

- Swallowing (pill)

- Snorting

- Injecting the powder that has been dissolved in water/alcohol

Because the "high" from the drug both starts and fades quickly, people often take repeated doses in a "binge and crash" pattern. In some cases, people take methamphetamine in a form

About This Chapter: Text under the heading "What Is Methamphetamine?" is excerpted from "Methamphetamine," National Institute on Drug Abuse (NIDA), June 2018; Text under the heading "What Is Yaba?" is excerpted from "Yaba Fast Facts," U.S. Department of Justice (DOJ), June 2003. Reviewed July 2018; Text under the heading "What Should I Do If Someone I Know Needs Help?" is excerpted from "MDMA (Ecstasy Or Molly)," National Institute on Drug Abuse (NIDA) for Teens, May 2017.

of binging known as a "run," giving up food and sleep while continuing to take the drug every few hours for up to several days.

What Is Its Origin?

Mexican drug trafficking organizations have become the primary manufacturers and distributors of methamphetamine to cities throughout the United States, including in Hawaii. Domestic clandestine laboratory operators also produce and distribute meth but usually on a smaller scale. The methods used depend on the availability of precursor chemicals. Currently, this domestic clandestinely produced meth is mainly made with diverted products that contain pseudoephedrine. Mexican methamphetamine is made with different precursor chemicals. The Combat Methamphetamine Epidemic Act (CMEA) of 2005 requires retailers of nonprescription products containing pseudoephedrine, ephedrine, or phenylpropanolamine to place these products behind the counter or in a locked cabinet. Consumers must show identification and sign a logbook for each purchase.

(Source: "Drugs Of Abuse," U.S. Drug Enforcement Administration (DEA).)

How Does Methamphetamine Affect The Brain?

Methamphetamine increases the amount of the natural chemical dopamine in the brain. Dopamine is involved in body movement, motivation, and reinforcement of rewarding behaviors. The drug's ability to rapidly release high levels of dopamine in reward areas of the brain strongly reinforces drug-taking behavior, making the user want to repeat the experience.

Short-Term Effects

Taking even small amounts of methamphetamine can result in many of the same health effects as those of other stimulants, such as cocaine or amphetamines. These include:

- Increased wakefulness and physical activity

- Decreased appetite

- Faster breathing

- Rapid and/or irregular heartbeat

- Increased blood pressure and body temperature

What Are Other Health Effects Of Methamphetamine?

Long-Term Effects

People who inject methamphetamine are at increased risk of contracting infectious diseases such as human immunodeficiency virus (HIV) and hepatitis B and C. These diseases are transmitted through contact with blood or other bodily fluids. Methamphetamine use can also alter judgment and decision-making leading to risky behaviors, such as unprotected sex, which also increases risk for infection.

Methamphetamine use may worsen the progression of human immunodeficiency virus (HIV) / acquired immunodeficiency syndrome (AIDS) and its consequences. Studies indicate that HIV causes more injury to nerve cells and more cognitive problems in people who have HIV and use methamphetamine than it does in people who have HIV and don't use the drug. Cognitive problems are those involved with thinking, understanding, learning, and remembering.

Long-term methamphetamine use has many other negative consequences, including:

- Extreme weight loss

- Severe dental problems ("meth mouth")

- Intense itching, leading to skin sores from scratching

- Anxiety

- Confusion

- Sleeping problems

- Violent behavior

- Paranoia—extreme and unreasonable distrust of others

- Hallucinations—sensations and images that seem real though they aren't

In addition, continued methamphetamine use causes changes in the brain's dopamine system that are associated with reduced coordination and impaired verbal learning. In studies of people who used methamphetamine over the long term, severe changes also affected areas of the brain involved with emotion and memory. This may explain many of the emotional and cognitive problems observed in those who use methamphetamine.

Although some of these brain changes may reverse after being off the drug for a year or more, other changes may not recover even after a long period of abstinence. A study even suggests that people who used methamphetamine have an increased the risk of developing Parkinson's disease, a disorder of the nerves that affects movement.

Are There Health Effects From Exposure To Secondhand Methamphetamine Smoke?

Researchers don't yet know whether people breathing in secondhand methamphetamine smoke can get high or have other health effects. What they do know is that people can test positive for methamphetamine after exposure to secondhand smoke. More research is needed in this area.

Can A Person Overdose On Methamphetamine?

Yes, a person can overdose on methamphetamine. An overdose occurs when the person uses too much of a drug and has a toxic reaction that results in serious, harmful symptoms or death. Methamphetamine overdose can lead to stroke, heart attack, or organ problems—such as kidney failure—caused by overheating. These conditions can result in death.

How Can A Methamphetamine Overdose Be Treated?

Because methamphetamine overdose often leads to a stroke, heart attack, or organ problems, first responders and emergency room doctors try to treat the overdose by treating these conditions, with the intent of:

- Restoring blood flow to the affected part of the brain (stroke)
- Restoring blood flow to the heart (heart attack)
- Treating the organ problems

Is Methamphetamine Addictive?

Yes, methamphetamine is highly addictive. When people stop taking it, withdrawal symptoms can include:

- Anxiety
- Fatigue
- Severe depression
- Psychosis
- Intense drug cravings

How Can People Get Treatment For Methamphetamine Addiction?

The most effective treatments for methamphetamine addiction so far are behavioral therapies, such as:

- Cognitive behavioral therapy (CBT), which helps patients recognize, avoid, and cope with the situations in which they are most likely to use drugs

- Motivational incentives, which uses vouchers or small cash rewards to encourage patients to remain drug-free

While research is underway, there are currently no government-approved medications to treat methamphetamine addiction.

Statistics And Trends*

Below are the tables showing the percentage of teens who use methamphetamine.

Table 46.1. Monitoring The Future Study: Trends In Prevalence Of Methamphetamine For 8th Graders, 10th Graders, And 12th Graders; 2017 (In Percent)

Drug	Time Period	8th Graders	10th Graders	12th Graders
Methamphetamine	Lifetime	0.70	0.90	1.10
	Past Year	0.50	0.40	0.60
	Past Month	0.20	0.20	0.30

Table 46.2. National Survey On Drug Use And Health: Trends In Prevalence Of Methamphetamine For Ages 12 Or Older, Ages 12–17, And Ages 18–25; 2016 (In Percent)

Drug	Time Period	Ages 12 Or Older	Ages 12–17	Ages 18–25
Methamphetamine	Lifetime	5.40	0.30	2.40
	Past Year	0.50	0.10	0.80
	Past Month	0.20	0.00	0.20

Text excerpted from "Methamphetamine," National Institute on Drug Abuse (NIDA).

What Is Yaba?

Yaba is a combination of methamphetamine (a powerful and addictive stimulant) and caffeine. Yaba, which means crazy medicine in Thai, is produced in Southeast and East Asia. The drug is popular in Asian communities in the United States and increasingly is available at raves and techno parties.

What Does Yaba Look Like?

Yaba is sold as tablets. These tablets are generally no larger than a pencil eraser. They are brightly colored, usually reddish-orange or green. Yaba tablets typically bear one of a variety of logos; R and WY are common logos.

How Is Yaba Used?

Yaba tablets typically are consumed orally. The tablets sometimes are flavored like candy (grape, orange, or vanilla). Another common method is called chasing the dragon. Users place the yaba tablet on aluminum foil and heat it from below. As the tablet melts, vapors rise and are inhaled. The drug also may be administered by crushing the tablets into powder, which is then snorted or mixed with a solvent and injected.

Who Uses Yaba?

It is difficult to determine the scope of yaba use in the United States because most data sources do not distinguish yaba from other forms of methamphetamine. Yaba has emerged as a drug of abuse in Asian communities in the United States, specifically in Northern California and in Los Angeles.

Yaba also is becoming increasingly popular at raves, techno parties, and other venues where the drug MDMA (3,4-methylenedioxymethamphetamine, typically called ecstasy) is used. Drug distributors deliberately market yaba to young people, many of whom have already tried MDMA. The bright colors and candy flavors of yaba tablets are examples of distributors' attempts to appeal to young people.

What Are The Risks?

Individuals who use yaba face the same risks as users of other forms of methamphetamine: rapid heart rate, increased blood pressure, and damage to the small blood vessels in the brain that can lead to stroke. Chronic use of the drug can result in inflammation of the heart lining. Overdoses can cause hyperthermia (elevated body temperature), convulsions, and death. Individuals who use yaba also may have episodes of violent behavior, paranoia, anxiety, confusion, and insomnia.

Although most users administer yaba orally, those who inject the drug expose themselves to additional risks, including contracting HIV, hepatitis B and C, and other blood-borne viruses (BBVs).

What Is It Called?

The most common names for yaba are crazy medicine and Nazi speed.

Is Yaba Illegal?

Yes, yaba is illegal because it contains methamphetamine, a Schedule II substance under the Controlled Substances Act (CSA). Schedule II drugs, which include cocaine and phencyclidine (PCP), have a high potential for abuse. Abuse of these drugs may lead to severe psychological or physical dependence.

What Should I Do If Someone I Know Needs Help?

If you, or a friend, are in crisis and need to speak with someone now:

- Call National Suicide Prevention Lifeline (NSPL) at 800-273-TALK (800-273-8255) (they don't just talk about suicide—they cover a lot of issues and will help put you in touch with someone close by)

If you need information on drug treatment and where you can find it, the Substance Abuse and Mental Health Services Administration (SAMHSA) can help.

- Call Substance Abuse Treatment Facility Locator at 800-662-HELP (800-662-4357)

- Visit the locator online at www.findtreatment.samhsa.gov

Chapter 47

Opiates: Heroin, Methadone, And Buprenorphine

Opiates are powerful drugs derived from the poppy plant that have been used for centuries to relieve pain. They include opium, heroin, morphine, and codeine. Even centuries after their discovery, opiates are still the most effective pain relievers available to physicians for treating pain. Although heroin has no medicinal use, other opiates, such as morphine and codeine, are used in the treatment of pain related to illnesses (for example, cancer) and medical and dental procedures. When used as directed by a physician, opiates are safe and generally do not produce addiction. But opiates also possess very strong reinforcing properties and can quickly trigger addiction when used improperly.

What Is Heroin?

Heroin is a highly addictive drug made from morphine, a psychoactive (mind-altering) substance that is extracted from the resin of the seed pod of the opium poppy plant. Heroin's color and look depend on how it is made and what else it may be mixed with. It can be white or brown powder or a black, sticky substance called "black tar heroin."

About This Chapter: Text in this chapter begins with excerpts from "Opiates," National Institute on Drug Abuse (NIDA) for Teens, June 25, 2018; Text under the heading "What Is Heroin?" is excerpted from "Heroin," National Institute on Drug Abuse (NIDA) for Teens, July 2017; Text under the heading "What Is Methadone?" is excerpted from "Methadone," Substance Abuse and Mental Health Services Administration (SAMHSA), September 28, 2015; Text under the heading "What Is Buprenorphine?" is excerpted from "Buprenorphine," Substance Abuse and Mental Health Services Administration (SAMHSA), May 31, 2016.; Text under the heading "What Should I Do If Someone I Know Needs Help?" is excerpted from "MDMA (Ecstasy Or Molly)," National Institute on Drug Abuse (NIDA) for Teens, May 2017.

Heroin is part of a class of drugs called opioids. Other opioids include some prescription pain relievers, such as codeine, oxycodone (OxyContin), and hydrocodone (e.g., Vicodin). These drugs are chemically similar to endorphins, which are opioid chemicals that the body makes naturally to relieve pain (such as after exercise).

Heroin use and overdose deaths have dramatically increased over the last decade. This increase is related to the growing number of people misusing prescription opioid pain relievers like OxyContin and Vicodin; many who become addicted to those drugs switch to heroin because it produces similar effects but is cheaper and easier to get. In fact, nearly 80 percent of people who use heroin report having first misused prescription opioids. However, only a small portion of people who misuse pain relievers switch to heroin. Both heroin and opioid pill use can lead to addiction and overdose.

How Heroin Is Used

Heroin is mixed with water and injected with a needle. It can also be sniffed, smoked, or snorted. Users sometimes combine it with other drugs, such as alcohol or cocaine (a "speedball"), which can be particularly dangerous and raise the risk of overdose.

What Happens To Your Brain When You Use Heroin?

When heroin enters the brain, it attaches to molecules on cells known as opioid receptors. These receptors are located in many areas of the brain and body, especially areas involved in the perception of pain and pleasure, as well as a part of the brain that regulates breathing.

Short-term effects of heroin include a rush of good feelings and clouded thinking. These effects can last for a few hours, and during this time people feel drowsy, and their heart rate and breathing slow down. When the drug wears off, people experience a depressed mood and often crave the drug to regain the good feelings.

Regular heroin use changes the functioning of the brain. Using heroin repeatedly can result in:

- **Tolerance:** More of the drug is needed to achieve the same "high."

- **Dependence:** The need to continue use of the drug to avoid withdrawal symptoms.

- **Addiction:** A devastating brain disease where, without proper treatment, people have trouble stopping using drugs even when they really want to and even after it causes terrible consequences to their health and other parts of their lives. Because of changes to how the brain functions after repeated drug use, people that are addicted crave the drug just to feel "normal."

What Happens To Your Body When You Use Heroin?

Opioid receptors are located in the brain, the brain stem, down the spinal cord, and in the lungs and intestines. Thus, using heroin can result in a wide variety of physical problems related to breathing and other basic life functions, some of which may be very serious. In 2011, more than 250,000 visits to a hospital emergency department involved heroin.

Heroin use can cause:

- Dry mouth
- Warm flushing skin
- Heavy feeling arms and legs
- Feeling sick to the stomach and throwing up
- Severe itching
- Clouded thinking
- Going "on the nod," switching back and forth between being conscious and semi-conscious
- Coma—a deep state of unconsciousness
- Dangerously slowed (or even stopped) breathing that can lead to overdose death
- Increased risk of human immunodeficiency virus (HIV) and hepatitis (a liver disease) through shared needles

Longer-term effects can include:

- Problems sleeping
- Damage to the tissues inside the nose for people who sniff or snort it
- Painful area of tissue filled with puss (an abscess)
- Infection of the heart
- Constipation and stomach cramping
- Liver and kidney disease
- Lung problems
- Mental health problems, such as depression
- Sexual problems for men
- Changes in menstrual cycles for women

Can You Overdose Or Die If You Use Heroin?

Yes, because heroin slows and sometimes stops breathing, its use does kill people—called a fatal overdose. Deaths from drug overdoses have been increasing since the early 1990s, fueled by increases in misuse of prescription opioids and, more recently, by a surge in heroin use. Nearly 13,000 people died in 2015 from heroin overdoses, with alarming increases among young people ages 15–24.

Signs of a possible heroin overdose are:

- Slow breathing
- Blue lips and fingernails
- Cold damp skin
- Shaking
- Vomiting or gurgling noise

People who are showing symptoms of overdose need urgent medical help. A drug called naloxone can be given to reverse the effects of heroin overdose and prevent death—but only if it is given in time. It is available in an easy-to-use nasal spray or autoinjector. It is often carried by emergency first responders, including police officers and emergency medical technicians (EMTs). In some states, doctors can now prescribe naloxone in advance to people who use heroin or prescription opioids and to their family members, so that in the event of an overdose, it can be given right away without waiting for emergency personnel (who may not arrive in time).

What Are The Other Risks Of Using Heroin?

In addition to the effects of the drug itself, heroin bought on the street often contains a mix of substances, including the dangerous opioid called fentanyl. Some of these substances can be toxic and can clog the blood vessels leading to the lungs, liver, kidney, or brain. This can cause permanent damage to those organs.

Also, sharing drug injection equipment or engaging in risky behaviors can increase the risk of being exposed to diseases such as HIV and hepatitis.

Is Heroin Addictive?

Yes, heroin can be very addictive. In 2015, about 591,000 people had a heroin use disorder. That means they had serious problems with the drug, including health issues, disability, and problems meeting responsibilities at work, school, or home. Of the people with heroin use disorder in 2015, 6,000 were teens and 155,000 were young adults.

Heroin enters the brain quickly, causing a fast, intense high. Using heroin repeatedly can cause people to develop tolerance to the drug. This means they need to take more and more of it to get the same effect. Eventually, they may need to keep taking the drug just to feel normal. It is estimated that about 23 percent of individuals who use heroin become addicted. For those who use heroin over and over again, addiction is more likely. Once a person becomes addicted to heroin, seeking and using the drug often becomes the main goal guiding their daily behavior.

When someone is addicted to heroin and stops using it, he or she may experience extremely uncomfortable and painful withdrawal symptoms, which is why it is so hard to quit. Those symptoms typically include:

- Muscle and bone pain
- Cold flashes with chills
- Throwing up
- Diarrhea
- Trouble sleeping
- Restlessness
- Kicking movements
- Strong craving for the drug

Fortunately, treatment can help an addicted person stop using and stay off heroin. Medicines can help with cravings that occur after quitting, helping a person to take control of their health and their lives.

Statistics And Trends*

Below are the tables showing the percentage of teens who use heroin.

Table 47.1. Trends In Prevalence Of Heroin For 8th Graders, 10th Graders, And 12th Graders (In Percent)

Drug	Time Period	8th Graders	10th Graders	12th Graders
Heroin	Lifetime	0.70	0.40	0.70
	Past Year	0.30	0.20	0.40
	Past Month	0.20	0.10	0.30

Table 47.2. National Survey On Drug Use And Health: Trends In Prevalence of Heroin For Ages 12 or Older, Ages 12–17, And Ages 18–25; 2016 (In Percent)

Drug	Time Period	Ages 12 Or Older	Ages 12–17	Ages 18–25
Heroin	Lifetime	1.80	0.10	1.60
	Past Year	0.40	0.10	0.70
	Past Month	0.20	0.00	0.30

Text excerpted from "Heroin," National Institute on Drug Abuse (NIDA)

What Is Methadone?

Methadone has been used for decades to treat people who are addicted to heroin and narcotic pain medicines. When taken as prescribed, it is safe and effective. It allows people to recover from their addiction and to reclaim active and meaningful lives. For optimal results, patients should also participate in a comprehensive medication-assisted treatment (MAT) program that includes counseling and social support.

How Does Methadone Work?

Methadone works by changing how the brain and nervous system respond to pain. It lessens the painful symptoms of opiate withdrawal and blocks the euphoric effects of opiate drugs such as heroin, morphine, and codeine, as well as semi-synthetic opioids like oxycodone and hydrocodone. Methadone is offered in pill, liquid, and wafer forms and is taken once a day. Pain relief from a dose of methadone lasts about 4–8 hours. As with all medications used in MAT, methadone is to be prescribed as part of a comprehensive treatment plan that includes counseling and participation in social support programs.

How Can A Patient Receive Methadone?

Patients taking methadone to treat opioid addiction must receive the medication under the supervision of a physician. After a period of stability (based on progress and proven, consistent compliance with the medication dosage), patients may be allowed to take methadone at home between program visits. By law, methadone can only be dispensed through an opioid treatment program (OTP) certified by SAMHSA.

The length of time in methadone treatment varies from person to person. Some patients may require treatment for years. Even if a patient feels that they are ready to stop methadone treatment, it must be stopped gradually to prevent withdrawal. Such a decision should be supervised by a doctor. Patients who develop a problem with methadone or have questions can access information through SAMHSA's Find Help (www.samhsa.gov/find-help) page.

Methadone Safety

Methadone can be addictive, so it must be used exactly as prescribed. This is particularly important for patients who are allowed to take methadone at home and aren't required to take medication under supervision at an OTP. Methadone medication is specifically tailored for the individual patient (as doses are often adjusted and readjusted) and is never to be shared with or given to others. Patients should share their complete health history with health providers to ensure the safe use of the medication.

Other medications may interact with methadone and cause heart conditions. Even after the effects of methadone wear off, the medication's active ingredients remain in the body for much longer. Taking more methadone can cause unintentional overdose.

The following tips can help achieve the best treatment results:

- Never use more than the amount prescribed, and always take at the times prescribed. If a dose is missed, or if it feels like it's not working, do not take an extra dose of methadone.

- Do not consume alcohol while taking methadone.

- Be careful driving or operating machinery on methadone.

- Call 911 if too much methadone is taken or if an overdose is suspected.

- Take steps to prevent children from accidentally taking methadone.

- Store methadone at room temperature and away from light.

- Dispose of unused methadone by flushing it down the toilet.

Side Effects Of Methadone

Side effects should be taken seriously, as some of them may indicate an emergency. Patients should stop taking methadone and contact a doctor or emergency services right away if they:

- Experience difficulty breathing or shallow breathing

- Feel lightheaded or faint

- Experience hives or a rash; swelling of the face, lips, tongue, or throat

- Feel chest pain

- Experience a fast or pounding heartbeat

- Experience hallucinations or confusion

Pregnant Or Breastfeeding Women And Methadone

Women who are pregnant or breastfeeding can safely take methadone. When withdrawal from an abused drug happens to a pregnant woman, it causes the uterus to contract and may bring on miscarriage or premature birth. Methadone's ability to prevent withdrawal symptoms helps pregnant women better manage their addiction while avoiding health risks to both mother and baby.

Undergoing methadone maintenance treatment while pregnant will not cause birth defects, but some babies may go through withdrawal after birth. This does not mean that the baby is addicted. Infant withdrawal usually begins a few days after birth but may begin 2–4 weeks after birth. Mothers taking methadone can still breastfeed. Research has shown that the benefits of breastfeeding outweigh the effect of the small amount of methadone that enters the breast milk. A woman who is thinking of stopping methadone treatment due to breastfeeding or pregnancy concerns should speak with her doctor first.

Training On Providing Methadone

Methadone as an opioid use disorder treatment is carefully regulated. MAT services professionals are required to acquire and maintain certifications to legally dispense and prescribe opioid dependency treatments.

What Is Buprenorphine?

Buprenorphine is used in medication-assisted treatment (MAT) to help people reduce or quit their use of heroin or other opiates, such as pain relievers like morphine.

Approved for clinical use in October 2002 by the U.S. Food and Drug Administration (FDA), buprenorphine represents the latest advance in MAT. Medications such as buprenorphine, in combination with counseling and behavioral therapies, provide a whole-patient approach to the treatment of opioid dependency. When taken as prescribed, buprenorphine is safe and effective.

Unlike methadone treatment, which must be performed in a highly structured clinic, buprenorphine is the first medication to treat opioid dependency that is permitted to be prescribed or dispensed in physician offices, significantly increasing treatment access. Under the Drug Addiction Treatment Act of 2000 (DATA 2000), qualified U.S. physicians can offer buprenorphine for opioid dependency in various settings, including in an office, community hospital, health department, or correctional facility.

SAMHSA-certified opioid treatment programs (OTPs) also are allowed to offer buprenorphine, but only are permitted to dispense treatment.

As with all medications used in MAT, buprenorphine is prescribed as part of a comprehensive treatment plan that includes counseling and participation in social support programs.

Buprenorphine offers several benefits to those with opioid dependency and to others for whom treatment in a methadone clinic is not preferred or is less convenient. The FDA has approved the following buprenorphine products:

- Bunavail (buprenorphine and naloxone) buccal film
- Suboxone (buprenorphine and naloxone) film
- Zubsolv (buprenorphine and naloxone) sublingual tablets
- Buprenorphine-containing transmucosal products for opioid dependency

Refer to the product websites for a complete listing of drug interactions, warnings, and precautions.

How Buprenorphine Works

Buprenorphine has unique pharmacological properties that help:

- Lower the potential for misuse
- Diminish the effects of physical dependency to opioids, such as withdrawal symptoms and cravings
- Increase safety in cases of overdose

Buprenorphine is an opioid partial agonist. This means that, like opioids, it produces effects such as euphoria or respiratory depression. With buprenorphine, however, these effects are weaker than those of full drugs such as heroin and methadone. Buprenorphine's opioid effects increase with each dose until at moderate doses they level off, even with further dose increases. This "ceiling effect" lowers the risk of misuse, dependency, and side effects.

Also, because of buprenorphine's long-acting agent, many patients may not have to take it everyday.

Side Effects Of Buprenorphine

Buprenorphine's side effects are similar to those of opioids and can include:

- Nausea, vomiting, and constipation
- Muscle aches and cramps
- Cravings
- Inability to sleep
- Distress and irritability
- Fever

Buprenorphine Misuse Potential

Because of buprenorphine's opioid effects, it can be misused, particularly by people who do not have an opioid dependency. Naloxone is added to buprenorphine to decrease the likelihood of diversion and misuse of the combination drug product. When these products are taken as sublingual tablets, buprenorphine's opioid effects dominate and naloxone blocks opioid withdrawals. If the sublingual tablets are crushed and injected, however, the naloxone effect dominates and can bring on opioid withdrawals.

Buprenorphine Safety

People should use the following precautions when taking buprenorphine:

- Do not take other medications without first consulting your doctor.
- Do not use illegal drugs, drink alcohol, or take sedatives, tranquilizers, or other drugs that slow breathing. Mixing large amounts of other medications with buprenorphine can lead to overdose or death.
- Do ensure that a physician monitors any liver-related health issues that you may have.

Pregnant Or Breastfeeding Women And Buprenorphine

Limited information exists on the use of buprenorphine in women who are pregnant and have an opioid dependency. But the few case reports available have not demonstrated any significant problems resulting from use of buprenorphine during pregnancy. The FDA classifies buprenorphine products as Pregnancy Category C medications, indicating that the risk of adverse effects has not been ruled out. In the United States, methadone remains the current standard of care for the use of MAT with pregnant women who have opioid dependency.

Treatment With Buprenorphine

The ideal candidates for opioid dependency treatment with buprenorphine:

- Have been objectively diagnosed with an opioid dependency
- Are willing to follow safety precautions for the treatment
- Have been cleared of any health conflicts with using buprenorphine
- Have reviewed other treatment options before agreeing to buprenorphine treatment

Before buprenorphine treatment begins, policies and procedures should be in place to guarantee patient privacy and the confidentiality of personally identifiable health information. Under the Confidentiality Regulation, Code of Federal Regulations (CFR), information relating to substance use and alcohol treatment must be handled with a higher degree of confidentiality than other medical information.

Buprenorphine treatment happens in three phases:

1. **The Induction Phase** is the medically monitored startup of buprenorphine treatment performed in a qualified physician's office or certified OTP using approved buprenorphine products. The medication is administered when a person with an opioid dependency has abstained from using opioids for 12–24 hours and is in the early stages of opioid withdrawal. It is important to note that buprenorphine can bring on acute withdrawal for patents who are not in the early stages of withdrawal and who have other opioids in their bloodstream.

2. **The Stabilization Phase** begins after a patient has discontinued or greatly reduced their misuse of the problem drug, no longer has cravings, and experiences few, if any, side effects. The buprenorphine dose may need to be adjusted during this phase. Because of the long-acting agent of buprenorphine, once patients have been stabilized, they can sometimes switch to alternate-day dosing instead of dosing every day.

3. **The Maintenance Phase** occurs when a patient is doing well on a steady dose of buprenorphine. The length of time of the maintenance phase is tailored to each patient and could be indefinite. Once an individual is stabilized, an alternative approach would be to go into a medically supervised withdrawal, which makes the

transition from a physically dependent state smoother. People then can engage in further rehabilitation—with or without MAT—to prevent a possible relapse.

Treatment of opioid dependency with buprenorphine is most effective in combination with counseling services, which can include different forms of behavioral therapy and self-help programs.

What Should I Do If Someone I Know Needs Help?

If you, or a friend, are in crisis and need to speak with someone now:

- Call National Suicide Prevention Lifeline (NSPL) at 800-273-TALK (800-273-8255) (they don't just talk about suicide—they cover a lot of issues and will help put you in touch with someone close by)

If you need information on drug treatment and where you can find it, the Substance Abuse and Mental Health Services Administration (SAMHSA) can help.

- Call Substance Abuse Treatment Facility Locator at 800-662-HELP (800-662-4357)

- Visit the locator online at www.findtreatment.samhsa.gov

Part Seven
Other Drug-Related Health Concerns

Chapter 48

The Medical Consequences Of Drug Abuse

People who suffer from addiction often have one or more accompanying medical issues, which may include lung or cardiovascular disease (CVD), stroke, cancer, and mental disorders. Imaging scans, chest X-rays*, and blood tests show the damaging effects of long-term drug abuse throughout the body. For example, research has shown that tobacco smoke causes cancer of the mouth, throat, larynx, blood, lungs, stomach, pancreas, kidney, bladder, and cervix. In addition, some drugs of abuse, such as inhalants, are toxic to nerve cells and may damage or destroy them either in the brain or the peripheral nervous system (PNS).

A type of high-energy radiation used to diagnose diseases by making pictures of the inside of the body.

> Drug use can have a wide range of short- and long-term, direct and indirect effects. These effects often depend on the specific drug or drugs used, how they are taken, how much is taken, the person's health, and other factors.
>
> Short-term effects can range from changes in appetite, wakefulness, heart rate, blood pressure, and/or mood to heart attack, stroke, psychosis, overdose, and even death. These health effects may occur after just one use.
>
> Longer-term effects can include heart or lung disease, cancer, mental illness, human immunodeficiency virus (HIV) / acquired immunodeficiency syndrome (AIDS), hepatitis, and others.
>
> (Source: "Health Consequences Of Drug Misuse," National Institute on Drug Abuse (NIDA).)

About This Chapter: This chapter includes text excerpted from "Drugs, Brains, And Behavior—The Science Of Addiction," National Institute on Drug Abuse (NIDA), July 2014. Reviewed July 2018.

Does Drug Abuse Cause Mental Disorders, Or Vice Versa?

Drug abuse and mental illness often coexist. In some cases, mental disorders such as anxiety, depression, or schizophrenia may precede addiction; in other cases, drug abuse may trigger or exacerbate those mental disorders, particularly in people with specific vulnerabilities.

How Can Addiction Harm Other People?

Beyond the harmful consequences for the person with the addiction, drug abuse can cause serious health problems for others. Three of the more devastating and troubling consequences of addiction are:

Negative Effects Of Prenatal Drug Exposure On Infants And Children

A mother's abuse of heroin or prescription opioids during pregnancy can cause a withdrawal syndrome (called neonatal abstinence syndrome, or NAS) in her infant. It is also likely that some drug-exposed children will need educational support in the classroom to help them overcome what may be subtle deficits in developmental areas such as behavior, attention, and thinking. Ongoing research is investigating whether the effects of prenatal drug exposure on the brain and behavior extend into adolescence to cause developmental problems during that time period.

Negative Effects Of Secondhand Smoke

Secondhand tobacco smoke, also called environmental tobacco smoke (ETS), is a significant source of exposure to a large number of substances known to be hazardous to human health, particularly to children. According to the Surgeon General's Report, The Health Consequences of Involuntary Exposure to Tobacco Smoke, involuntary exposure to secondhand smoke increases the risks of heart disease and lung cancer in people who have never smoked by 25–30 percent and 20–30 percent, respectively.

Increased Spread Of Infectious Diseases

Injection of drugs such as heroin, cocaine, and methamphetamine currently accounts for about 12 percent of new acquired immunodeficiency syndrome (AIDS) cases. Injection drug use is also a major factor in the spread of hepatitis C, a serious, potentially fatal liver disease. Injection drug use is not the only way that drug abuse contributes to the spread of infectious diseases. All drugs of abuse cause some form of intoxication, which interferes with judgment and increases the likelihood of risky sexual behaviors. This, in turn, contributes to the spread of human immunodeficiency virus (HIV) / acquired immunodeficiency syndrome (AIDS), hepatitis B and C, and other sexually transmitted diseases (STDs).

What Are Some Effects Of Specific Abused Substances?

- **Nicotine** is an addictive stimulant found in cigarettes and other forms of tobacco. Tobacco smoke increases a user's risk of cancer, emphysema, bronchial disorders, and CVD. The mortality rate associated with tobacco addiction is staggering. Tobacco use killed approximately 100 million people during the 20th century, and, if current smoking trends continue, the cumulative death toll for this century has been projected to reach 1 billion.

- **Alcohol** consumption can damage the brain and most body organs. Areas of the brain that are especially vulnerable to alcohol-related damage are the cerebral cortex (largely responsible for our higher brain functions, including problem-solving and decision making), the hippocampus (important for memory and learning), and the cerebellum (important for movement coordination).

- **Marijuana** is the most commonly abused illegal substance. This drug impairs short-term memory and learning, the ability to focus attention, and coordination. It also increases heart rate, can harm the lungs, and can increase the risk of psychosis in those with an underlying vulnerability.

- **Prescription medications**, including opioid pain relievers (such as OxyContin® and Vicodin®), antianxiety sedatives (such as Valium® and Xanax®), and attention deficit hyperactivity disorder (ADHD) stimulants (such as Adderall® and Ritalin®), are commonly misused to self-treat for medical problems or abused for purposes of getting high or (especially with stimulants) improving performance. However, misuse or abuse of these drugs (that is, taking them other than exactly as instructed by a doctor and for the purposes prescribed) can lead to addiction and even, in some cases, death. Opioid pain relievers, for instance, are frequently abused by being crushed and injected or snorted, greatly raising the risk of addiction and overdose.

Unfortunately, there is a common misperception that because medications are pre-scribed by physicians, they are safe even when used illegally or by another person than they were prescribed for.

- **Inhalants** are volatile substances found in many household products, such as oven clean-ers, gasoline, spray paints, and other aerosols, that induce mind-altering effects; they are frequently the first drugs tried by children or young teens. Inhalants are extremely toxic and can damage the heart, kidneys, lungs, and brain. Even a healthy person can suffer heart failure and death within minutes of a single session of prolonged sniffing of an inhalant.

- **Cocaine** is a short-acting stimulant, which can lead users to take the drug many times in a single session (known as a "binge"). Cocaine use can lead to severe medical conse-quences related to the heart and the respiratory, nervous, and digestive systems.

- **Amphetamines**, including methamphetamine, are powerful stimulants that can pro-duce feelings of euphoria and alertness. Methamphetamine's effects are particularly long-lasting and harmful to the brain. Amphetamines can cause high body temperature and can lead to serious heart problems and seizures.

- **MDMA (3,4-methylenedioxymethamphetamine)**, also known as Ecstacy or "Molly," produces both stimulant and mind-altering effects. It can increase body temperature, heart rate, blood pressure, and heart-wall stress. MDMA may also be toxic to nerve cells.

- **Lysergic acid diethylamide (LSD)** is one of the most potent hallucinogenic, or percep-tion-altering, drugs. Its effects are unpredictable, and abusers may see vivid colors and images, hear sounds, and feel sensations that seem real but do not exist. Users also may have traumatic experiences and emotions that can last for many hours.

- **Heroin** is a powerful opioid drug that produces euphoria and feelings of relaxation. It slows respiration, and its use is linked to an increased risk of serious infectious diseases, especially when taken intravenously. People who become addicted to opioid pain reliev-ers sometimes switch to heroin instead, because it produces similar effects and may be cheaper or easier to obtain.

- **Steroids**, which can also be prescribed for certain medical conditions, are abused to increase muscle mass and to improve athletic performance or physical appearance. Seri-ous consequences of abuse can include severe acne, heart disease, liver problems, stroke, infectious diseases, depression, and suicide.

- **Drug combinations.** A particularly dangerous and common practice is the combining of two or more drugs. The practice ranges from the coadministration of legal drugs, like alcohol and nicotine, to the dangerous mixing of prescription drugs, to the deadly combination of heroin or cocaine with fentanyl (an opioid pain medication). Whatever the context, it is critical to realize that because of drug-drug interactions, such practices often pose significantly higher risks than the already harmful individual drugs.

Chapter 49

Mental And Substance Use Disorders

Mental and substance use disorders (SUDs) affect people from all walks of life and all age groups. These illnesses are common, recurrent, and often serious, but they are treatable and many people do recover. Learning about some of the most common mental and substance use disorders can help people recognize their signs and to seek help.

According to National Survey on Drug Use and Health (NSDUH), an estimated 43.6 million (18.1%) Americans ages 18 and up experienced some form of mental illness. In the past year, 20.2 million adults (8.4%) had a substance use disorder. Of these, 7.9 million people had both a mental disorder and substance use disorder, also known as co-occurring mental and substance use disorders. Various mental and substance use disorders have prevalence rates that differ by gender, age, race, and ethnicity.

Mental Disorders

Mental disorders involve changes in thinking, mood, and/or behavior. These disorders can affect how we relate to others and make choices. Mental disorders take many different forms, with some rooted in deep levels of anxiety, extreme changes in mood, or reduced ability to focus or behave appropriately. Others involve unwanted, intrusive thoughts and some may result in auditory and visual hallucinations or false beliefs about basic aspects of reality. Reaching a level that can be formally diagnosed often depends on a reduction in a person's ability to function as a result of the disorder.

Anxiety disorders are the most common type of mental disorders, followed by depressive disorders. Different mental disorders are more likely to begin and occur at different stages in

About This Chapter: This chapter includes text excerpted from "Mental And Substance Use Disorders," Substance Abuse and Mental Health Services Administration (SAMHSA), September 20, 2017.

life and are thus more prevalent in certain age groups. Lifetime anxiety disorders generally have the earliest age of first onset, most commonly around age 6. Other disorders emerge in childhood, approximately 11 percent of children 4–17 years of age (6.4 million) have been diagnosed with attention deficit hyperactivity disorder (ADHD) as of 2011. Schizophrenia spectrum and psychotic disorders emerge later in life, usually in early adulthood. Not all mental health issues first experienced during childhood or adolescence continue into adulthood, and not all mental health issues are first experienced before adulthood. Mental disorders can occur once, reoccur intermittently, or be more chronic in nature. Mental disorders frequently co-occur with each other and with substance use disorders. Because of this and because of variation in symptoms even within one type of disorder, individual situations and symptoms are extremely varied.

Serious Mental Illness

Serious mental illness among people ages 18 and older is defined at the federal level as having, at any time during the past year, a diagnosable mental, behavior, or emotional disorder that causes serious functional impairment that substantially interferes with or limits one or more major life activities. Serious mental illnesses include major depression, schizophrenia, and bipolar disorder, and other mental disorders that cause serious impairment. In 2014, there were an estimated 9.8 million adults (4.1%) ages 18 and up with a serious mental illness in the past year. People with serious mental illness are more likely to be unemployed, arrested, and/or face inadequate housing compared to those without mental illness.

Serious Emotional Disturbance (SED)

The term serious emotional disturbance is used to refer to children and youth who have had a diagnosable mental, behavioral, or emotional disorder in the past year, which resulted in functional impairment that substantially interferes with or limits the child's role or functioning in family, school, or community activities. A Centers for Disease Control and Prevention (CDC) review of population-level information found that estimates of the number of children with a mental disorder range from 13–20 percent, but current national surveys do not have an indicator of SED.

Substance Use Disorders

Substance use disorders (SUDs) occur when the recurrent use of alcohol and/or drugs causes clinically significant impairment, including health problems, disability, and failure to meet major responsibilities at work, school, or home. In 2014, about 21.5 million Americans ages 12 and older (8.1%) were classified with a substance use disorder in the past year. Of those, 2.6 million had problems with both alcohol and drugs, 4.5 million had problems with drugs but not alcohol, and 14.4 million had problems with alcohol only.

Alcohol Use Disorder (AUD)*

Excessive alcohol use can increase a person's risk of developing serious health problems in addition to those issues associated with intoxication behaviors and alcohol withdrawal symptoms. According to the Centers for Disease Control and Prevention (CDC), excessive alcohol use causes 88,000 deaths a year.

Many Americans begin drinking at an early age. In 2012, about 24 percent of eighth graders and 64 percent of twelfth graders used alcohol in the past year.

Excessive drinking can put you at risk of developing an alcohol use disorder (AUD) in addition to other health and safety problems. Genetics have also been shown to be a risk factor for the development of an AUD.

To be diagnosed with an AUD, individuals must meet certain diagnostic criteria. Some of these criteria include problems controlling intake of alcohol, continued use of alcohol despite problems resulting from drinking, development of a tolerance, drinking that leads to risky situations, or the development of withdrawal symptoms. The severity of an AUD—mild, moderate, or severe—is based on the number of criteria met.

Tobacco Use Disorder*

According to the CDC, more than 480,000 deaths each year are caused by cigarette smoking. Tobacco use and smoking do damage to nearly every organ in the human body, often leading to lung cancer, respiratory disorders, heart disease, stroke, and other illnesses.

In 2014, an estimated 66.9 million Americans aged 12 or older were current users of a tobacco product (25.2%). Young adults aged 18–25 had the highest rate of current use of a tobacco product (35%), followed by adults aged 26 or older (25.8%), and by youths aged 12–17 (7%).

In 2014, the prevalence of current use of a tobacco product was 37.8 percent for American Indians or Alaska Natives, 27.6 percent for whites, 26.6 percent for blacks, 30.6 percent for Native Hawaiians or other Pacific Islanders, 18.8 percent for Hispanics, and 10.2 percent for Asians.

Cannabis Use Disorder (CUD)*

Marijuana is the most-used drug after alcohol and tobacco in the United States. According to Substance Abuse and Mental Health Services Administration (SAMHSA) data:

- In 2014, about 22.2 million people ages 12 and up reported using marijuana during the past month.

- Also in 2014, there were 2.6 million people in that age range who had used marijuana for the first time within the past 12 months. People between the ages of 12 and 49 report first using the drug at an average age of 18.5.

In the past year, 4.2 million people ages 12 and up met criteria for a SUD based on marijuana use.

Marijuana's immediate effects include distorted perception, difficulty with thinking and problem solving, and loss of motor coordination. Long-term use of the drug can contribute to respiratory infection, impaired memory, and exposure to cancer-causing compounds. Heavy marijuana use in youth has also been linked to increased risk for developing mental illness and poorer cognitive functioning.

Some symptoms of cannabis use disorder include disruptions in functioning due to cannabis use, the development of tolerance, cravings for cannabis, and the development of withdrawal symptoms, such as the inability to sleep, restlessness, nervousness, anger, or depression within a week of ceasing heavy use.

Stimulant Use Disorder*

Stimulants increase alertness, attention, and energy, as well as elevate blood pressure, heart rate, and respiration. They include a wide range of drugs that have historically been used to treat conditions, such as obesity, attention deficit hyperactivity disorder and, occasionally, depression. Like other prescription medications, stimulants can be diverted for illegal use. The most commonly abused stimulants are amphetamines, methamphetamine, and cocaine. Stimulants can be synthetic (such as amphetamines) or can be plant-derived (such as cocaine). They are usually taken orally, snorted, or intravenously.

In 2014, an estimated 913,000 people ages 12 and older had a stimulant use disorder because of cocaine use, and an estimated 476,000 people had a stimulant use disorder as a result of using other stimulants besides methamphetamines. In 2014, almost 569,000 people in the United States ages 12 and up reported using methamphetamines in the past month.

Symptoms of stimulant use disorders include craving for stimulants, failure to control use when attempted, continued use despite interference with major obligations or social functioning, use of larger amounts over time, development of tolerance, spending a great deal of time to obtain and use stimulants, and withdrawal symptoms that occur after stopping or reducing use, including fatigue, vivid and unpleasant dreams, sleep problems, increased appetite, or irregular problems in controlling movement.

Hallucinogen Use Disorder*

Hallucinogens can be chemically synthesized (as with lysergic acid diethylamide or LSD) or may occur naturally (as with psilocybin mushrooms, peyote). These drugs can produce visual and auditory hallucinations, feelings of detachment from one's environment and oneself, and distortions in time and perception.

In 2014, approximately 246,000 Americans had a hallucinogen use disorder. Symptoms of hallucinogen use disorder include craving for hallucinogens, failure to control use when attempted, continued use despite interference with major obligations or social functioning, use of larger amounts over time, use in risky situations like driving, development of tolerance, and spending a great deal of time to obtain and use hallucinogens.

Opioid Use Disorder*

Opioids reduce the perception of pain but can also produce drowsiness, mental confusion, euphoria, nausea, constipation, and, depending upon the amount of drug taken, can depress respiration. Illegal opioid drugs, such as heroin and legally available pain relievers such as oxycodone and hydrocodone can cause serious health effects in those who misuse them. Some people experience a euphoric response to opioid medications, and it is common that people misusing opioids try to intensify their experience by snorting or injecting them. These methods increase their risk for serious medical complications, including overdose. Other users have switched from prescription opiates to heroin as a result of availability and lower price. Because of variable purity and other chemicals and drugs mixed with heroin on the black market, this also increases risk of overdose. Overdoses with opioid pharmaceuticals led to almost 17,000 deaths in 2011. Since 1999, opiate overdose deaths have increased 265 percent among men and 400 percent among women.

In 2014, an estimated 1.9 million people had an opioid use disorder related to prescription pain relievers and an estimated 586,000 had an opioid use disorder related to heroin use.

Symptoms of opioid use disorders include strong desire for opioids, inability to control or reduce use, continued use despite interference with major obligations or social functioning, use of larger amounts over time, development of tolerance, spending a great deal of time to obtain and use opioids, and withdrawal symptoms that occur after stopping or reducing use, such as negative mood, nausea or vomiting, muscle aches, diarrhea, fever, and insomnia.

Text excerpted from "Substance Use Disorders," Substance Abuse and Mental Health Services Administration (SAMHSA)

Co-Occurring Mental And Substance Use Disorders

The coexistence of both a mental health and a substance use disorder is referred to as co-occurring disorders. According to NSDUH, approximately 7.9 million adults had co-occurring disorders in 2014. During the past year, for those adults surveyed who experienced substance use disorders and any mental illness, rates were highest among adults ages 26–49 (42.7%). For adults with past-year serious mental illness and co-occurring substance use disorders, rates were highest among those ages 18–25 (35.3%) in 2014.

Co-Occurring Disorders*

Co-occurring disorders were previously referred to as dual diagnoses. According to Substance Abuse and Mental Health Services Administration's (SAMHSA) 2014 National Survey on Drug Use and Health (NSDUH), approximately 7.9 million adults in the United States had co-occurring disorders in 2014.

People with mental health disorders are more likely than people without mental health disorders to experience an alcohol or substance use disorder. Co-occurring disorders can be difficult to diagnose due to the complexity of symptoms, as both may vary in severity. In many cases, people receive treatment for one disorder while the other disorder remains untreated. This may occur because both mental and substance use disorders can have biological, psychological, and social components. Other reasons may be inadequate provider training or screening, an overlap of symptoms, or that other health issues need to be addressed first. In any case, the consequences of undiagnosed, untreated, or undertreated co-occurring disorders can lead to a higher likelihood of experiencing homelessness, incarceration, medical illnesses, suicide, or even early death.

People with co-occurring disorders are best served through integrated treatment. With integrated treatment, practitioners can address mental and substance use disorders at the same time, often lowering costs and creating better outcomes. Increasing awareness and building capacity in service systems are important in helping identify and treat co-occurring disorders. Early detection and treatment can improve treatment outcomes and the quality of life for those who need these services.

Text excerpted from "Co-Occurring Disorders," Substance Abuse and Mental Health Services Administration (SAMHSA)

Treatment For Co-Occurring Mental And Substance Use Disorders*

People with a mental disorder are more likely to experience a substance use disorder (SUD) and people with a SUD are more likely to have a mental disorder when compared with the general population. According to the National Survey of Substance Abuse Treatment Services (N-SSATS), about 45 percent of Americans seeking SUD treatment have been diagnosed as having a co-occurring mental and SUD.

SAMHSA supports an integrated treatment approach to treating co-occurring mental and SUDs. Integrated treatment requires collaboration across disciplines. Integrated treatment planning addresses both mental health and substance abuse, each in the context of the other disorder. Treatment planning should be client-centered, addressing clients' goals and using treatment strategies that are acceptable to them.

Integrated treatment or treatment that addresses mental and substance use conditions at the same time is associated with lower costs and better outcomes such as:

- Reduced substance use

- Improved psychiatric symptoms and functioning

- Decreased hospitalization

- Increased housing stability

- Fewer arrests

- Improved quality of life

Text excerpted from "Behavioral Health Treatments And Services," Substance Abuse and Mental Health Services Administration (SAMHSA)

Prevention Of Substance Abuse And Mental Illness

Mental and substance use disorders can have a powerful effect on the health of individuals, their families, and their communities. In 2014, an estimated 9.8 million adults aged 18 and older in the United States had a serious mental illness, and 1.7 million of which were aged 18 to 25. Also 15.7 million adults (aged 18 or older) and 2.8 million youth (aged 12–17) had a major depressive episode during the past year. In 2014, an estimated 22.5 million Americans aged 12 and older self-reported needing treatment for alcohol or illicit drug use, and 11.8 million adults self-reported needing mental health treatment or counseling in the past year. These disorders are among the top conditions that cause disability and carry a high burden of disease in the United States, resulting in significant costs to families, employers, and publicly funded health systems. By 2020, mental and substance use disorders will surpass all physical diseases as a major cause of disability worldwide.

In addition, drug and alcohol use can lead to other chronic diseases such as diabetes and heart disease. Addressing the impact of substance use alone is estimated to cost Americans more than $600 billion each year.

Preventing mental and/or substance use disorders and related problems in children, adolescents, and young adults is critical to Americans' behavioral and physical health. Behaviors and symptoms that signal the development of a behavioral disorder often manifest two to four years before a disorder is present. In addition, people with a mental health issue are more likely to use alcohol or drugs than those not affected by a mental illness. Results from the 2014 NSDUH report showed that of those adults with any mental illness, 18.2 percent had a substance use disorder, while those adults with no mental illness only had a 6.3 percent rate of substance use disorder in the past year. If communities and families can intervene early, behavioral health disorders might be prevented, or symptoms can be mitigated.

(Source: "Prevention Of Substance Abuse And Mental Illness," Substance Abuse and Mental Health Services Administration (SAMHSA).)

Chapter 50

Substance Abuse, Depression, And Suicide

Research has suggested that depressive symptoms are linked to the initiation of drug taking in adolescents. A study by researchers at the University of Southern California (USC) examined negative urgency—or acting rashly during periods of extreme negative emotion—as the mechanism linking depressive symptoms and substance abuse initiation.

Ninth-graders in two Los Angeles public high schools completed confidential surveys assessing negative urgency, depression levels, use of a variety of drugs, and other emotional health behaviors. Students' depressive symptom levels were found to be associated with lifetime use of cigarettes and other forms of tobacco, marijuana, alcohol, inhalants, and prescription painkillers, and negative urgency was linked to the adolescents' depression levels and age of first use and lifetime use of alcohol. These findings suggest that emotional vulnerability increases the likelihood of trying a variety of drugs in early adolescence. Interventions that target emotional coping mechanisms and the reduction of negative urgency may be useful in preventing early drug use, warranting further study.

Substance Use And Suicide

One of the reasons alcohol and/or drug misuse significantly affects suicide rates is the disinhibition that occurs when a person is intoxicated. Although less is known about the

About This Chapter: Text in this chapter begins with excerpts from "Depressive Symptoms And Drug Abuse In Adolescents," National Institute on Drug Abuse (NIDA), January 6, 2015; Text under the heading "Substance Use And Suicide" is excerpted from "Substance Use And Suicide: A Nexus Requiring A Public Health Approach," Substance Abuse and Mental Health Services Administration (SAMHSA), 2016; Text under the heading "Alcohol And Other Drug Abuse Increase Youth Suicide Rates" is excerpted from "Does Alcohol And Other Drug Abuse Increase The Risk For Suicide?" U.S. Department of Health and Human Services (HHS), May 7, 2008. Reviewed July 2018.

relationship between suicide risk and other drug use, the number of substances used seems to be more predictive of suicide than the types of substances used. However, the research on this subject is limited, and the relationship between drug misuse and suicide risk is even less developed. More research is needed on the association between different drugs, drug combinations, and self-medication on suicidal behavior.

Surveillance data nevertheless reveal that a diagnosis of alcohol misuse or dependence is associated with a suicide risk that is 10 times greater than the suicide risk in the general population, and individuals who inject drugs are at about 14 times greater risk for suicide.

Alcohol Use Amplifies Suicide Risk

- Between 40–60 percent of those who die by suicide are intoxicated at the time of death
- 18–66 percent who die by suicide have some alcohol in their blood at the time of death
- Middle- or older-aged alcoholics at greater risk than younger alcoholics
- Alcohol use disorders are a significant risk factor for "medically serious" suicide attempts
- 25–30 percent suicides are by those with a diagnosis of alcohol abuse or dependence
  - Among alcohol dependents, 7–15 percent individuals complete suicide
- Risk factors among alcoholics include:
  - Family history of alcoholism
  - Early onset of drinking and alcohol dependence
  - Higher alcohol intake

(Source: "Substance Use Disorders And Suicide," U.S. Department of Veterans Affairs (VA).)

Acute alcohol intoxication may substantially increase the risk of suicide by decreasing inhibitions and increasing depressed mood. The acute effects of alcohol intoxication act as important proximal risk factors for suicidal behavior among individuals with alcohol use disorders and those without. Mechanisms responsible for alcohol's ability to increase the proximal risk for suicidal behavior include alcohol's ability to:

1. increase psychological distress,

2. increase aggressiveness,

3. propel suicidal ideation into action through suicide-specific alcohol expectancies (e.g., alcohol may supply the motivation to complete the action, the user may believe that alcohol will assist in completing suicide painlessly), and

4. constrict cognition, which impairs the generation and implementation of alternative coping strategies.

Alcohol And Other Drug Abuse Increase Youth Suicide Rates

A number of national surveys have helped shed light on the relationship between alcohol and other drug use and suicidal behavior. A review of minimum-age drinking laws and suicides among youths age 18–20 found that lower minimum-age drinking laws were associated with higher youth suicide rates. In a large study following adults who drink alcohol, suicide ideation was reported among persons with depression. In another survey, persons who reported that they had made a suicide attempt during their lifetime were more likely to have had a depressive disorder, and many also had an alcohol and/or substance abuse disorder. In a study of all nontraffic injury deaths associated with alcohol intoxication, over 20 percent were suicides.

In studies that examine risk factors among people who have completed suicide, substance use and abuse occurs more frequently among youth and adults, compared to older persons. For particular groups at risk, such as American Indians and Alaskan Natives, depression and alcohol use and abuse are the most common risk factors for completed suicide. Alcohol and substance abuse problems contribute to suicidal behavior in several ways. Persons who are dependent on substances often have a number of other risk factors for suicide. In addition to being depressed, they are also likely to have social and financial problems. Substance use and abuse can be common among persons prone to be impulsive, and among persons who engage in many types of high-risk behaviors that result in self-harm. Fortunately, there are a number of effective prevention efforts that reduce risk for substance abuse in youth, and there are effective treatments for alcohol and substance use problems. Researchers are currently testing treatments specifically for persons with substance abuse problems who are also suicidal, or have attempted suicide in the past.

Chapter 51

Drug Use And Infectious Diseases

Drug use is linked to risky behaviors such as needle sharing and unsafe sex and can also weaken the immune system. This combination greatly increases the likelihood of contracting human immunodeficiency virus (HIV), hepatitis, and other infectious diseases.

Why Are Cocaine Users At Risk For Contracting HIV/AIDS And Hepatitis?

Drug intoxication and addiction can compromise judgment and decision making and potentially lead to risky sexual behavior, including trading sex for drugs, and needle sharing. This increases a cocaine user's risk for contracting infectious diseases such as human immunodeficiency virus (HIV) and hepatitis C (HCV). There are no vaccines to prevent HIV or HCV infections.

Studies that examine patterns of HIV infection and progression have demonstrated that cocaine use accelerates HIV infection. Research indicates that cocaine impairs immune cell function, promotes replication of the HIV virus, and potentiates the damaging effects of HIV on different types of cells in the brain and spinal cord, resulting in further damage. Studies also suggest that cocaine use accelerates the development of NeuroAIDS, neurological conditions associated with HIV infection. Symptoms of NeuroAIDS include memory loss, movement problems, and vision impairment.

Cocaine users with HIV often have advanced progression of the disease, with increased viral load and accelerated decreases in cluster of differentiation 4+ (CD4+) cell counts. Infection

About This Chapter: This chapter includes text excerpted from "HIV, Hepatitis, And Other Infectious Diseases," National Institute on Drug Abuse (NIDA), March 2017.

with HIV increases risk for coinfection with HCV, a virus that affects the liver. Coinfection can lead to serious illnesses—including problems with the immune system and neurologic conditions. Liver complications are very common, with many coinfected individuals dying of

New HIV Infections[a]

- In 2015, 6 percent (2,392) of the 39,513 diagnoses of HIV in the United States were attributed to IDU and another 3 percent (1,202) to male-to-male sexual contact[b] and IDU.

- Of the HIV diagnoses attributed to IDU in 2015,[c] 59 percent (1,412) were among men, and 41 percent (980) were among women.

- Of the HIV diagnoses attributed to IDU in 2015, 38 percent (901) were among blacks/African Americans, 40 percent (951) were among whites, and 19 percent (443) were among Hispanics/Latinos.[d]

- If current rates continue, 1 in 23 women who inject drugs and 1 in 36 men who inject drugs will be diagnosed with HIV in their lifetime.

- Of the 18,303 AIDS diagnoses in 2015, 10 percent (1,804) were attributed to IDU, and another 4 percent (761) were attributed to male-to-male sexual contact and IDU.

Living With HIV

- At the end of 2013, an estimated 103,100 men in the United States were living with HIV attributed to IDU. Of these, 5 percent were undiagnosed. An estimated 68,200 women were living with HIV attributed to IDU, and 5 percent were undiagnosed.

- Among PWID who were diagnosed with HIV in 2014, 82 percent of males and 83 percent of females were linked to care within 3 months.[e]

- Among PWID diagnosed with HIV in 2012 or earlier, 49 percent of males and 56 percent of females were retained in HIV care at the end of 2013.[e]

[a]HIV and AIDS diagnoses indicate when a person is diagnosed with HIV or AIDS, not when the person was infected.

[b]The term male-to-male sexual contact is used in CDC surveillance systems to indicate a behavior that transmits HIV infection, not how individuals self-identify in terms of their sexuality.

[c]Unless otherwise indicated, the numbers include infections attributed to IDU only, not those attributed to IDU and male-to-male sexual contact.

[d]Hispanics/Latinos can be of any race.

[e]Based on 32 states and the District of Columbia (the areas with complete lab reporting by December 2015).

(Source: "HIV And Injection Drug Use," Centers for Disease Control and Prevention (CDC).)

chronic liver disease and cancer. Although the link between injection drug use and HIV/HCV is well established, more studies are needed to understand the molecular mechanisms underlying this increased risk of coinfection in noninjecting substance users.

The interaction of substance use, HIV, and hepatitis may accelerate disease progression. For example, HIV speeds the course of HCV infection by accelerating the progression of hepatitis-associated liver disease. Research has linked HIV/HCV coinfection with increased mortality when compared to either infection alone. Substance use and coinfection likely negatively influence HIV disease progression and the ability of the body to marshal an immune response.

Patients with HIV/HCV coinfection can benefit from substance abuse treatment and antiretroviral therapies, when closely monitored. Antiretroviral treatment is not effective for everyone and can have significant side effects, necessitating close medical supervision. Testing for HIV and HCV is recommended for any individual who has ever injected drugs, since the disease is highly transmissible via injection.

Why Does Heroin Use Create Special Risk For Contracting HIV/AIDS And Hepatitis B And C (HBV/HCV)?

Heroin use increases the risk of being exposed to HIV, viral hepatitis, and other infectious agents through contact with infected blood or body fluids (e.g., semen, saliva) that results from the sharing of syringes and injection paraphernalia that have been used by infected individuals or through unprotected sexual contact with an infected person. Snorting or smoking does not eliminate the risk of infectious disease like hepatitis and HIV/AIDS because people under the influence of drugs still engage in risky sexual and other behaviors that can expose them to these diseases.

People who inject drugs (PWIDs) are the highest risk group for acquiring hepatitis C (HCV) infection and continue to drive the escalating HCV epidemic. Each PWID infected with HCV is likely to infect 20 other people. Of the 30,500 new HCV infections occurring in the United States in 2014, most cases occurred among PWID.

Hepatitis B (HBV) infection in PWIDs was reported to be as high as 25 percent in the United States in 2014, which is particularly disheartening since an effective vaccine that protects against HBV infection is available. There is currently no vaccine available to protect against HCV infection.

Drug use, viral hepatitis and other infectious diseases, mental illnesses, social dysfunctions, and stigma are often co-occurring conditions that affect one another, creating more complex health challenges that require comprehensive treatment plans tailored to meet all of a patient's needs. For example, National Institute on Drug Abuse (NIDA)-funded research has found that substance use disorder treatment, along with HIV prevention and community-based outreach programs, can help people who use drugs change the behaviors that put them at risk for contracting HIV and other infectious diseases. They can reduce drug use and drug-related risk behaviors such as needle sharing and unsafe sexual practices and, in turn, reduce the risk of exposure to HIV/AIDS and other infectious diseases.

Are People Who Abuse Methamphetamine At Risk For Contracting HIV/AIDS And Hepatitis B And C?

Methamphetamine abuse raises the risk of contracting or transmitting HIV and hepatitis B and C—not only for individuals who inject the drug but also for noninjecting methamphetamine abusers. Among injecting drug users, HIV and other infectious diseases are spread primarily through the reuse or sharing of contaminated syringes, needles, or related paraphernalia. But regardless of how methamphetamine is taken, its intoxicating effects can alter judgment and inhibition and lead people to engage in unsafe behaviors like unprotected sex.

Methamphetamine abuse is associated with a culture of risky sexual behavior, both among men who have sex with men and in heterosexual populations, a link that may be attributed to the fact that methamphetamine and related stimulants can increase libido. (Although paradoxically, long-term methamphetamine abuse may be associated with decreased sexual functioning, at least in men.) The combination of injection practices and sexual risk-taking may result in HIV becoming a greater problem among methamphetamine abusers than among other drug abusers, and some epidemiologic reports are already showing this trend. For example, while the link between HIV infection and methamphetamine abuse has not yet been established for heterosexuals, data show an association between methamphetamine abuse and the spread of HIV among men who have sex with men.

Methamphetamine abuse may also worsen the progression of HIV disease and its consequences. In animal studies, methamphetamine has been shown to increase viral replication. Clinical studies in humans suggest that current methamphetamine users taking highly active antiretroviral therapy (HAART) to treat HIV may be at greater risk of developing AIDS than nonusers, possibly as a result of poor medication adherence. Methamphetamine abusers with HIV also have shown greater neuronal injury and cognitive impairment due to HIV, compared with those who do not abuse the drug.

NIDA-funded research has found that, through drug abuse treatment, prevention, and community-based outreach programs, drug abusers can change their HIV risk behaviors. Drug abuse and drug-related risk behaviors, such as needle sharing and unsafe sexual practices, can be reduced significantly, thus decreasing the risk of exposure to HIV and other infectious diseases. Therefore, drug abuse treatment is HIV prevention.

Steroids And Other Appearance And Performance Enhancing Drugs (APEDs) And Hepatitis And HIV Risks

Appearance and performance enhancing drugs (APEDs) are most often used by males to improve appearance by building muscle mass or to enhance athletic performance. Although they may, directly and indirectly, have effects on a user's mood, they do not produce a euphoric high, which makes APEDs distinct from other drugs such as cocaine, heroin, and marijuana. However, users may develop a substance use disorder, defined as continued use despite adverse consequences.

Anabolic-androgenic steroids (AAS), the best studied class of APEDs (and the main subject of this report) can boost a user's confidence and strength, leading users to overlook the severe, long lasting, and in some cases, irreversible damage they can cause. They can lead to early heart attacks, strokes, liver tumors, kidney failure, and psychiatric problems. In addition, stopping use can cause depression, often leading to resumption of use. Because steroids are often injected, users who share needles or use nonsterile injecting techniques are also at risk

Public health strategies are important to prevent the spread of disease among persons who use drugs. For example, outreach programs, in the community and on the streets, make available to persons who use drugs prevention and risk reduction, testing, and referral services. Recommended approaches, immunizations, and screening, can protect the health of a person who uses drugs through medical interventions, while evidence-based behavioral interventions help prevent sexual and injection transmission by addressing risky behaviors.

(Source: "Strategies For Disease Prevention," Centers for Disease Control and Prevention (CDC).)

for contracting dangerous infections such as viral hepatitis and HIV. Steroids are popularly associated with doping by elite athletes, but since the 1980s, their use by male nonathlete weightlifters has exceeded their use by competitive athletes. Their use is closely associated with disordered male body image—most specifically, muscle dysmorphia.

Chapter 52

Substance Abuse And Sexual Health

According to the Surgeon General's Report "Facing Addiction in America," the misuse of substances such as alcohol and drugs is a growing problem in the United States. Although substance misuse can occur at any age, the teenage and young adult years are particularly critical at-risk periods. Research shows that the majority of adults who meet the criteria for having a substance use disorder (SUD) started using substances during their teen and young adult years. Teen substance use is also associated with sexual risk behaviors that put young people at risk for human immunodeficiency virus (HIV), sexually transmitted diseases (STDs), and pregnancy. To address these issues, more needs to be done to lessen risks and increase protective factors for teens.

What We Know

Studies conducted among teens have identified an association between substance use and sexual risk behaviors such as ever having sex, having multiple sex partners, not using a condom, and pregnancy before the age of 15 years of age. Researchers have found that as the frequency of substance use increases, the likelihood of sex and the number of sex partners also increases. In addition, studies show that sexual risk behaviors increase in teens who use alcohol, and are highest among students who use marijuana, cocaine, prescription drugs (such as sedatives, opioids, and stimulants), and other illicit drugs. Teens who reported no substance use are the least likely to engage in sexual risk-taking. According to the National Youth Risk Behavior Survey

About This Chapter: Text in this chapter begins with excerpts from "Substance Use And Sexual Risk Behaviors Among Teens," Centers for Disease Control and Prevention (CDC), April 14, 2017; Text under the heading "Date Rape Drugs" is excerpted from "What Are Date Rape Drugs And How Do You Avoid Them?" National Institute on Drug Abuse (NIDA) for Teens, March 16, 2015.

(YRBS), 41 percent of high school students have ever had intercourse and 30 percent of high school students are currently sexually active. Of the students who are currently sexually active, 21 percent drank alcohol or used drugs before last sexual intercourse.

Fast Facts

- Of the students who are currently sexually active, 21 percent drank alcohol or used drugs before last sexual intercourse

- 30 percent of high school students are currently sexually active

- 41 percent of high school students have ever had intercourse

---

Risk Factors And Prevention Activities

Substance use and sexual risk behaviors share some common underlying factors that may predispose teens to these behaviors. Because substance use clusters with other risk behaviors, it is important to learn whether precursors can be determined early to help identify youth who are most at risk. Primary prevention approaches that are most effective are those that address common risk factors. Prevention programs for substance use and sexual risk behaviors should include a focus on individuals, peers, families, schools, and communities. When students' school environments are supportive and their parents are engaged in their lives, they are less likely to use alcohol and drugs and engage in sexual behaviors that put them at risk for HIV, STDs, or pregnancy.

Substance use is associated with behaviors that put teens at risk for HIV, STDs, and pregnancy

Common risk factors for substance use and sexual risk behaviors include:

- Extreme economic deprivation (poverty, overcrowding)

- Family history of the problem behavior, family conflict, and family management problems

- Favorable parental attitudes towards the problem behavior and/or parental involvement in the problem behavior

- Lack of positive parent engagement

- Association with substance using peers

- Alienation and rebelliousness

- Lack of school connectedness

For primary prevention activities targeting substance use and sexual risk behaviors to be effective, they should include:

- School-based programs that promote social and emotional competence

- Peer-led drug and alcohol resistance programs

- Parenting skills training

- Parent engagement

- Family support programs

What Centers For Disease Control And Prevention Is Doing

The Centers for Disease Control and Prevention (CDC) is engaging in a variety of efforts to develop strategies to combat substance use and sexual risk behaviors among teens. Some efforts include:

- Conducting further analysis of existing data from the YRBS, School Health Policies and Practices Study (SHPPS), and School Health Profiles (Profiles).

- Improving YRBS questions pertaining to prescription opioids and other substances.

- Conducting a three-year demonstration project called Teens Linked to Care (TLC). The project is supported by the Hilton Foundation and the CDC Foundation, and assesses the ability of rural communities to integrate substance use prevention and sexual risk prevention program activities in school-based settings.

- Researching the topic of teen substance use and its association with a variety of risks and behaviors.

- Conducting an analysis of local and state policies on teen substance use prevention.

Date Rape Drugs

You may have been warned that sometimes people secretly slip drugs into other people's drinks to take advantage of them sexually. These drugs are called "date rape drugs." Date rape, also known as "drug-facilitated sexual assault," is any type of sexual activity that a person does not agree to. It may come from someone you know, someone may have just met, and/or someone thought you could trust.

Date rape drugs can make people become physically weak or pass out. This is why people who want to rape someone use them—because they leave individuals unable to protect themselves. Many of these drugs have no color, smell, or taste, and people often do not know that they've taken anything. Many times people who have been drugged (usually girls or women, but not always) are unable to remember what happened to them.

The Dangerous Three

The three most common date rape drugs are Rohypnol® (flunitrazepam), GHB (gamma-hydroxybutyric acid), and ketamine.

1. **Rohypnol** (also known as roofies, forget-me-pill, and R-2) is a type of prescription pill known as a benzodiazepine—it's chemically similar to drugs such as Valium or Xanax, but unlike these drugs, it is not approved for medical use in this country.

   • It has no taste or smell and is sometimes colorless when dissolved in a drink.

   • People who take it can feel very sleepy and confused and forget what happens after its effects kick in.

   • It can also cause weakness and trouble breathing, and can make it difficult for those who have taken it to move their body.

   • The effects of Rohypnol can be felt within 30 minutes of being drugged and can last for several hours.

   • To prevent misuse of Rohypnol, the manufacturer changed the pill to look like an oblong olive green tablet with a speckled blue core. When dissolved in light-colored drinks, the new pills dye the liquid blue and alert people that their drink has been tampered with. Unfortunately, generic versions of Rohypnol may not contain the blue dye.

2. **GHB** (also known as cherry meth, scoop, and goop) is a type of drug that acts as a central nervous system (CNS) depressant and is prescribed for the treatment of narcolepsy (a sleep disorder).

   • It can cause a person to throw up; it can also slow their heart rate and make it hard to breathe.

   • At high doses, it can result in a coma or death.

   • It's a tasteless, odorless drug that can be a powder or liquid. It's colorless when dissolved in a drink.

- Mixing it with alcohol makes these effects worse.

- GHB can take effect in 15–30 minutes, and the effects may last for 3–6 hours.

3. **Ketamine** (also known as cat valium, k-hole, and purple) is a dissociative anesthetic. That means it distorts perceptions of sight and sound, and makes a person feel detached from their environment and themselves. It also reduces pain and overall feeling. Like other anesthetic drugs, it's used during surgical procedures in both humans and animals.

- It's a tasteless, odorless drug that can be a powder or liquid.

- It can cause hallucinations and make people feel totally out of it.

- It can also increase heartbeat, raise blood pressure, and cause nausea.

- The effects of ketamine may last for 30–60 minutes.

All Drugs Lower Your Defenses

It's important to remember that all drugs affect how well your mind and body operate. In fact, alcohol is linked to far more date rapes than the drugs we've mentioned here. And nearly all drugs of abuse make people vulnerable to being taken advantage of—by impairing their judgment, reducing their reaction time, and clouding their thinking. And as disgusting as it is to think about, when you don't have your wits about you, someone may take that as an opportunity to push themselves on you.

How Can You Avoid Date Rape Drugs?

If you're at a party where people are drinking alcohol, you should be aware that there could be predators hoping to make you drunk or vulnerable. No matter what you're drinking, even if it's soda or juice, people can slip drugs in your drinks—so pour all drinks yourself and never leave them unattended (even if you have to take them into the bathroom with you). Also, be sure to stick with your friends. There's safety in numbers. But even if you leave your drink or leave your friends behind, know this for certain: if you are drugged and taken advantage of, it's not your fault. People who date rape other people are committing a crime.

Chapter 53

Substance Abuse And Pregnancy

When you are pregnant, you are not just "eating for two." You also breathe and drink for two, so it is important to carefully consider what you give to your baby. If you smoke, use alcohol or take illegal drugs, so does your unborn baby. First, don't smoke. Smoking during pregnancy passes nicotine and cancer-causing drugs to your baby. Smoke also keeps your baby from getting nourishment and raises the risk of stillbirth or premature birth. Don't drink alcohol. There is no known safe amount of alcohol a woman can drink while pregnant. Alcohol can

---

Risks Of Stillbirth From Substance Use In Pregnancy

- Tobacco use—1.8 to 2.8 times greater risk of stillbirth, with the highest risk found among the heaviest smokers

- Marijuana use—2.3 times greater risk of stillbirth

- Evidence of any stimulant, marijuana, or prescription pain reliever use—2.2 times greater risk of stillbirth

- Passive exposure to tobacco—2.1 times greater risk of stillbirth

(Source: "Substance Use In Women," National Institute on Drug Abuse (NIDA).)

About This Chapter: Text in this chapter begins with excerpts from "Pregnancy And Substance Abuse," MedlinePlus, National Institutes of Health (NIH), January 3, 2017; Text under the heading "Substance Use While Pregnant And Breastfeeding" is excerpted from "Substance Use In Women," National Institute on Drug Abuse (NIDA), June 2018; Text under the heading "Unique Needs Of Pregnant Women With Substance Use Disorders (SUDs)" is excerpted from "Principles Of Drug Addiction Treatment: A Research-Based Guide (Third Edition)," National Institute on Drug Abuse (NIDA), January 2018.

cause lifelong physical and behavioral problems in children, including fetal alcohol syndrome (FAS). Don't use illegal drugs. Using illegal drugs may cause underweight babies, birth defects, or withdrawal symptoms after birth. If you are pregnant and you smoke, drink alcohol or do drugs, get help. Your healthcare provider can recommend programs to help you quit. You and your baby will be better off.

Substance Use While Pregnant And Breastfeeding

Substance use during pregnancy can be risky to the woman's health and that of her children in both the short and long term. Use of some substances can increase the risk of miscarriage and can cause migraines, seizures, or high blood pressure in the mother, which may affect the baby. In addition, the risk of stillbirth is two to three times greater in women who smoke tobacco or marijuana, take prescription pain relievers, or use illegal drugs during pregnancy. In one study of dispensaries, nonmedical personnel at marijuana dispensaries were recommending marijuana to pregnant women for nausea, but medical experts warn against it. Given the risks some substances may have on the unborn baby, it is important for the women to ask their doctor or pharmacist about any medicines they use or plan on using.

When a woman uses substances regularly during pregnancy, the baby may go through withdrawal after birth, a condition called neonatal abstinence syndrome (NAS). Research has shown that NAS can occur with a pregnant woman's use of opioids, alcohol, caffeine, and some prescription sedatives. The type and severity of a baby's withdrawal symptoms depend on the drug(s) used, how long and how often the mother used, how her body breaks down the drug, and if the baby was born full term or prematurely.

Also, substance use by the pregnant mother can lead to long-term and even fatal effects, including:

- Low birth weight

- Birth defects

- Small head size

- Premature birth

- Sudden infant death syndrome

- Developmental delays

- Problems with learning, memory, and emotional control

Some substances, such as marijuana, alcohol, nicotine, and certain medicines, can be found in breast milk. However, little is known about the long-term effects on a child who is exposed to these substances through the mother's milk. Scientists do know that teens who use drugs while their brains are still developing could be damaging their brain's learning abilities. Therefore, similar risks for brain problems could exist for drug-exposed babies. Given the potential of all drugs to affect a baby's developing brain, women who are breastfeeding should talk with a healthcare provider about all of their substance use.

Unique Needs Of Pregnant Women With Substance Use Disorders (SUDs)

Using drugs, alcohol, or tobacco during pregnancy exposes not just the woman but also her developing fetus to the substance and can have potentially deleterious and even long-term effects on exposed children. Smoking during pregnancy can increase risk of stillbirth, infant mortality, sudden infant death syndrome (SIDS), preterm birth, respiratory problems, slowed fetal growth, and low birth weight. Drinking during pregnancy can lead to the child developing fetal alcohol spectrum disorders (FASDs), characterized by low birth weight and enduring cognitive and behavioral problems.

Symptoms of drug withdrawal in a newborn can develop immediately or up to 14 days after birth and can include:

• Blotchy skin coloring	• Rapid breathing
• Diarrhea	• Increased heart rate
• Excessive or high-pitched crying	• Seizures
• Abnormal sucking reflex	• Sleep problems
• Fever	• Slow weight gain
• Hyperactive reflexes	• Stuffy nose and sneezing
• Increased muscle tone	• Sweating
• Irritability	• Trembling
• Poor feeding	• Vomiting

(Source: "Substance Use In Women," National Institute on Drug Abuse (NIDA).)

Prenatal use of some drugs, including opioids, may cause a withdrawal syndrome in newborns called neonatal abstinence syndrome (NAS). Babies with NAS are at greater risk of seizures, respiratory problems, feeding difficulties, low birth weight, and even death. Research has established the value of evidence-based treatments for pregnant women (and their babies), including medications. For example, although no medications have been U.S. Food and Drug Administration (FDA)-approved to treat opioid dependence in pregnant women, methadone maintenance combined with prenatal care and a comprehensive drug treatment program can improve many of the detrimental outcomes associated with untreated heroin abuse. However, newborns exposed to methadone during pregnancy still require treatment for withdrawal symptoms. Another medication option for opioid dependence, buprenorphine, has been shown to produce fewer NAS symptoms in babies than methadone, resulting in shorter infant hospital stays. In general, it is important to closely monitor women who are trying to quit drug use during pregnancy and to provide treatment as needed.

Chapter 54

Substance Abuse And Military Families

Active-duty and retired members of the armed forces are not immune to the substance use problems that affect the rest of society. The stresses of deployment during wartime and the unique culture of the military account for some differences between substance use in military members and civilians. Zero-tolerance policies and stigma pose difficulties in identifying and treating substance use problems in military personnel, as does lack of confidentiality that deters many who need treatment from seeking it.

Those with multiple deployments, combat exposure, and related injuries are at greatest risk of developing substance use problems. They are more apt to engage in new-onset heavy weekly drinking and binge drinking, to suffer alcohol- and drug-related problems, and start smoking or relapse to smoking. Like civilians, they risk addiction to opioid pain medicines prescribed after an injury. The National Institute of Drug Abuse (NIDA) continues to examine the trends in substance use in specific populations, including military personnel, and search for better methods for preventing and treating substance use disorders that are specific to these populations.

About This Chapter: Text in this chapter begins with excerpts from "Military," National Institute on Drug Abuse (NIDA), April 2016; Text beginning with the heading "Substance Use Disorders (SUDs) In The U.S. Department Of Veterans Affairs (VA) And The U.S. Department Of Defense (DoD)" is excerpted from "VA/DoD Clinical Practice Guideline For The Management Of Substance Use Disorders," U.S. Department of Veterans Affairs (VA), December 2015; Text under the heading "Homelessness Among Veterans In Substance Abuse Treatment" is excerpted from "Twenty-One Percent Of Veterans In Substance Abuse Treatment Were Homeless," Substance Abuse and Mental Health Services Administration (SAMHSA), January 7, 2014. Reviewed July 2018.

Substance Use Disorders (SUDs) In The U.S. Department Of Veterans Affairs (VA) And The U.S. Department of Defense (DoD)

Substance use disorders (SUDs) commonly co-occurs with and complicates other conditions or issues. These conditions or issues maybe health-related, such as other mental health conditions, or may be societal, such as homelessness, criminal justice involvement, or unemployment. For instance, among veterans with posttraumatic stress disorder (PTSD), co-occurring SUD was common and found to be associated with an increase in mortality. The association was especially pronounced for young veterans, including those who served in Iraq and Afghanistan.

Furthermore, it was found that roughly 33 percent and 22 percent of homeless veterans had spent money on alcohol and drugs, respectively, in the past month; however, there was no significant association found between the source of income (e.g., VA disability compensation) and the amount spent on alcohol and drugs. Among Iraq or Afghanistan veterans who were first-time users of U.S. Department of Veterans Affairs (VA) healthcare between October 15, 2001, and September 30, 2009, and followed through January 1, 2010, SUD diagnoses were associated with being male, less than 25 years of age, and exposed to combat. Of those with an SUD diagnosis, 55–75 percent also received diagnoses for PTSD or depression.

- There are an estimated 23.4 million veterans in the United States, and about 2.2 million military service members and 3.1 million immediate family members.
- Approximately 50 percent of returning service members who need treatment for mental health conditions seek it, but only slightly more than half who receive treatment receive adequate care.
- Between 2004 and 2006, 7.1 percent of U.S. veterans met the criteria for a substance use disorder.
- The Army suicide rate reached an all-time high in 2012.
- In the 5 years from 2005–2009, more than 1,100 members of the Armed Forces took their own lives, an average of 1 suicide every 36 hours.
- Mental and substance use disorders caused more hospitalizations among U.S. troops in 2009 than any other cause.

(Source: "Veterans And Military Families," Substance Abuse and Mental Health Services Administration (SAMHSA).)

Management Of Substance Use Disorders In The U.S. Department of Defense Healthcare Settings

The U.S. Department of Defense (DoD) substance abuse programs are command and medical programs that emphasize readiness and personal responsibility. These programs are designed to provide services which are proactive and responsive to the needs of the DoD workforce by emphasizing alcohol and other substance abuse deterrence, prevention, education, and rehabilitation. The implementation of alcohol and other substance risk reduction and prevention strategies are designed to provide effective alcohol and other substance abuse prevention and education at all levels of command, and encourage commanders to provide alcohol and drug-free leisure activities. The ultimate goal of DoD substance use programs is to improve readiness and to restore to duty those substance-impaired service members who have the potential for continued military service.

In the DoD, active-duty service members who are involved in the abuse of alcohol or use of illicit substances are encouraged to voluntarily refer themselves for care and treatment to a substance use program. However, if a service member screens positive for the use of illicit drugs during a mandatory unit urinalysis, regulations require that the service member enroll into a substance abuse program and be processed for possible separation from the military. The service member's commander intervenes early for all personnel assigned to his/her command suspected of being alcohol and/or substance abusers. Service members, who fail to participate adequately in substance use programs or to respond successfully to rehabilitation, may be faced with administrative separation from the military.

After enrollment into substance abuse programs, all active-duty service members will have a treatment team convene with the patient, clinician, and command representative to review the treatment plan and goals. Recognizing the importance of medical readiness, the Health Insurance Portability and Accountability Act (HIPAA) specifically exempts some communication between clinicians and commanders. Regulations require that active-duty personnel enrolled in rehabilitation and referral services have an individualized aftercare plan designed to identify the continued support of the patient with monthly monitoring (minimally) during the first year after in a patient treatment.

Homelessness Among Veterans In Substance Abuse Treatment

U.S. military veterans are a large portion of homeless adults. There is a possibility that the number of homeless veterans may grow as the total number of veterans increases due to military conflicts. One challenge faced by many homeless veterans is substance abuse. About 70 percent of homeless veterans have a substance abuse problem. Homelessness among substance-abusing veterans can be a barrier to treatment. Targeting homeless veterans in need of treatment so that they can receive support through outreach services, case management, and housing assistance can improve their chances of entering treatment and experiencing positive treatment outcomes.

Chapter 55

Substance Abuse And Violence

What Is The Relation Between Drugs And Gangs?

Street gangs, outlaw motorcycle gangs (OMGs), and prison gangs are the primary distributors of illegal drugs on the streets of the United States. Gangs also smuggle drugs into the United States and produce and transport drugs within the country. Street gang members convert powdered cocaine into crack cocaine and produce most of the phencyclidine (PCP) available in the United States. Gangs, primarily OMGs, also produce marijuana and methamphetamine. In addition, gangs increasingly are involved in smuggling large quantities of cocaine and marijuana and lesser quantities of heroin, methamphetamine, and 3,4-methylenedioxymethamphetamine (MDMA), also known as ecstasy, into the United States from foreign sources of supply. Gangs primarily transport and distribute powdered cocaine, crack cocaine, heroin, marijuana, methamphetamine, MDMA, and PCP in the United States.

Located throughout the country, street gangs vary in size, composition, and structure. Large, nationally affiliated street gangs pose the greatest threat because they smuggle, produce, transport, and distribute large quantities of illicit drugs throughout the country and are extremely violent. Local street gangs in rural, suburban, and urban areas pose a low but growing threat. Local street gangs transport and distribute drugs within very specific areas. These gangs often imitate the larger, more powerful national gangs in order to gain respect from rivals.

Some gangs collect millions of dollars per month selling illegal drugs, trafficking weapons, operating prostitution rings, and selling stolen property. Gangs launder proceeds by investing

About This Chapter: Text beginning with the heading "What Is The Relation Between Drugs And Gangs?" is excerpted from "Drugs And Gangs Fast Facts," U.S. Department of Justice (DOJ), July 1, 2009. Reviewed July 2018; Text under the heading "Drugs And Love And Violence" is excerpted from "Love And Drugs And Violence," National Institute on Drug Abuse (NIDA) for Teens, February 16, 2016.

in real estate, recording studios, motorcycle shops, and construction companies. They also operate various cash-based businesses, such as barbershops, music stores, restaurants, catering services, tattoo parlors, and strip clubs, in order to commingle drug proceeds with funds generated through legitimate commerce.

What Is The Extent Of Gang Operation And Crime In The United States?

There are at least 21,500 gangs and more than 731,000 active gang members in the United States. Gangs conduct criminal activity in all 50 states and U.S. territories. Although most gang activity is concentrated in major urban areas, gangs also are proliferating in rural and suburban areas of the country as gang members flee increasing law enforcement pressure in urban areas or seek more lucrative drug markets. This proliferation in nonurban areas increasingly is accompanied by violence and is threatening society in general.

According to a U.S. Department of Justice (DOJ) survey, 20 percent of students aged 12 through 18 reported that street gangs had been present at their school during the previous 6 months. More than a quarter (28%) of students in urban schools reported a street gang presence, and 18 percent of students in suburban schools and 13 percent in rural schools reported the presence of street gangs. Public schools reported a much higher percentage of gang presence than private schools.

What Are The Dangers Associated With Gang Activity?

Large street gangs readily employ violence to control and expand drug distribution activities, targeting rival gangs and dealers who neglect or refuse to pay extortion fees. Members also use violence to ensure that members adhere to the gang's code of conduct or to prevent a member from leaving. In November 2004, a 19-year-old gang member in Fort Worth, Texas, was sentenced to 30 years in prison for fatally shooting a childhood friend who wanted to leave their local street gang. Authorities throughout the country report that gangs are responsible for most of the serious violent crime in the major cities of the United States. Gangs engage in an array of criminal activities including assault, burglary, drive-by shooting, extortion, homicide, identification fraud, money laundering, prostitution operations, robbery, sale of stolen property, and weapons trafficking.

What Are Some Signs That Young People May Be Involved In Gang Activity?

Changes in behavior such as skipping school, hanging out with different friends or, in certain places, spray-painting graffiti and using hand signals with friends can indicate gang affiliation. In addition, individuals who belong to gangs often dress alike by wearing clothing of the same color, wearing bandannas, or even rolling up their pant legs in a certain way. Some gang members wear certain designer labels to show their gang affiliation. Gang members often have

---

Dating violence is controlling, abusive, and aggressive behavior in a romantic relationship. It can happen in straight or gay relationships. It can include verbal, emotional, physical, or sexual abuse, or a combination.

The researchers found that teens treated in the emergency department for an injury related to dating violence were more likely to be girls than boys. There were also differences in the types of drugs used before a dating violence incident versus nondating violence incidents.

For example, some youth tended to use alcohol alone or in combination with marijuana just before a nondating violence incident occurred and tended to abuse prescription sedatives (Xanax or Valium) and/or opioids (like Vicodin and OxyContin) before a dating violence incident occurred.

This study tells us that the drug of choice may be different for boys and girls, and that girls are more likely than boys to experience dating violence. The drugs used may also be different depending on the situation (for example, being at home versus being at a bar or club). But more research is needed to learn how different drugs may make us more or less aggressive or more likely to be the victim of someone else who is using drugs or alcohol. Understanding more about this, and how gender and substance use factor into dating violence (and nondating violence), will help public health educators develop programs to help teens who may end up in violent situations.

(Source: "Drug Use And Violence: An Unhappy Relationship," National Institute on Drug Abuse (NIDA).)

---

tattoos. Also, because gang violence frequently is glorified in rap music, young people involved in gangs often try to imitate the dress and actions of rap artists. Finally, because substance abuse is often a characteristic of gang members, young people involved in gang activity may exhibit signs of drug or alcohol use.

Drugs And Love And Violence

It sounds like the name of a new reality show, right? But in real life, there is a connection between people in abusive dating relationships, and drugs and alcohol.

Actually, it's a two-way street. Drugs and alcohol increase the risk for dating violence, and people who are victims of dating violence are at increased risk for using drugs and alcohol.

Being drunk or drugged can make someone more likely to physically or emotionally hurt a person they're in a relationship with. Drugs and alcohol make it harder to keep your emotions in check and to make the right choices. They also make it easier to act impulsively without thinking through the consequences. And the people on the receiving end of that abuse are more likely to turn to drugs and alcohol to cope with the depression and anxiety that result from being victimized.

Abuse between teens in a romantic relationship is known as teen dating violence. It happens when one person intentionally hurts the other—or when they both do it to each other. Dating violence can be emotional, physical, and/or sexual, and it also includes stalking. It can be with a current or former partner. It can happen in person or electronically. And it has real consequences for a person's health, today and in the future.

Abusive relationships don't always start out that way. Often, they start with teasing, or periods of jealousy or being controlling. But as with many unhealthy behaviors, over time it can get worse. For nearly 10 percent of high school students surveyed by the Centers for Disease Control and Prevention (CDC) in 2013, "worse" means that in the last year they were hit, slapped, or physically hurt by their partner.

The best way to avoid teen dating violence (for those of you allowed to date!) is by having healthy relationships. This doesn't mean there isn't any conflict in the relationship, because that isn't realistic—even for the most in-love people ever. It means both people learning how to resolve their differences respectfully. That can make all the difference.

Chapter 56

Drugged Driving

Use of illicit* drugs or misuse of prescription drugs can make driving a car unsafe—just like driving after drinking alcohol. Drugged driving puts the driver, passengers, and others who share the road at risk.

"Illicit" refers to use of illegal drugs, including marijuana according to federal law, and misuse of prescription drugs

Why Is Drugged Driving Dangerous?

The effects of specific drugs differ depending on how they act in the brain. For example, marijuana can slow reaction time, impair judgment of time and distance, and decrease coordination. Drivers who have used cocaine or methamphetamine can be aggressive and reckless when driving. Certain kinds of sedatives, called benzodiazepines, can cause dizziness and drowsiness. All of these impairments can lead to vehicle crashes. Research studies have shown negative effects of marijuana on drivers, including an increase in lane weaving, poor reaction time, and altered attention to the road. Use of alcohol with marijuana made drivers more impaired, causing even more lane weaving.

It is difficult to determine how specific drugs affect driving because people tend to mix various substances, including alcohol. But we do know that even small amounts of some drugs can have a measurable effect. As a result, some states have zero-tolerance laws for drugged driving. This means a person can face charges for driving under the influence (DUI) if there is any amount of drug in the blood or urine. It's important to note that many states are waiting for research to better define blood levels that indicate impairment, such as those they use with alcohol.

About This Chapter: This chapter includes text excerpted from "Drugged Driving," National Institute on Drug Abuse (NIDA), June 2016.

How Many People Take Drugs And Drive?

According to the National Survey on Drug Use and Health (NSDUH), 20.7 million people aged 16 or older drove under the influence of alcohol in the past year and 11.8 million drove under the influence of illicit drugs. NSDUH findings also show that men are more likely than women to drive under the influence of drugs or alcohol. And a higher percentage of young adults aged 18–25 drive after taking drugs or drinking than do adults 26 or older.

Which Drugs Are Linked To Drugged Driving?

After alcohol, marijuana is the drug most often found in the blood of drivers involved in crashes. Tests for detecting marijuana in drivers measure the level of delta-9-tetrahydrocannabinol (THC), marijuana's mind-altering ingredient, in the blood. But the role that marijuana plays in crashes is often unclear. THC can be detected in body fluids for days or even weeks after use, and it is often combined with alcohol. The risk associated with marijuana in combination with alcohol, cocaine, or benzodiazepines appears to be greater than that for either drug by itself.

How Marijuana Affects Driving

In recent years, state actions to legalize the use of marijuana for medical and recreational use have increased concern over potential risks of driving impaired by marijuana. Other than alcohol, it is the drug that is most frequently detected in drivers' systems after a vehicle crash, as well as the general driving population.

National Highway Traffic Safety Administration's (NHTSA) Crash Risk Study, the largest of its kind ever conducted, assessed whether marijuana use by drivers is associated with greater risk of crashes. The survey found that marijuana users are more likely to be involved in crashes, but that the increased risk may be due in part because marijuana users are more likely to be in groups at higher risk of crashes. In particular, marijuana users are more likely to be young men—a group already at high risk.

We know that marijuana can be dangerous when combined with driving. Studies show that marijuana impairs psychomotor skills, lane tracking, and cognitive functions, but it is still unclear the extent to which it contributes to the occurrence of vehicle crashes. Some studies have attempted to estimate the risk of driving after marijuana use, but these remain inconclusive in terms of predicting real-world crash risk.

(Source: "Drug-Impaired Driving," National Highway Traffic Safety Administration (NHTSA).)

Several studies have shown that drivers with THC in their blood were roughly twice as likely to be responsible for a deadly crash or be killed than drivers who hadn't used drugs or alcohol. However, a large National Highway Traffic Safety Administration (NHTSA) study found no significant increased crash risk traceable to marijuana after controlling for drivers' age, gender, race, and presence of alcohol. More research is needed.

Along with marijuana, prescription drugs are also commonly linked to drugged driving crashes. A 2010 nationwide study of deadly crashes found that about 47 percent of drivers who tested positive for drugs had used a prescription drug, compared to 37 percent of those had used marijuana and about 10 percent of those who had used cocaine. The most common prescription drugs found were pain relievers. However, the study didn't distinguish between medically-supervised and illicit use of the prescription drugs.

How Often Does Drugged Driving Cause Crashes?

It's hard to measure how many crashes are caused by drugged driving. This is because:

- A good roadside test for drug levels in the body doesn't yet exist.

- Police don't usually test for drugs if drivers have reached an illegal blood alcohol level because there's already enough evidence for a DUI charge.

- Many drivers who cause crashes are found to have both drugs and alcohol or more than one drug in their system, making it hard to know which substance had the greater effect.

One NHTSA study found that in 2009, 18 percent of drivers killed in a crash tested positive for at least one drug. A 2010 study showed that 11 percent of deadly crashes involved a drugged driver.

Why Is Drugged Driving A Problem In Teens And Young Adults?

Teen drivers are less experienced and are more likely than older drivers to underestimate or not recognize dangerous situations. They are also more likely to speed and allow less distance between vehicles. When lack of driving experience is combined with drug use, the results can be tragic. Car crashes are the leading cause of death among young people aged 16–19 years.

A 2011 survey of middle and high school students showed that, in the 2 weeks before the survey, 12 percent of high school seniors had driven after using marijuana, compared to around

9 percent who had driven after drinking alcohol. A study of college students with access to a car found that 1 in 6 had driven under the influence of a drug other than alcohol at least once in the past year. Marijuana was the most common drug used, followed by cocaine and prescription pain relievers.

What Steps Can People Take To Prevent Drugged Driving?

Because drugged driving puts people at a higher risk for crashes, public health experts urge people who use drugs and alcohol to develop social strategies to prevent them from getting behind the wheel of a car while impaired. Steps people can take include:

- Offering to be a designated driver
- Appointing a designated driver to take all car keys
- Getting a ride to and from parties where there are drugs and alcohol
- Discussing the risks of drugged driving with friends in advance

Part Eight
Treatment For Addiction

Chapter 57

Dealing With Drug Addiction

What Is Drug Addiction?

Drug addiction is a chronic disease characterized by compulsive, or uncontrollable, drug seeking and use despite harmful consequences and changes in the brain, which can be long lasting. These changes in the brain can lead to the harmful behaviors seen in people who use drugs. Drug addiction is also a relapsing disease. Relapse is the return to drug use after an attempt to stop.

The path to drug addiction begins with the voluntary act of taking drugs. But over time, a person's ability to choose not to do so becomes compromised. Seeking and taking the drug becomes compulsive. This is mostly due to the effects of long-term drug exposure on brain function. Addiction affects parts of the brain involved in reward and motivation, learning and memory, and control over behavior. Addiction is a disease that affects both the brain and behavior.

Can Drug Addiction Be Treated?

Yes, but it's not simple. Because addiction is a chronic disease, people can't simply stop using drugs for a few days and be cured. Most patients need long-term or repeated care to stop using completely and recover their lives.

Addiction treatment must help the person do the following:

- Stop using drugs
- Stay drug-free
- Be productive in the family, at work, and in society

About This Chapter: This chapter includes text excerpted from "Treatment Approaches For Drug Addiction," National Institute on Drug Abuse (NIDA), January 2018.

Principles Of Effective Treatment

Based on scientific research since the mid-1970s, the following key principles should form the basis of any effective treatment program:

- Addiction is a complex but treatable disease that affects brain function and behavior.
- No single treatment is right for everyone.
- People need to have quick access to treatment.
- Effective treatment addresses all of the patient's needs, not just his or her drug use.
- Staying in treatment long enough is critical.
- Counseling and other behavioral therapies are the most commonly used forms of treatment.
- Medications are often an important part of treatment, especially when combined with behavioral therapies.
- Treatment plans must be reviewed often and modified to fit the patient's changing needs.
- Treatment should address other possible mental disorders.
- Medically assisted detoxification is only the first stage of treatment.
- Treatment doesn't need to be voluntary to be effective.
- Drug use during treatment must be monitored continuously.
- Treatment programs should test patients for human immunodeficiency virus (HIV) / acquired immunodeficiency syndrome (AIDS), hepatitis B and C, tuberculosis (TB), and other infectious diseases as well as teach them about steps they can take to reduce their risk of these illnesses.

What Are Treatments For Drug Addiction?

There are many options that have been successful in treating drug addiction, including:

- Behavioral counseling
- Medication
- Medical devices and applications used to treat withdrawal symptoms or deliver skills training
- Evaluation and treatment for co-occurring mental health issues such as depression and anxiety
- Long-term followup to prevent relapse

A range of care with a tailored treatment program and follow-up options can be crucial to success. Treatment should include both medical and mental health services as needed. Follow-up care may include community- or family-based recovery support systems.

How Are Medications And Devices Used In Drug Addiction Treatment?

Medications and devices can be used to manage withdrawal symptoms, prevent relapse, and treat co-occurring conditions.

Withdrawal. Medications and devices can help suppress withdrawal symptoms during detoxification. Detoxification is not in itself "treatment," but only the first step in the process. Patients who do not receive any further treatment after detoxification usually resume their drug use. One study of treatment facilities found that medications were used in almost 80 percent of detoxifications. In November 2017, the U.S. Food and Drug Administration (FDA) granted a new indication to an electronic stimulation device, NSS-2 Bridge, for use in helping reduce opioid withdrawal symptoms. This device is placed behind the ear and sends electrical pulses to stimulate certain brain nerves.

Relapse prevention. Patients can use medications to help re-establish normal brain function and decrease cravings. Medications are available for treatment of opioid (heroin, prescription pain relievers), tobacco (nicotine), and alcohol addiction. Scientists are developing other medications to treat stimulant (cocaine, methamphetamine) and cannabis (marijuana) addiction. People who use more than one drug, which is very common, need treatment for all of the substances they use.

- **Opioids.** Methadone (Dolophine®, Methadose®), buprenorphine (Suboxone®, Subutex®, Probuphine®, Sublocade™), and naltrexone (Vivitrol®) are used to treat opioid addiction. Acting on the same targets in the brain as heroin and morphine, methadone and buprenorphine suppress withdrawal symptoms and relieve cravings. Naltrexone blocks the effects of opioids at their receptor sites in the brain and should be used only in patients who have already been detoxified. All medications help patients reduce drug seeking and related criminal behavior and help them become more open to behavioral treatments. A National Institute on Drug Abuse (NIDA) study found that once treatment is initiated, both a buprenorphine/naloxone combination and an extended-release naltrexone formulation are similarly effective in treating opioid addiction. Because full detoxification is necessary for treatment with naloxone, initiating treatment among active users was difficult, but once detoxification was complete, both medications had similar effectiveness.

- **Tobacco.** Nicotine replacement therapies have several forms, including the patch, spray, gum, and lozenges. These products are available over the counter. The U.S. Food and Drug Administration (FDA) has approved two prescription medications for nicotine addiction: bupropion (Zyban®) and varenicline (Chantix®). They work differently in the brain, but both help prevent relapse in people trying to quit. The medications are more effective when combined with behavioral treatments, such as group and individual therapy as well as telephone quitlines.

- **Alcohol.** Three medications have been FDA-approved for treating alcohol addiction and a fourth, topiramate, has shown promise in clinical trials (large-scale studies with people). The three approved medications are as follows:

  - **Naltrexone** blocks opioid receptors that are involved in the rewarding effects of drinking and in the craving for alcohol. It reduces relapse to heavy drinking and is highly effective in some patients. Genetic differences may affect how well the drug works in certain patients.

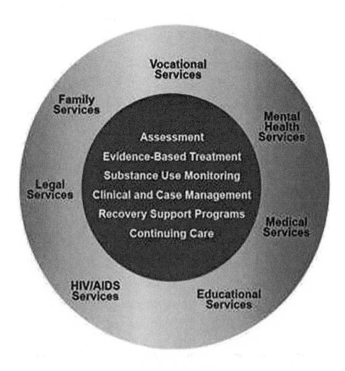

Figure 57.1. Drug Addiction Treatment Components

- **Acamprosate (Campral®)** may reduce symptoms of long-lasting withdrawal, such as insomnia, anxiety, restlessness, and dysphoria (generally feeling unwell or unhappy). It may be more effective in patients with severe addiction.

- **Disulfiram (Antabuse®)** interferes with the breakdown of alcohol. Acetaldehyde builds up in the body, leading to unpleasant reactions that include flushing (warmth and redness in the face), nausea, and irregular heartbeat if the patient drinks alcohol. Compliance (taking the drug as prescribed) can be a problem, but it may help patients who are highly motivated to quit drinking.

- **Co-occurring conditions.** Other medications are available to treat possible mental health conditions, such as depression or anxiety, that may be contributing to the person's addiction.

How Are Behavioral Therapies Used To Treat Drug Addiction?

Behavioral therapies help patients:

- Modify their attitudes and behaviors related to drug use

- Increase healthy life skills

- Persist with other forms of treatment, such as medication

Patients can receive treatment in many different settings with various approaches.

Outpatient behavioral treatment includes a wide variety of programs for patients who visit a behavioral health counselor on a regular schedule. Most of the programs involve individual or group drug counseling, or both. These programs typically offer forms of behavioral therapy such as:

- **Cognitive behavioral therapy (CBT),** which helps patients recognize, avoid, and cope with the situations in which they are most likely to use drugs

- **Multidimensional family therapy (MDFT)**—developed for adolescents with drug abuse problems as well as their families—which addresses a range of influences on their drug abuse patterns and is designed to improve overall family functioning

- **Motivational interviewing,** which makes the most of people's readiness to change their behavior and enter treatment

- **Motivational incentives (contingency management),** which uses positive reinforcement to encourage abstinence from drugs

Treatment is sometimes intensive at first, where patients attend multiple outpatient sessions each week. After completing intensive treatment, patients transition to regular outpatient treatment, which meets less often and for fewer hours per week to help sustain their recovery. In September 2017, the FDA permitted marketing of the first mobile application, reSET®, to help treat substance use disorders. This application is intended to be used with outpatient treatment to treat alcohol, cocaine, marijuana, and stimulant substance use disorders. In September 2017, the FDA permitted marketing of the first mobile application, reSET®, to help treat substance use disorders. This application is intended to be used with outpatient treatment to treat alcohol, cocaine, marijuana, and stimulant substance use disorders.

Inpatient or residential treatment can also be very effective, especially for those with more severe problems (including co-occurring disorders). Licensed residential treatment facilities offer 24-hour structured and intensive care, including safe housing and medical attention. Residential treatment facilities may use a variety of therapeutic approaches, and they are generally aimed at helping the patient live a drug-free, crime-free lifestyle after treatment. Examples of residential treatment settings include:

- **Therapeutic communities**, which are highly structured programs in which patients remain at a residence, typically for 6–12 months. The entire community, including treatment staff and those in recovery, act as key agents of change, influencing the patient's attitudes, understanding, and behaviors associated with drug use.

- **Shorter-term residential treatment**, which typically focuses on detoxification as well as providing initial intensive counseling and preparation for treatment in a community-based setting

- **Recovery housing**, which provides supervised, short-term housing for patients, often following other types of inpatient or residential treatment. Recovery housing can help people make the transition to an independent life—for example, helping them learn how to manage finances or seek employment, as well as connecting them to support services in the community.

How Many People Get Treatment For Drug Addiction?

According to Substance Abuse and Mental Health Services Administration's (SAMHSA) National Survey on Drug Use and Health (NSDUH), 22.5 million people (8.5% of the U.S.

population) aged 12 or older needed treatment for an illicit* drug or alcohol use problem in 2014. Only 4.2 million (18.5% of those who needed treatment) received any substance use treatment in the same year. Of these, about 2.6 million people received treatment at specialty treatment programs.

*The term "illicit" refers to the use of illegal drugs, including marijuana according to federal law, and misuse of prescription medications.

Chapter 58

Substance Abuse Treatment

The treatment system for substance use disorders (SUDs) comprises multiple service components, including the following:

- Individual and group counseling

- Inpatient and residential treatment

- Intensive outpatient treatment

- Partial hospital programs

- Case or care management

- Medication

- Recovery support services

- 12-step fellowship

- Peer supports

A person accessing treatment may not need to access every one of these components, but each plays an important role. These systems are embedded in a broader community and the support provided by various parts of that community also play an important role in supporting the recovery of people with substance use disorders.

About This Chapter: This chapter includes text excerpted from "Treatments For Substance Use Disorders," Substance Abuse and Mental Health Services Administration (SAMHSA), June 13, 2018.

Principles Of Effective Treatment And Treatment Planning

Treatment can occur in a variety of settings but most treatment for substance use disorders has traditionally been provided in specialty substance use disorder treatment programs. For this reason, the majority of research has been performed within these specialty settings.

The National Institute on Drug Abuse (NIDA) has detailed the evidence-based principles of effective treatment for adolescents with substance use disorders that apply regardless of the particular setting of care or type of substance use disorder treatment program:

1. Adolescent substance use needs to be identified and addressed as soon as possible.
2. Adolescents can benefit from a drug abuse intervention even if they are not addicted to a drug.
3. Routine annual medical visits are an opportunity to ask adolescents about drug use.
4. Legal interventions and sanctions or family pressure may play an important role in getting adolescents to enter, stay in, and complete treatment.
5. Substance use disorder treatment should be tailored to the unique needs of the adolescent.
6. Treatment should address the needs of the whole person, rather than just focusing on his or her drug use.
7. Behavioral therapies are effective in addressing adolescent drug use.
8. Families and the community are important aspects of treatment.
9. Effectively treating substance use disorders in adolescents requires also identifying and treating any other mental health conditions they may have.
10. Sensitive issues such as violence and child abuse or risk of suicide should be identified and addressed.
11. It is important to monitor drug use during treatment.
12. Staying in treatment for an adequate period of time and continuity of care afterward are important.
13. Testing adolescents for sexually transmitted diseases like human immunodeficiency virus (HIV), as well as hepatitis B and C, is an important part of drug treatment.

The goals of substance use disorder treatment are similar to those of treatments for other serious, often chronic, illnesses: reduce the major symptoms of the illness, improve health and social function, and teach and motivate patients to monitor their condition and manage threats of relapse. Substance use disorder treatment can be provided in inpatient or outpatient settings, depending on the needs of the patient, and typically incorporates a combination of behavioral therapies, medications, and Recovery Support Services. However, unlike treatments for most other medical illnesses, substance use disorder treatment has traditionally been provided in programs (both residential and outpatient) outside of the mainstream healthcare system. The intensity of the treatment regimens offered can vary substantially across program types.

(Source: "Early Intervention, Treatment, And Management Of Substance Use Disorders," Office of the Surgeon General (OGS).)

Individual And Group Counseling

Counseling can be provided at the individual or group level. Individual counseling often focuses on reducing or stopping substance use, skill building, adherence to a recovery plan, and social, family, and professional/educational outcomes. Group counseling is often used in addition to individual counseling to provide social reinforcement for pursuit of recovery.

Counselors provide a variety of services to people in treatment for substance use disorders including assessment, treatment planning, and counseling. These professionals provide a variety of therapies. Some common therapies include:

- **Cognitive behavioral therapy (CBT)** teaches individuals in treatment to recognize and stop negative patterns of thinking and behavior. For instance, cognitive behavioral therapy might help a person be aware of the stressors, situations, and feelings that lead to substance use so that the person can avoid them or act differently when they occur.

- **Contingency management** is designed to provide incentives to reinforce positive behaviors, such as remaining abstinent from substance use.

- **Motivational enhancement therapy (MET)** helps people with substance use disorders to build motivation and commit to specific plans to engage in treatment and seek recovery. It is often used early in the process to engage people in treatment.

- **12-step facilitation therapy** seeks to guide and support engagement in 12-step programs such as Alcoholics Anonymous (AA) or Narcotics Anonymous (NA).

Some forms of counseling are tailored to specific populations. For instance, young people need a different set of treatment services to guide them towards recovery. Treatments for youth often involve a family component. Two models for youth that are often used in combination and have been supported by Substance Abuse and Mental Health Services Administration (SAMHSA) grants are the Adolescent Community Reinforcement Approach (ACRA) and Assertive Continuing Care (ACC). ACRA uses defined procedures to build skills and support engagement in positive activities. ACC provides intensive follow-up and home-based services to prevent relapse and is delivered by a team of professionals.

Inpatient And Residential Settings

Treatment can be provided in inpatient or residential sessions. This happens within specialty substance use disorder treatment facilities, facilities with a broader behavioral health focus, or by specialized units within hospitals. Longer-term residential treatment has lengths of stay that can be as long as 6–12 months and is relatively uncommon. These programs focus on helping individuals change their behaviors in a highly structured setting. Shorter-term residential treatment is much more common, and typically has a focus on detoxification (also known as medically managed withdrawal) as well as providing initial intensive treatment, and preparation for a return to community-based settings.

An alternative to inpatient or residential treatment is partial hospitalization or intensive outpatient treatment. These programs have people attend very intensive and regular treatment sessions multiple times a week early in their treatment for an initial period. After completing partial hospitalization or intensive outpatient treatment, individuals often step down into regular outpatient treatment which meets less frequently and for fewer hours per week to help sustain their recovery.

Treating Criminal Justice-Involved Drug Abusers And Addicted Individuals

Often, drug abusers come into contact with the criminal justice system earlier than other health or social systems, presenting opportunities for intervention and treatment prior to, during, after, or in lieu of incarceration. Research has shown that combining criminal justice sanctions with drug treatment can be effective in decreasing drug abuse and related crime. Individuals under legal coercion tend to stay in treatment longer and do as well as or better than those not under legal pressure. Studies show that for incarcerated individuals with drug problems, starting drug abuse treatment in prison and continuing the same treatment upon release—in other words, a seamless continuum of services—results in better outcomes: less drug use and less criminal behavior.

(Source: "Principles Of Drug Addiction Treatment: A Research-Based Guide," National Institute on Drug Abuse (NIDA).)

Medications

Using medication to treat substance use disorders is often referred to as medication-assisted treatment (MAT). In this model, medication is used in combination with counseling and behavioral therapies. Medications can reduce the cravings and other symptoms associated with withdrawal from a substance by occupying receptors in the brain associated with using that drug (agonists or partial agonists), block the rewarding sensation that comes with using a substance (antagonists), or induce negative feelings when a substance is taken. MAT is has been primarily used for the treatment of opioid use disorder but is also used for alcohol use disorder (AUD) and the treatment of some other substance use disorders.

Medications For Alcohol Use Disorders

Medications also exist that can assist in the treatment of alcohol use disorder. Acamprosate is a medication that reduces symptoms of protracted withdrawal and has been shown to help individuals with alcohol use disorders who have achieved abstinence go on to maintain abstinence for several weeks to months. Naltrexone, a medication used to block the effects of opioids, has also been used to reduce craving in those with alcohol use disorders. Disulfiram is another medication which changes the way the body metabolizes alcohol, resulting in an unpleasant reaction that includes flushing, nausea, and other unpleasant symptoms if a person takes the medication and then consumes alcohol.

Medications For Tobacco Use Disorders

There are three medications approved by the U.S. Food and Drug Administration (FDA) to treat tobacco use disorders (cigarette smoking). Nicotine replacement medications assist with reducing nicotine withdrawal symptoms including anger and irritability, depression, anxiety, and decreased concentration. Because nicotine delivered through chewing of gum containing nicotine, via transdermal patch, or in lozenges has a slower onset of action than does the systemic delivery of nicotine through smoked tobacco; these medications have little effect on craving for cigarettes. These medications are available over-the-counter. However, the nicotine inhaler and nasal spray deliver nicotine more rapidly to the brain and so are available only by prescription. Bupropion is a medication originally developed and approved as an anti-depressant that was also found to help people to quit smoking. This medication can be used at the same dose for either cigarette smoking or depression treatment (or both). Varenicline is a nicotine partial agonist that reduces craving for cigarettes and has been helpful in smoking cessation for many. Bupropion and varenicline are prescription medications.

Medication For Opioid Use Disorders

Medication-assisted treatment with methadone, buprenorphine, or extended-release injectable naltrexone plays a critical role in the treatment of opioid use disorders. According to the latest survey of opioid treatment providers more than 300,000 people received some form of medication-assisted treatment for an opioid use disorder in 2011.

Opioid agonist therapies with methadone or buprenorphine reduce the effects of opioid withdrawal and reduce cravings. They have been shown to increase retention in treatment and reduce risk behaviors that lead to transmission of HIV and viral hepatitis such as using opioids by injection. Medication-assisted treatment with extended-release injectable naltrexone reduces the risk of relapse to opioid use and helps control cravings. Extended-release injectable naltrexone is particularly useful for people exiting a controlled setting where abstinence has been enforced such as jail or residential rehabilitation or in situations where maintenance with an opioid agonist is not available or appropriate. People who misuse prescription opioids benefit from medication-assisted treatment as much as people abusing heroin. There are no other FDA-approved medications for the treatment of other substance use disorders.

Recovery Support Services

Recovery support services are nonclinical services that are used with treatment to support individuals in their recovery goals. These services are often provided by peers, or others who are already in recovery. Recovery support can include:

- Transportation to and from treatment and recovery-oriented activities

- Employment or educational supports

- Specialized living situations

- Peer-to-peer services, mentoring, coaching

- Spiritual and faith-based support

- Parenting education

- Self-help and support groups

- Outreach and engagement

- Staffing drop-in centers, clubhouses, respite/crisis services, or warmlines (peer-run listening lines staffed by people in recovery themselves)

- Education about strategies to promote wellness and recovery

Peer Supports

Peers are individuals in recovery who can use their own experiences to help others working towards recovery. Peer supports are a critical component of the substance use disorder treatment system. Many people who work in the treatment system as counselors or case managers are in recovery, and peers are central to many recovery support efforts.

Peers also play a powerful role as a part of mutual-support groups. These groups, including Alcoholics Anonymous (AA) or Narcotics Anonymous (NA) and other 12-step programs, provide peer support for ending or reducing substance use. They provide an international support network which is relied upon by many people in recovery from substance use disorders. Mutual-support groups are often intentionally incorporated into treatment plans and can provide a ready community for individuals who are trying to change their lifestyles to get away from alcohol and other drugs. While mutual-support groups do not work for everyone and are not a necessary part of recovery, they are a fundamental component of the SUD treatment system, even if they are not considered formal treatment.

Chapter 59

When A Family Member Is Dealing With Substance Abuse

What Is Substance Abuse?

Alcoholism and drug dependence and addiction, known as substance use disorders (SUDs), are complex problems. People with these disorders once were thought to have a character defect or moral weakness; some people mistakenly still believe that. However, most scientists and medical researchers now consider dependence on alcohol or drugs to be a long-term illness, like asthma, hypertension (high blood pressure), or diabetes. Most people who drink alcohol drink very little, and many people can stop taking drugs without a struggle. However, some people develop a substance use disorder—use of alcohol or drugs that is compulsive or dangerous (or both).

Why Do Some People Develop A Problem But Others Don't?

Substance use disorder (SUD) is an illness that can affect anyone: rich or poor, male or female, employed or unemployed, young or old, and any race or ethnicity. Nobody knows for sure exactly what causes it, but the chance of developing a substance use disorder depends partly on genetics—biological traits passed down through families. A person's environment, psychological traits, and stress level also play major roles by contributing to the use of alcohol or drugs. Researchers have found that using drugs for a long-time changes the brain in

About This Chapter: This chapter includes text excerpted from "What Is Substance Abuse Treatment?" Substance Abuse and Mental Health Services Administration (SAMHSA), 2014. Reviewed July 2018.

important, long-lasting ways. It is as if a switch in the brain turned on at some point. This point is different for every person, but when this switch turns on, the person crosses an invisible line and becomes dependent on the substance. People who start using drugs or alcohol early in life run a greater risk of crossing this line and becoming dependent. These changes in the brain remain long after a person stops using drugs or drinking alcohol.

Who Provides Treatment?

Many different kinds of professionals provide treatment for substance use disorders. In most treatment programs, the main caregivers are specially trained individuals certified or licensed as substance abuse treatment counselors. About half these counselors are people who are in recovery themselves. Many programs have staff from several different ethnic or cultural groups. Most treatment programs assign patients to a treatment team of professionals. Depending on the type of treatment, teams can be made up of social workers, counselors, doctors, nurses, psychologists, psychiatrists, or other professionals.

What Will Happen First?

Everyone entering treatment receives a clinical assessment. A complete assessment of an individual is needed to help treatment professionals offer the type of treatment that best suits him or her. The assessment also helps program counselors work with the person to design an effective treatment plan. Although clinical assessment continues throughout a person's treatment, it starts at or just before a person's admission to a treatment program. The counselor will begin by gathering information about the person, asking many questions such as those about the person, asking many questions.

The counselor may invite you, as a family member, to answer questions and express your own concerns as well. Be honest—this is not the time to cover up your loved one's behavior. The counselor needs to get a full picture of the problem to plan and help implement the most effective treatment. It is particularly important for the counselor to know whether your family member has any serious medical problems or whether you suspect that he or she may have an emotional problem. You may feel embarrassed answering some of these questions or have difficulty completing the interview, but remember: the counselor is there to help you and your loved one. The treatment team uses the information gathered to recommend the best type of treatment. No one type of treatment is right for everyone; to work, the treatment needs to meet your family member's individual needs.

After the assessment, a counselor or case manager is assigned to your family member. The counselor works with the person (and possibly his or her family) to develop a treatment plan.

This plan lists problems, treatment goals, and ways to meet those goals. Based on the assessment, the counselor may refer your family member to a physician to decide whether he or she needs medical supervision to stop alcohol or drug use safely.

What Actually Happens In Treatment Programs?

Although treatment programs differ, the basic ingredients of treatment are similar. Most programs include many or all elements presented below.

Assessment

All treatment programs begin with a clinical assessment of a person's individual treatment needs. This assessment helps in the development of an effective treatment plan.

Medical Care

Programs in hospitals can provide this care on site. Other outpatient or residential programs may have doctors and nurses come to the program site for a few days each week, or a person may be referred to other places for medical care. Medical care typically include screening and treatment for human immunodeficiency virus (HIV) / acquired immunodeficiency syndrome (AIDS), hepatitis, tuberculosis (TB), and women's health issues.

A Treatment Plan

The treatment team, along with the person in treatment, develops a treatment plan based on the assessment. A treatment plan is a written guide to treatment that includes the person's goals, treatment activities designed to help him or her meet those goals, ways to tell whether a goal has been met, and a timeframe for meeting goals. The treatment plan helps both the person in treatment and treatment program staff stay focused and on track. The treatment plan is adjusted over time to meet changing needs and ensure that it stays relevant.

Group And Individual Counseling

At first, individual counseling generally focuses on motivating the person to stop using drugs or alcohol. Treatment then shifts to helping the person stay drug and alcohol-free. The counselor attempts to help the person:

- See the problem and become motivated to change

385

- Change his or her behavior

- Repair damaged relationships with family and friends

- Build new friendships with people who don't use alcohol or drugs

- Create a recovery lifestyle

Group counseling is different in each program, but group members usually support and try to help one another cope with life without using drugs or alcohol. They share their experiences, talk about their feelings and problems, and find out that others have similar problems. Groups also may explore spirituality and its role in recovery.

Individual Assignments

People in treatment may be asked to read certain things (or listen to audio tapes), to complete written assignments (or record them on audiotapes), or to try new behaviors.

Education About Substance Use Disorder (SUD)

People learn about the symptoms and the effects of alcohol and drug use on their brains and bodies. Education groups use videotapes or audiotapes, lectures, or activities to help people learn about their illness and how to manage it.

Life Skills Training

This training can include learning and practicing employment skills, leisure activities, social skills, communication skills, anger management, stress management, goal setting, and money and time management.

Testing For Alcohol Or Drug Use

Program staff members regularly take urine samples from people for drug testing. Some programs are starting to test saliva instead of urine. They also may use a Breathalyzer™ to test people for alcohol use.

Relapse Prevention Training

Relapse prevention training teaches people how to identify their relapse triggers, how to cope with cravings, how to develop plans for handling stressful situations, and what to do if they relapse. A trigger is anything that makes a person crave a drug. Triggers often are connected to the person's past use, such as a person he or she used drugs with, a time or place, drug use paraphernalia (such as syringes, a pipe, or a bong), or a particular situation or emotion.

Orientation To Self-Help Groups

Participants in self-help groups support and encourage one another to become or stay drug and alcohol-free. Twelve-step programs are perhaps the best known of the self-help groups.

Treatment For Mental Disorders

Many people with a substance use disorder also have emotional problems such as depression, anxiety, or posttraumatic stress disorder. Adolescents in treatment also may have behavior problems, conduct disorder, or attention deficit hyperactivity disorder. Treating both the substance use and mental disorders increases the chances that the person will recover. Some counselors think people should be alcohol and drug-free for at least 3–4 weeks before a treatment professional can identify emotional illness correctly. The program may provide mental healthcare, or it may refer a person to other sites for this care. Mental healthcare often includes the use of medications, such as antidepressants.

Family Education And Counseling Services

This education can help you understand the disease and its causes, effects, and treatment. Programs provide this education in many ways: lectures, discussions, activities, and group meetings. Some programs provide counseling for families or couples.

Family counseling is especially critical in treatment for adolescents. Parents need to be involved in treatment planning and follow-up care decisions for the adolescent. Family members also need to participate as fully as possible in the family counseling the program offers.

Medication

Many programs use medications to help in the treatment process. Although no medications cure dependence on drugs or alcohol, some do help people stay abstinent and can be lifesaving.

Follow-Up Care (Also Called Continuing Care)

Even when a person has successfully completed a treatment program, the danger of returning to alcohol or drug use (called a "slip" or relapse) remains. The longer a person stays in treatment, including follow-up, the more likely he or she is to stay in recovery. Once a person has completed basic treatment, a program will offer a follow-up care program at the treatment facility or will refer him or her to another site. Most programs recommend that a person stay in follow-up care for at least 1 year. Adolescents often need follow-up care for a longer period.

Just For You

Now that your family member is in treatment, things are starting to change. Some of the tension and turmoil that probably were part of your life may be starting to ease. But the first weeks of treatment are stressful. Each family member is adjusting to changes, starting to deal with past conflicts, and establishing new routines. Amid all these changes, it is important that you take good care of yourself—get enough sleep, eat right, rest, exercise, and talk to supportive friends and relatives. Your church, mosque, synagogue, temple, or other spiritual organization also may be a good source of support.

Recovery is not just an adjustment for the person in treatment—it also is an adjustment for you. For the past few years, you may have assumed roles or taken care of tasks that were your loved one's responsibilities. Now, as time passes, you and he or she may need to learn new ways of relating to each other and learn different ways of sharing activities and chores. If you are the parent of an adolescent in treatment, you will need to be closely involved in treatment planning and treatment activities. You may need to adjust your life and family relationships to allow for the extra time this involvement will take.

You may have many questions about how your family member will behave in these early stages of recovery. Everyone acts differently. Some people are very happy to be getting treatment at last; others suffer a great deal while they adjust to a new life and attempt to live it without alcohol and drugs. They may be sad, angry, or confused. It is important for you to realize that these are normal reactions and to get support for yourself. Al-Anon is the best-known and most available resource for family members and friends of alcoholics. Al-Anon was founded 50 years ago to provide support for those living with someone with alcoholism. Alateen, for older children and adolescents, was founded somewhat later on. Many family members of people who use drugs also participate in Al-Anon or Alateen. These meetings are free and available in most communities.

Your community also may have Nar-Anon meetings. This group was founded for families and friends of those using drugs. Other groups also may be helpful, such as Co-Dependents Anonymous (CoDA) and Adult Children of Alcoholics (ACoA). The treatment program should be able to give you schedules of local meetings of all these groups.

Many treatment professionals consider substance use disorders family diseases. To help the whole family recover and cope with the many changes going on, you may be asked to take part in treatment. This approach may involve going to a family education program or to counseling for families or couples.

It is important to remember the following points as you and your family member recover:

- You are participating in treatment for yourself, not just for the sake of the person who used substances.

- Your loved one's recovery, sobriety, or abstinence does not depend on you.

- Your family's recovery does not depend on the recovery of the person who used substances.

- You did not cause your family member's substance use disorder. It is not your fault.

You still may have hurt feelings and anger from the past that need to be resolved. You need support to understand and deal with these feelings, and you need to support your loved one's efforts to get well.

Family-Based Approaches

Family-based approaches to treating adolescent substance abuse highlight the need to engage the family, including parents, siblings, and sometimes peers, in the adolescent's treatment. Involving the family can be particularly important, as the adolescent will often be living with at least one parent and be subject to the parent's controls, rules, and/or supports. Family-based approaches generally address a wide array of problems in addition to the young person's substance problems, including family communication and conflict; other co-occurring behavioral, mental health, and learning disorders; problems with school or work attendance; and peer networks. Research shows that family-based treatments are highly efficacious; some studies even suggest they are superior to other individual and group treatment approaches.

(Source: "Principles Of Adolescent Substance Use Disorder Treatment: A Research-Based Guide," National Institute on Drug Abuse (NIDA).)

What If I Need Help With Basic Living Issues?

You may need very practical help while your family member is in treatment. If your family member is the sole financial provider and unable to work because he or she is in treatment, how will the bills get paid? If your family member is the primary caregiver for children or an elderly adult, how will these needs be met? The treatment program may be able to help you arrange disability leave or insurance through your loved one's employer. Ask the counselor about different types of assistance that may be available to help you meet various needs. Most treatment programs work with other community programs. These programs may include food pantries, clothing programs, transportation assistance, child care, adult day care, legal assistance, financial counseling, and healthcare services. Your family may be eligible for help from programs that help those in recovery.

I'm Afraid It Won't Work

Treatment is just the first step to recovery. During this process family members sometimes have mixed feelings. You may feel exhausted, angry, relieved, worried, and afraid that, if this doesn't work, nothing will. You may feel as if you are walking on eggshells and that, if you do something wrong, you may cause your loved one to relapse. It is important for you to remember that you cannot cause a relapse—only the person who takes a drug or picks up a drink is responsible for that.

No one can predict whether your family member will recover, or for how long, but many people who receive treatment do get better. The longer people stay in treatment the more likely they will remain drug and alcohol free. About half the people who complete treatment for the first time continue to recover.

Of course, this means that about half will return to drinking alcohol and using drugs (called relapse) before they finally give them up for good. Adolescents are even more likely to use drugs or alcohol or both again. It is not uncommon for a person to need to go through treatment more than one time. Often the person needs to return to treatment quickly to prevent a slip or relapse from leading to a chronic problem. It is important for you to understand that relapse is often a part of the recovery process. Do not be discouraged if your family member uses alcohol or drugs again. Many times relapses are short and the person continues to recover.

A treatment program may involve you in relapse prevention planning and may help you learn what to do if your family member relapses. Your family member will benefit if you do not drink or use drugs around him or her, especially in the first months after his or her treatment begins. When you choose not to use drugs or alcohol, you help your loved one avoid triggers. As you both begin to understand and accept the illness, the risk of relapse decreases. The changes in attitudes, behaviors, and values that you both are learning and practicing will become part of your new recovering lifestyle.

Chapter 60

Helping A Friend With A Substance Abuse Problem

Help A Friend In Need

Figuring out what to do when a friend or someone you know is having trouble with drugs or alcohol can be tricky. You want to help, but you might not know how to bring it up. Here are some tips.

- **Listen.** If he talks to you, just be there for him. Admitting a problem—never mind talking to someone about it—is really hard. Listen to what he has to say about his drug use without making judgments.

- **Encourage.** Suggest that she talk to an adult she trusts—a coach or teacher, a school counselor, a relative, or a doctor.

- **Share.** Maybe your friend doesn't see his or her drug use as a bad thing. But plenty of real scientific information about what drugs can do to a person is on the National Institute on Drug Abuse (NIDA) website. Once your friend understands how drugs affect the brain, body, and life, it might open their eyes.

- **Inform.** When he's ready to make a change and seek treatment, help him find a doctor, therapist, support group, or treatment program. You can use Substance Abuse and Mental Health Services Administration's (SAMHSA) Substance Abuse Treatment Facility Locator or call 800-662-HELP (800-662-4357).

About This Chapter: Text under the heading "Help A Friend In Need" is excerpted from "How To Help A Friend In Need," National Institute on Drug Abuse (NIDA) for Teens, September 24, 2009. Reviewed July 2018; Text under the heading "Things To Say And Do" is excerpted from "Real Teens Ask: How Can I Help My Friend?" National Institute on Drug Abuse (NIDA) for Teens, July 20, 2010. Reviewed July 2018.

- **Support.** Don't give up on your friend, even if she isn't ready to get help. Keep reaching out. Encourage them to get treatment, and support them along the way—that's the best way to help someone you care about who is struggling with addiction.

Things To Say And Do

Here are some ideas of things to say and do:

What To Do

- Find out if your friend is experimenting with drugs, or if he may be addicted. Neither one is good—but you may need more support if your friend is addicted.

- Understand that addiction is a brain disease. Just like you wouldn't expect someone with cancer to be able to heal herself without a doctor's help, the right treatment, and support from family and friends, you can't expect your friend to heal herself.

- Know that it's never easy for anyone to admit that they have a drug problem. You'll need to be patient—and not give up easily.

- Listen, encourage, share, and support. Sounds easy, right? But it's so hard.

- By the way, it's tough having a friend with addiction issues. So, if you need some support, visit www.al-anon.org.

What To Say

- Just telling your friend that you're concerned can be a big help. Your friend may not want to talk about it, and the effects of drugs on the brain may keep him from "hearing" you or acting on your advice.

- Assure your friend you are there for her and that she is not alone. People with drug problems often have gotten in with the wrong crowd—and they don't want to turn away from these so-called friends for fear of being alone.

- Suggest that he speak to a trusted adult who will keep it confidential. Maybe there's a family friend who could help.

- Turn to a professional for immediate help if the problem looks to be too big for you to handle alone, or if you're worried your friend may have suicidal thoughts that she could act on.

- Use SAMHSA's Substance Abuse Treatment Facility Locator (www.findtreatment. samhsa.gov) or call 800-662-HELP (800-662-4357) to tap into a support network where you can find immediate and confidential help 24/7. They' can also direct you to local treatment options.

When the people we care about and have lots in common with make bad choices, it can be frustrating, confusing, and a little depressing. Still, we should be there for our friends—and also try to be a good role models for them by making smart choices ourselves.

> There are many ways to help and support your friend, but in the end, it will need to be your friend's decision. And just by asking us this question, it's easy to see you're a good friend. Sometimes our friends won't appreciate advice they don't want to hear—especially if they're using drugs—but telling the truth to help someone close to you is part of being a real friend, even when it's hard to do.

Chapter 61

Recovery: The Many Paths To Wellness

Like any other chronic health condition, substance use disorders (SUDs) can go into remission. Among individuals with substance use disorders, this commonly involves the person stopping substance use, or at least reducing it to a safer level—for example, a student who was binge drinking several nights a week during college but reduced his alcohol consumption to one or two drinks a day after graduation. In general healthcare, treatments that reduce major disease symptoms to normal or "subclinical" levels are said to produce remission, and such treatments are thereby considered effective. However, serious substance use disorders are chronic conditions that can involve cycles of abstinence and relapse, possibly over several years following attempts to change. Thus, sustaining remission among those seriously affected typically requires a personal program of sustained recovery management.

For some people with substance use disorders, especially those whose problems are not severe, remission is the end of a chapter in their life that they rarely think about later, if at all. But for others, particularly those with more severe substance use disorders, remission is a component of a broader change in their behavior, outlook, and identity. That change process becomes an ongoing part of how they think about themselves and their experience with substances. Such people describe themselves as being "in recovery."

Various definitions of individual recovery have been offered nationally and internationally. Although they differ in some respects, all of these recovery definitions describe personal changes that are well beyond simply stopping substance use. As such, they are conceptually broader than "abstinence" or "remission." For example, the Betty Ford Institute (BFI)

About This Chapter: This chapter includes text excerpted from "Chapter 5 Recovery: The Many Paths To Wellness," Office of the Surgeon General (OGS), October 4, 2015.

Consensus Panel defined recovery as "a voluntarily maintained lifestyle characterized by sobriety, personal health, and citizenship." Similarly, the Substance Abuse and Mental Health Services Administration (SAMHSA) defines recovery as "a process of change through which individuals improve their health and wellness, live a self-directed life, and strive to reach their full potential.

Recovery-Related Values And Beliefs

When people talk about the recovery movement, they often invoke a set of values and beliefs that may be embraced by individuals with substance use disorders, families, treatment professionals, and even entire healthcare systems. Some examples of these values and beliefs include:

- People who suffer from substance use disorders (recovering or not) have essential worth and dignity.

- The shame and discrimination that prevents many individuals from seeking help must be vigorously combated.

- Recovery can be achieved through diverse pathways and should be celebrated.

- Access to high-quality treatment is a human right, although recovery is more than treatment.

- People in recovery and their families have valuable experiences and encouragement to offer others who are struggling with substance use.

Recovery-Oriented Systems Of Care

Increasingly, Recovery Support Services (RSS) are being organized into a framework for infusing the entire health and social service system with recovery-related beliefs, values, and approaches. This transformation has been described as:

...a shift away from crisis-oriented, deficit-focused, and professionally-directed models of care to a vision of care that is directed by people in recovery, emphasizes the reality and hope of long-term recovery, and recognizes the many pathways to healing for people with addiction and mental health challenges.

Recovery-Oriented Systems of Care (ROSC) embrace the idea that severe substance use disorders are most effectively addressed through a chronic care management model that includes longer term, outpatient care; recovery housing; and recovery coaching and management checkups. Recovery-oriented systems are designed to be easy to navigate for people seeking help, transparent in their operations, and responsive to the cultural diversity of the communities they serve. Treatment in recovery-oriented systems is offered as one component in a range of other services, including recovery supports. Treatment professionals act in a partnership/consultation role, drawing upon each person's goals and strengths, family supports, and community resources.

National Recovery Month

Every September, SAMHSA sponsors Recovery Month to increase awareness and understanding of mental and substance use disorders and celebrate the people who recover.

(Source: "National Recovery Month," Substance Abuse and Mental Health Services Administration (SAMHSA).)

Recovery Supports

Even after a year or 2 of remission is achieved—through treatment or some other route—it can take 4–5 more years before the risk of relapse drops below 15 percent, the level of risk that people in the general population have of developing a substance use disorder in their lifetime. As a result, similar to other chronic conditions, a person with a serious substance use disorder often requires ongoing monitoring and management to maintain remission and to provide early re-intervention should the person relapse. Recovery support services refer to the collection of community services that can provide emotional and practical support for continuing remission as well as daily structure and rewarding alternatives to substance use.

Mutual Aid Groups

Mutual aid groups are perhaps the best known type of RSS, and they share a number of features. The members share a problem or status and they value experiential knowledge—learning from each other's experiences is a central element—and they focus on personal-change goals. The groups are voluntary associations that charge no fees and are self-led by the members.

Mutual aid groups focused on substance use differ from other RSS in important respects. First, they have been in existence longer, having originally been created by American Indians in the 18th century after the introduction of alcohol to North America by Europeans. The best-known mutual aid group, Alcoholics Anonymous (AA), was founded in 1935. Second, mutual aid groups advance specific pathways to recovery, in contrast to the general supports provided by other RSS. For example, an experienced AA member will help new members learn and incorporate AA's specific approach to recovery. In contrast, recovery coaches will support a variety of recovery options and support services, of which AA may be one of many. Third, mutual aid groups have their own self-supporting ecosystem that interacts with, but is fundamentally independent of, other health and social service systems. In contrast, other RSS are often part of formal health and social service systems.

Recovery Coaching

Voluntary and paid recovery coach positions are a new development in the addiction field. Coaches do not provide "treatment" per se, but they often help individuals discharging from treatment to connect to community services while addressing any barriers or problems that may hinder the recovery process. A recovery coach's responsibilities may include providing strategies to maintain abstinence, connecting people to recovery housing and social services, and helping people develop personal skills that maintain recovery. Recovery coaches may or may not be in recovery themselves, but in either case they do not presume that the same path toward recovery will work for everyone they coach. Some community-based recovery organizations offer training programs for recovery coaches, but no national standardized approach to training coaches has been developed.

Recovery Housing

Recovery-supportive houses provide both a substance-free environment and mutual support from fellow recovering residents. Many residents stay in recovery housing during and/or after outpatient treatment, with self-determined residency lasting for several months to years. Residents often informally share resources with each other, giving advice borne of experience about how to access healthcare, find employment, manage legal problems, and interact with the social service system. Some recovery houses are connected with affiliates of the National Alliance of Recovery Residences (NARR), a nonprofit organization that serves 25 regional affiliate organizations that collectively support more than 25,000 persons in recovery across over 2,500 certified recovery residences. A leading example of recovery-supportive houses is Oxford Houses, which are peer-run, self-sustaining, substance-free residences that host 6–10 recovering individuals per house and require that all members maintain abstinence.

Recovery Management

Recovery-oriented care often use long-term recovery management protocols, such as recovery management check-ups (RMCs), and telephone case monitoring. The RMC model for substance use disorders draws heavily from monitoring and early re-intervention protocols used for other chronic diseases, such as diabetes and hypertension. With the core components of tracking, assessment, linkage, engagement, and retention, patients are monitored quarterly for several years following an initial treatment. If a relapse occurs, the patient is connected with the necessary services and encouraged to remain in treatment. The main assumption is that early detection and treatment of relapse will improve long-term outcomes.

Recovery-Based Education

High school and college environments can be difficult for students in recovery because of perceived and actual high levels of substance use among other students, peer pressure to engage in substance use, and widespread availability of alcohol and drugs. The emergence of high school and collegiate recovery support programs is an important response to this challenge in that they provide recovery-supportive environments, recovery norms, and peer engagement with other students in recovery.

Recovery High Schools

Recovery high schools help students in recovery focus on academic learning while simultaneously receiving RSS. Such schools support abstinence and student efforts to overcome personal issues that may compromise academic performance or threaten continued recovery. The earliest known program opened in 1979, and the number slowly increased to approximately 35 schools in 15 states by 2015. A study of 17 recovery high schools found that most had small and rapidly changing enrollments, ranging from 12–25 students. Rates of abstinence from "all alcohol and other drugs" increased from 20 percent during the 90 days before enrolling to 56 percent since enrolling. Students' opinions of the schools were positive, with 87 percent reporting overall satisfaction. A study of graduates from one recovery high school found that 39 percent reported no drug or alcohol use in the past 30 days and more than 90 percent had enrolled in college.

Recovery In Colleges

Collegiate recovery support programs vary in number and type of RSS. Most provide some combination of recovery residence halls or recovery-specific wings, counseling services, on-site mutual aid group meetings, and other educational and social supports. These services are provided within an environment that facilitates social role modeling of sobriety and connection among recovering peers. The programs often require participants to demonstrate 3–6 months with no use of alcohol and drugs as a requirement for admission. Recovering college peers may help these new students effectively manage the environmental risks present on many college

Emerging Treatment Technologies

Technological advancements are changing not only the face of healthcare generally, but also the treatment of substance use disorders. In this regard, approximately 20 percent of substance use disorder treatment programs have adopted electronic health record (EHR) systems. With the growing adoption of EHRs, individuals and their providers can more easily access and share treatment records to improve coordination of care.

The use of telehealth to deliver healthcare, provide health information or education, and monitor the effects of care, has also rapidly increased. Telehealth can be facilitated through a variety of media, including smartphones, the Internet, video conferencing, wireless communication, and streaming media. It offers alternative, cost-effective care options for individuals living in rural or remote areas or when physically traveling to a healthcare facility poses significant challenges.

Several studies have been conducted on technology-assisted screening, assessment, and brief intervention for substance use disorders. Many of these studies focus on Internet-based assessments and brief interventions for at-risk, college-age populations. Examples of evaluated tools include the Check Your Drinking screener, electronic alcohol screening and brief intervention (e-SBI) Drinker's Check-up, alcohol electronic Check-Up to Go (e-CHUG), and Marijuana eCHECKUP TO GO. Other studies assessed interventions that can be implemented in general healthcare settings, including Project Quit Using Drugs Intervention Trial (QUIT), a brief intervention in a primary care setting that also includes follow-up coaching calls for individuals who have been identified through screening as engaging in risky drug use, and use of kiosks in emergency departments to screen for alcohol and drug use. In the latter study, patients in the emergency department were found to be significantly more likely to disclose their substance use at a kiosk compared to a healthcare professional or other interviewer. Other studies focus on telephone-based assessments and brief interventions related to alcohol and drug use, including DIAL, and a telephone-based monitoring and brief counseling intervention.

Preliminary evidence shows that Web- and telephone-based assessments and brief interventions are superior to no treatment in reducing substance use, and often result in similar or improved outcomes when compared to alternative brief intervention options.

(Source: "Early Intervention, Treatment, And Management Of Substance Use Disorders," Office of the Surgeon General (OGS).)

campuses. Participants in collegiate recovery programs often have significant accompanying mental health problems, such as depression or an eating disorder, in addition to their substance use disorder, which can complicate recovery. Nevertheless, observational data from two model programs suggest that rates of return to use (defined as any use of alcohol or other substance) are only 4–13 percent in any given semester.

Part Nine
If You Need More Information

Chapter 62

National Organizations For Drug Information

Action on Smoking and Health (ASH)

1250 Connecticut Ave. N.W.
Seventh Fl.
Washington, DC 20006
Phone: 202-659-4310
Website: www.ash.org
E-mail: info@ash.org

Al-Anon

1600 Corporate Landing Pkwy
Virginia Beach, VA 23454-5617
Toll-Free: 888-425-2666
Phone: 757-563-1600
Fax: 757-563-1656
Website: al-anon.org
E-mail: wso@al-anon.org

Alcoholics Anonymous (AA)

AA World Services, Inc.
475 Riverside Dr. W. 120th St.
11th Fl.
New York, NY 10115
Phone: 212-870-3400
Website: www.aa.org

Bureau of Alcohol, Tobacco, Firearms, and Explosives (ATF)

99 New York Ave. N.E.
Washington, DC 20226
Toll-Free: 800-800-3855
Phone: 202-648-7080
Website: www.atf.gov

About This Chapter: Resources in this chapter were compiled from several sources deemed reliable; all contact information was verified and updated in July 2018.

Campaign for Tobacco-Free Kids
1400 I St. N.W.
Ste. 1200
Washington, DC 20005
Phone: 202-296-5469
Fax: 202-296-5427
Website: www.tobaccofreekids.org

Center for Substance Abuse Prevention (CSAP)
Substance Abuse and Mental Health
Services Administration (SAMHSA)
5600 Fishers Ln.
Rockville, MD 20857
Toll-Free: 877-SAMHSA-7
(877-726-4727)
Phone: 240-276-2420
Website: www.samhsa.gov/about-us/who-we-are/offices-centers/csap

Center of Alcohol Studies
Rutgers, the State University of New Jersey
607 Allison Rd.
Piscataway, NJ 08854
Phone: 848-445-2190
Fax: 732-445-3500
Website: alcoholstudies.rutgers.edu

Center on Addiction
633 Third Ave.
19th Fl.
New York, NY 10017-6706
Phone: 212-841-5200
Fax: 212-956-8020
Website: www.centeronaddiction.org

Centers for Disease Control and Prevention (CDC)
1600 Clifton Rd.
Atlanta, GA 30329-4027
Toll-Free: 800-CDC-INFO (800-232-4636)
Toll-Free TTY: 888-232-6348
Website: www.cdc.gov

Co-Anon Family Groups
P.O. Box 3664
Gilbert, AZ 85299
Phone: 480-442-3869
Website: www.co-anon.org

Cocaine Anonymous World Services
21720 S. Wilmington Ave.
Ste. 304
Long Beach, CA 90810-1641
Phone: 310-559-5833
Fax: 310-559-2554
Website: www.ca.org
E-mail: cawso@ca.org

Do It Now Foundation (Drug Information)
P.O. Box 27921
Tempe, AZ 85285
Website: www.doitnow.org

Families Anonymous
701 Lee St.
Ste. 670
Des Plaines, IL 60016
Toll-Free: 800-736-9805
Phone: 847-294-5877
Fax: 847-294-5837
Website: www.familiesanonymous.org
E-mail: famanon@FamiliesAnonymous.org

Hazelden Foundation

P.O. Box 11
Center City, MN 55012-0011
Toll-Free: 866-261-3734
Phone: 651-231-4000
Website: www.hazelden.org
E-mail: info@hazelden.org

Higher Education Center for Alcohol And Drug Misuse Prevention and Recovery

325 Stillman Hall
1947 College Rd.
Columbus, OH 43210
Phone: 614-292-5572
Website: www.hecaod.osu.edu
E-mail: hecaod@osu.edu

Nar-Anon Family Groups

23110 Crenshaw Blvd.
Ste. A
Torrance, CA 90505
Toll-Free: 800-477-6291
Phone: 310-534-8188
Website: www.nar-anon.org
E-mail: wso@nar-anon.org

Narcotics Anonymous (NA)

P.O. Box 9999
Van Nuys, CA 91409
Phone: 818-773-9999
Fax: 818-700-0700
Website: www.na.org

National Asian Pacific American Families Against Drug Abuse (NAPAFASA)

340 E. Second St.
Ste. 409
Los Angeles, CA 90012
Phone: 213-625-5795
Website: www.napafasa.org
E-mail: info@napafasa.org

National Association for Children of Alcoholics (NACoA)

10920 Connecticut Ave.
Ste. 100
Kensington, MD 20895
Toll-Free: 888-55-4COAS (888-554-2627)
Phone: 301-468-0985
Fax: 301-468-0987
Website: www.nacoa.net
E-mail: nacoa@nacoa.org

National Council on Alcoholism and Drug Dependence (NCADD)

217 Bdwy.
Ste. 712
New York, NY 10007
Toll-Free: 800-NCA-CALL
(800-622-2255)
Phone: 212-269-7797
Fax: 212-269-7510
Website: www.ncadd.org
E-mail: national@ncadd.org

National Criminal Justice Reference Service (NCJRS)

P.O. Box 6000
Rockville, MD 20849-6000
Toll-Free: 800-851-3420
Phone: 202-836-6998
TTY: 301-240-6310
Fax: 301-240-5830
Website: www.ncjrs.gov
E-mail: responsecenter@ncjrs.gov

National Drug Intelligence Center (NDIC)

U.S. Department of Justice (DOJ)
950 Pennsylvania Ave. N.W.
Washington, DC 20530-0001
Phone: 202-514-2000
Toll-Free TTY: 800-877-8339
Website: www.justice.gov/archive/ndic

National Institute on Alcohol Abuse and Alcoholism (NIAAA)

5635 Fishers Ln.
MSC 9304
Bethesda, MD 20892
Toll-Free: 888-MY-NIAAA (888-69-64222)
Phone: 301-443-3860
Website: www.niaaa.nih.gov

National Institute on Drug Abuse (NIDA)

6001 Executive Blvd.
Rm. 5213
Bethesda, MD 20892
Phone: 301-443-1124
Website: www.drugabuse.gov
E-mail: information@nida.nih.gov

National Institute of Justice (NIJ)

810 Seventh St. N.W.
Washington, DC 20531
Toll-Free: 800-851-3420 (National Criminal Justice Reference Service)
Phone: 202-307-2942
TTY: 301-240-6310
Website: www.nij.gov/about/pages/contact.aspx

National Parents Resource Institute for Drug Education (PRIDE)

4 W. Oak St.
Fremont, MI 49412
Toll-Free: 800-668-9277
Phone: 231-924-1662
Fax: 231-924-5663
E-mail: info@pridyouthprograms.org

National Survey on Drug Use and Health (NSDUH)

Substance Abuse and Mental Health Services Administration (SAMHSA)
5600 Fishers Ln.
Rockville, MD 20857
Toll-Free: 800-848-4079
Website: www.samhsa.gov/about-us/who-we-are/offices-centers/cbhsq

The Nemours Foundation

10140 Centurion Pkwy N.
Jacksonville, FL 32256
Phone: 904-697-4100
Website: www.nemours.org

Office of Safe and Healthy Students (OSHS)

U.S. Department of Education (ED)
400 Maryland Ave. S.W.
Rm. 3E-245
Washington, DC 20202-6450
Phone: 202-453-6777
Fax: 202-453-6742
Website: www.ed.gov/offices/OESE/SDFS
E-mail: OESE@ed.gov

Partnership for a Drug-Free Kids

352 Park Ave. S.
Ninth Fl.
New York, NY 10010
Toll-Free: 855-DRUGFREE
(855-378-4373)
Phone: 212-922-1560
Fax: 212-922-1570
Website: www.drugfree.org

Phoenix House

164 W. 74th St.
New York, NY 10023
Website: www.phoenixhouse.org

Pride Surveys

2140 Newmarket Pkwy S.E.
Ste. 116
Marietta, GA 30067
Toll-Free: 800-279-6361
Fax: 770-726-9327
Website: www.pridesurveys.com

Students Against Destructive Decisions (SADD)

1440 G St.
Washington, D.C. 20005
Phone: 508-481-3568
Website: www.sadd.org
E-mail: info@sadd.org

Substance Abuse and Mental Health Services Administration (SAMHSA)

5600 Fishers Ln.
Rockville, MD 20857
Toll-Free: 877-SAMHSA-7
(877-726-4727)
Phone: 240-276-2130
Toll-Free TTY: 800-487-4889
Website: www.samhsa.gov

U.S. Drug Enforcement Administration (DEA)

Office of Diversion Control
8701 Morrissette Dr.
Springfield, VA 22152
Toll-Free: 800-882-9539
Phone: 202-307-1000
Website: www.dea.gov
E-mail: ODLL@usdoj.gov

U.S. Food and Drug Administration (FDA)

10903 New Hampshire Ave.
Silver Spring, MD 20993
Toll-Free: 888-INFO-FDA (888-463-6332)
Website: www.fda.gov

Chapter 63

Substance Abuse Hotlines And Helplines

Al-Anon/Alateen Information Line
Toll-Free: 800-344-2666
Monday–Friday, 8:00 a.m. to 6:00 p.m. ET

Alcohol and Drug Abuse Hotline
Toll-Free: 800-729-6686

Alcohol and Drug Helpline
WellPlace
Toll-Free: 800-821-4357

Alcohol Hotline
Adcare Hospital
Toll-Free: 800-331-2900
7 days a week, 24 hours a day

Alcohol Treatment Referral Hotline
Toll-Free: 800-252-6465

Center for Substance Abuse Treatment (CSAT)
Substance Abuse and Mental Health Services Administration (SAMHSA)
Toll-Free: 800-662-HELP (800-662-4357)
Toll-Free TDD: 800-487-4889

Cocaine Anonymous (CA)
Toll-Free: 800-347-8998

Families Anonymous (FA)
Toll-Free: 800-736-9805

Girls and Boys Town National Hotline
Toll-Free: 800-448-3000
Toll-Free TDD: 800-448-1833

Marijuana Anonymous (MA)
Toll-Free: 800-766-6779

About This Chapter: Resources in this chapter were compiled from several sources deemed reliable; all contact information was verified and updated in July 2018.

NAMI Information Helpline

Nation's Voice on Mental Illness
Toll-Free: 800-950-NAMI (800-950-6264)
Monday–Friday, 10:00 a.m. to 6:00 p.m. ET

Narconon International Helpline

Toll-Free: 855-775-8441

National Center for Victims of Crime

Toll-Free: 855-4-VICTIM
(855-484-2846)

National Child Abuse Hotline

Childhelp USA
Toll-Free: 800-4-A-CHILD
(800-422-4453)

National Clearinghouse for Alcohol and Drug Information (NCADI)

Toll-Free: 800-729-6686
24 hours a day, 7 days a week

National Council on Alcoholism and Drug Dependence Hopeline

Toll-Free: 800-622-2255
24 hours a day, 7 days a week

National Domestic Violence Hotline

Toll-Free: 800-799-7233
Toll-Free TTY: 800-787-3224

National Helpline for Substance Abuse

Toll-Free: 800-262-2463

National Institute on Drug Abuse (NIDA) Hotline

Toll-Free: 800-662-4357

National Organization for Victim Assistance (NOVA)

Toll-Free: 800-TRY-NOVA
(800-879-6682)
Monday–Friday, 9:00 a.m. to 5:00 p.m. ET

National Runaway Safeline

Toll-Free: 800-RUNAWAY
(800-786-2929)

National Sexual Assault Hotline

Rape, Abuse, and Incest National Network
(RAINN)
Toll-Free: 800-656-HOPE (800-656-4673)

National Suicide Hopeline

Toll-Free: 800-SUICIDE (800-784-2433)
7 days a week, 24 hours a day

National Suicide Prevention Lifeline

Toll-Free: 800-273-TALK (800-273-8255)
Toll-Free TDD: 800-799-4889

Stop It Now!

Toll-Free: 888-PREVENT (888-773-8368)
Limited phone hours; also online at www.
stopitnow.org

Chapter 64

State-By-State List Of Alcohol And Drug Referral Phone Numbers

Alabama

Department of Mental Health (DMH)
Toll-Free: 800-367-0955
Phone: 334-242-3454
Fax: 334-242-0725
Website: www.mh.alabama.gov

Alaska

Department of Health and Social Services (DHSS)
Phone: 907-465-3370
Fax: 907-465-2185
Website: dhss.alaska.gov/dbh

American Samoa

American Samoa Government
Department of Human and Social Services
Phone: 684-633-2609
Fax: 684-633-7449
Website: www.americansamoa.gov/services

Arizona

Department of Health Services
Toll-Free: 800-867-5808
Phone: 602-542-1025
Fax: 602-364-4558
Website: www.azdhs.gov

Colorado

Department of Human Services (DHS)
Phone: 303-866-7400
Fax: 303-866-7481
Website: www.colorado.gov/pacific/cdhs/contact-us-5
E-mail: cdhs_communications@state.co.us

Connecticut

Department of Mental Health and Addiction Services (DMHAS)
Toll-Free: 800-446-7348
Phone: 860-418-7000
TTY: 860-418-6707
Website: www.ct.gov/dmhas

About This Chapter: Resources in this chapter were compiled from several sources deemed reliable; all contact information was verified and updated in July 2018.

Delaware

Health and Social Services (DHHS)
Division of Substance Abuse and Mental
Health (DSAMH)
Toll-Free: 800-652-2929
Phone: 302-255-9399
Fax: 302-255-4427
Website: www.dhss.delaware.gov/dhss/
dsamh/contact.html

District of Columbia

Behavioral Health Addiction Prevention
and Recovery Administration (APRA)
Department of Behavioral Health
Phone: 202-727-8857
Fax: 202-777-0092
Website: www.dbh.dc.gov

Florida

Substance Abuse Program Office
Department of Children and Families
Toll-Free: 800-962-2873
Phone: 850-487-1111
Fax: 850-922-4996
Website: www.dcf.state.fl.us; www.
myflfamilies.com

Georgia

Department of Behavioral Health and
Developmental Disabilities (DBHDD)
Office of Public Affairs
Toll-Free: 800-436-7442
Phone: 404-657-2331
Fax: 404-657-2256
Website: mhddad.dhr.georgia.gov

Guam

Behavioral Health and Wellness Center
(GBHWC)
Department of Mental Health and
Substance Abuse
Toll-Free: 800-222-1222
Phone: 671-647-5330
Fax: 671-649-6948
Website: www.gbhwc.guam.gov

Hawaii

Alcohol and Drug Abuse Division
Department of Health
Phone: 808-692-7506
Fax: 808-692-7521
Website: health.hawaii.gov/substance-abuse

Illinois

Department of Human Services
Toll-Free: 800-843-6154
Toll-Free TTY: 866-324-5553
Website: www.dhs.state.il.us/page.aspx?

Indiana

Division of Mental Health and Addiction
(DMHA)
Family and Social Services Administration
(FSSA)
Toll-Free: 800-457-8283
Fax: 317-233-3472
Website: www.in.gov/fssa/dmha/index.htm

Iowa

Division of Behavioral Health
Department of Public Health
Toll-Free: 866-834-9671
Phone: 515-281-7689
Toll-Free TTY: 800-735-2942
Website: idph.iowa.gov

Kansas

Department for Children and Families (DCF)
Toll-Free: 888-369-4777
Phone: 785-296-6807
TTY: 785-296-1491
Website: www.dcf.ks.gov/Pages/Default.aspx

Kentucky

Cabinet for Health and Family Services (CHFS)
Toll-Free: 800-372-2973
Phone: 502-564-5497
Fax: 502-564-9523
Website: chfs.ky.gov/Pages/index.aspx
E-mail: CHFS.Listens@ky.gov

Louisiana

Department of Health
Toll-Free: 877-664-2248
Phone: 225-342-9500
Fax: 225-342-5568
Website: ldh.la.gov

Maine

Office of Substance Abuse and Mental Health Services (SAMHS)
Toll-Free: 800-499-0027
Phone: 207-287-2595
Fax: 207-287-9152
Toll-Free TTY: 888-568-1112
Website: www.maine.gov/dhhs/samhs
E-mail: osa.ircosa@maine.gov

Maryland

Department of Health
Toll-Free: 877-463-3464
Phone: 410-767-6500
Website: health.maryland.gov/pages/index.aspx

Massachusetts

Bureau of Substance Abuse Services (BSAS)
Department of Public Health
Toll-Free: 800-327-5050
Phone: 617-624-5111
Toll-Free TTY: 888-448-8321
Website: www.mass.gov/orgs/bureau-of-substance-addiction-services

Michigan

Department of Health and Human Services (DHSS)
Toll-Free: 855-ASK-MICH (855-275-6424)
Phone: 517-373-3740
Fax: 517-335-2121
Toll-Free TTY: 800-649-3777
Website: www.michigan.gov/mdhhs
E-mail: MDCH-BSAAS@michigan.gov

Minnesota

Alcohol and Drug Abuse Division
Department of Human Services
Phone: 651-431-2460
Fax: 651-431-7449
Website: mn.gov/dhs/general-public/about-dhs/contact-us/division-addresses.jsp
E-mail: dhs.adad@state.mn.us

Mississippi

Department of Mental Health (DMH)
Toll-Free: 877-210-8513
Phone: 601-359-1288
Fax: 601-359-6295
TDD: 601-359-6230
Website: www.dmh.ms.gov

Missouri

Department of Mental Health (DMH)
Toll-Free: 800-364-9687
Phone: 573-751-4122
Fax: 573-751-8224
Website: dmh.mo.gov
E-mail: dbhmail@dmh.mo.gov

Montana

Addictive and Mental Disorders Division
(AMDD)
Department of Public Health and Human
Services
Phone: 406-444-3964
Fax: 406-444-4435
Website: www.dphhs.mt.gov/amdd

Nevada

Division of Public and Behavioral Health
(DPBH)
Department of Health and Human Services
Phone: 775-684-4200
Fax: 775-684-4211
Website: dpbh.nv.gov
E-mail: dpbh@health.nv.gov

New Hampshire

Bureau of Drug and Alcohol Services
(BDAS)
Department of Health and Human Services
Toll-Free: 800-804-0909
Phone: 603-271-6738
Website: www.dhhs.nh.gov/dcbcs/bdas

New Jersey

Department of Human Services (DHS)
Toll-Free: 800-238-2333
Toll-Free TTY: 877-294-4356
Website: www.nj.gov/health

New Mexico

Behavioral Health Services Division (BHSD)
Department of Human Services
Phone: 505-476-9266
Fax: 505-476-9277
Website: www.hsd.state.nm.us/Behavioral_
health_services_division.aspx

New York

Office of Alcoholism and Substance Abuse
Services (OASAS)
Phone: 518-473-3460
Website: oasas.ny.gov
E-mail: communications@oasas.ny.gov

North Carolina

Mental Health, Developmental Disabilities
and Substance Abuse Services
Toll-Free: 800-662-7030
Phone: 919-733-7011
Fax: 919-733-4556
Website: www.ncdhhs.gov/divisions/
mhddsas
E-mail: contactdmh@dhhs.nc.gov

North Dakota

Behavioral Health Division
Department of Human Services (DHS)
Toll-Free: 800-472-2622
Phone: 701-328-8920
Fax: 701-328-8969
Website: www.nd.gov/dhs/services/
mentalhealth
E-mail: dhsbhd@nd.gov

Ohio

Department of Mental Health and
Addiction Services (MHAS)
Toll-Free: 877-275-6364
Phone: 614-466-2596
Website: mha.ohio.gov

Oklahoma

Department of Mental Health and
Substance Abuse Services (DMHSAS)
Toll-Free: 800-522-9054
Phone: 405-248-9200
Fax: 405-248-9321
Website: ok.gov/odmhsas

Oregon

Addictions and Mental Health Services
(AMH)
Health Systems Division (HSD)
Toll-Free: 800-527-5772
Phone: 503-945-5772
Website: www.oregon.gov/oha/HSD/Pages/
index.aspx

Pennsylvania

Department of Drug and Alcohol Programs
(DDAP)
Phone: 717-736-7459
Fax: 717-787-6285
Website: www.ddap.pa.gov/pages/default.
aspx

Puerto Rico

Office of Quality of the Administration
of Health Services and Against Addiction
(ASSMCA)
Phone: 787-763-7575
Websites: www.assmca.pr.gov; www.
samhsa.gov/capt/about-capt/state-tribe-
jurisdiction-contacts/puerto-rico

Rhode Island

Department of Behavioral Healthcare,
Developmental Disabilities and Hospitals
(BHDDH)
Phone: 401-462-3201
Fax: 401-462-3204
Website: www.bhddh.ri.gov

South Carolina

Department of Alcohol and Other Drug
Abuse Services (DAODAS)
Phone: 803-896-5555
Fax: 803-896-5557
Website: www.daodas.sc.gov

South Dakota

Division of Rehabilitation Services (DRS)
Department of Human Services (DHS)
Phone: 605-773-3195
Fax: 605-773-5483
Website: dhs.sd.gov

Tennessee

Department of Mental Health and
Substance Abuse Services (DMHSAS)
Toll-Free: 800-560-5767
Phone: 615-532-6500
Website: www.tn.gov/behavioral-health.
html
E-mail: OCA.TDMHSAS@tn.gov

Texas

Mental Health and Substance Abuse
Division (MHSA)
Department of State Health Service
(DSHS)
Toll-Free: 888-963-7111
Phone: 512-776-7111
Fax: 512-206-5714
Toll-Free TTY: 800-735-2989
Website: www.dshs.state.tx.us/sa/default.
shtm
E-mail: customer.service@dshs.texas.gov

Utah

Division of Substance Abuse and Mental
Health (DSAMH)
Department of Human Services (DHS)
Toll-Free: 800-273-8255
Phone: 801-538-4171
Website: www.dsamh.utah.gov
E-mail: dhsinfo@utah.gov

Vermont

Alcohol and Drug Abuse Programs
Department of Health
Toll-Free: 800-464-4343
Phone: 802-651-1550
Fax: 802-865-7754
Website: www.healthvermont.gov

Virgin Islands

Department of Health
Phone: 340-774-4888
Fax: 340-774-4701
Website: www.samhsa.gov/capt/about-capt/
state-tribe-jurisdiction-contacts/u.s.-virgin-
islands

Virginia

Department of Behavioral Health and
Developmental Services (DBHDS)
Phone: 804-786-3921
Fax: 804-371-6638
Website: www.dbhds.virginia.gov

Washington

Department of Social and Health Services
(DSHS)
Toll-Free: 800-737-0617
Website: www.dshs.wa.gov
E-mail: askdshs@dshs.wa.gov

West Virginia

Bureau for Behavioral Health and Health
Facilities (BBHHF)
Phone: 304-356-4811
Fax: 304-558-1008
Website: dhhr.wv.gov/bhhf/Pages/default.
aspx

Wisconsin

Bureau of Prevention, Treatment, and
Recovery, Division of Care and Treatment
Services
Department of Health Services
Phone: 608-266-2717
Website: www.dhs.wisconsin.gov/dcts/bptr.
htm
E-mail: DHSWEBMAILDCTS@dhs.
wisconsin.gov

Wyoming

Behavioral Health Division
Department of Health
Toll-Free: 866-571-0944
Phone: 307-777-7656
Website: health.wyo.gov/behavioralhealth

Chapter 65

Additional Reading About Substance Abuse

Web-Based Additional Sources For Substance Abuse

Alcohol Use Disorder (AUD)
The Mayo Clinic
Website: www.mayoclinic.org/diseases-conditions/alcohol-use-disorder/symptoms-causes/syc-20369243?DSECTION=all

Learn The Link—Drugs And HIV
National Institute on Drug Abuse (NIDA)
Website: www.drugabuse.gov/news-events/public-education-projects/learn-link-drugs-hiv

Glaucoma And Marijuana Use
National Eye Institute (NEI)
Website: nei.nih.gov/news/statements/marij

Heroin
National Institute on Drug Abuse (NIDA)
Website: www.drugabuse.gov/publications/research-reports/heroin/scope-heroin-use-in-united-states

---

About This Chapter: The mobile apps listed in this chapter were compiled from several sources deemed reliable. Inclusion does not constitute endorsement, and there is no implication associated with omission. All website information was verified and updated in July 2018.

Marijuana: Facts For Teens

National Institute on Drug Abuse (NIDA)
Website: www.drugabuse.gov/publications/marijuana-facts-teens/letter-to-teens

PEERx

National Institute on Drug Abuse (NIDA)
Website: teens.drugabuse.gov/peerx

Prescription Drug Abuse

The Nemours Foundation
Website: kidshealth.org/en/teens/prescription-drug-abuse.html

Smoking And Asthma

The Nemours Foundation
Website: kidshealth.org/en/teens/smoking-asthma.html

Marijuana Facts & Figures

Office of National Drug Control Policy (ONDCP)
Website: www.whitehousedrugpolicy.org/drugfact/marijuana/marijuana_ff.html

Mobile Apps For Substance Abuse

AnxietyCoach

AnxietyCoach is as a comprehensive self-help tool for a wide variety of worries, fears, obsessions, and compulsions. By helping a teen overcome these things, it may prevent them from self-medication with prescription or other drug abuse.
Website: itunes.apple.com/us/app/anxietycoach/id565943257?mt=8

Flipd

Flipd is a simple and distraction blocker that prevents you from getting off task. Backed by research, Flipd is proven to help you to stay focused, improve your attention, and increase productivity thanks to its effective lock screen. Stay connected and remove distractions with Flipd.
Website: play.google.com/store/apps/details?id=com.flipd.app&hl=en_IN

The Mindfulness App

The Mindfulness App is designed for both beginners and experienced meditators, so everyone has something to gain. The focus is to help you become more present in your daily life, which is important in early recovery. The app features statistics, guided and silent meditations and health app integration.
Website: play.google.com/store/apps/details?id=se.lichtenstein.mind.en&hl=en_IN

No More! Quit Your Addictions

No More! supports you daily in overcoming any weakness which is holding you back from becoming a better person. It does not matter if you are trying to overcome a serious addiction like drinking, smoking, gambling, or trying to improve your life.
Website: play.google.com/store/apps/details?id=com.leoncvlt.nomore

Nomo—Sobriety Clocks

Nomo can be a great tool for people who are supporting someone through recovery. The clock function can mark emotional turning points, and you have the choice of sharing any feelings of fear, joy, or shame that you are experiencing in the "encouragement" section of the app, which helps you feel less alone in your recovery.
Website: itunes.apple.com/us/app/nomo-sobriety-clocks/id566975787?mt=8

Nudge

Nudge organizes all of your tracking programs, including Moves, Runkeeper, and Apple Health, to help you meet your diet or weight loss goals. Through the app you can link up with social clubs and receive advice, support, and inspiration from other users. It also connects you with a personal coach if you need more support and motivation.
Websites: play.google.com/store/apps/details?id=com.nudgeyourself.nudge&hl=en_IN

Pear reSET

Pear reSET is the first mobile medical application approved by the U.S. Food and Drug Administration (FDA) to help treat substance use disorders. The digital therapy app consists of a specialized, 12-week program schedule that includes weekly check-ins. Currently, it is only available for download to individuals who are over the age of 17 and have a prescription from a clinician. It guides the users through a series of engaging lessons that help guide them through recovery. Users complete the lessons at their own pace and take a quiz after completing each lesson to receive virtual rewards.
Website: itunes.apple.com/us/app/pear-reset/id1096230845?mt=8

Quit That

Quit That tracks the progress you've made by quitting anything, from coffee and junk food to heroin and meth. It tracks the days and hours since you stopped and also how much money you've saved. There's no limit to the number of bad habits or addictions you can track and, thankfully, no ads or tiresome prompts to deal with.
Website: itunes.apple.com/us/app/quit-that!-track-how-long/id909400800?mt=8

Recoverize

Recoverize motivates users with daily AA and NA readings, recovery stories, a chat room, speaker tapes, a meditation mode, and more. Users can keep track of their sober time when they create an account and find recovery events near them.
Website: play.google.com/store/apps/details?id=com.idmlsd8910ji2ky1ypqx5a

421

Sober Grid

Sober Grid allows you to create online profiles and interact, support, and engage with other people in recovery using a platform similar to Facebook. You can also use the app to create anonymous check-ins about whether you're sober or not, your mood, and what's going on. These daily connections with others in the recovery community can help you remain clean and sober. If you turn on the GPS locator, you can find other sober people nearby.

Website: play.google.com/store/apps/details?id=com.sobergrid&hl=en_IN

SoberTool

SoberTool is an easy way to track your clean and sober days. The app includes daily motivational messages and reminders to keep you on target. You can earn rewards by hitting different milestones for the time that you have stayed sober. The app even calculates your estimated savings from staying sober.

Websites: play.google.com/store/apps/details?id=com.osu.cleanandsobertoolboxandroid

Squirrel Recovery: Addiction

Squirrel Recovery allows you to set up a support circle with other people in recovery from substance addictions (its focus). The people in your circle know from your answers how you are doing and can respond accordingly to offer support and encouragement when you need it most. The app tracks the number of days of your sobriety and rewards you with "coins" as you rack up more sober days.

Website: play.google.com/store/apps/details?id=com.capstone2015.sobrietysupport&hl=en

Strides

Strides holds you accountable and charts your progress toward your goals. You can track anything: sobriety, eating healthy, meditating, exercising, and much more. Strides lets you set 4 customizable types of trackers. Choose "target" if you want to reach a goal by a certain date; "habit" if you want to build a good habit or break a bad one; "average" to track an average value over time; and "milestones" to keep track of your pace to complete a project. This app is great if you want to set goals and see your progress.

Website: itunes.apple.com/us/app/strides-habit-tracker/id672401817?mt=8

WEconnect—Recovery Aftercare

WEconnect supports recovery aftercare for alcohol and drug addiction populations by helping you stay accountable to your new, healthy routine, creating healthy habits, keeping you connected to and encouraging communication with your private support network, and you earn rewards along the way that enhance your recovery!

Website: itunes.apple.com/us/app/weconnect-recovery-aftercare/id1175036419?mt=8

Yonder

Yonder app helps you plan your next adventure. When you are in recovery, it is extremely helpful to stay busy. Going outside and enjoying the outdoors is an excellent way to keep your mind and body healthy. Whether you're already someone who likes to adventure, or you just want to travel more, this app allows you to plan adventures like hikes, kayaking trips, rock climbing, and more.

Website: play.google.com/store/apps/details?id=com.yonder.android&hl=en

Index

Index

Page numbers that appear in *Italics* refer to tables or illustrations. Page numbers that have a small 'n' after the page number refer to citation information shown as Notes. Page numbers that appear in **Bold** refer to information contained in boxes within the chapters.

H

X

Y

Z